Emergent Health Communication Scholarship from and about African American, Latino/a/x, and American Indian/Alaskan Native Peoples

I0888107

This book presents research by African American, Latino/a/x, and Alaskan Indian/Native American (AI/AN) communication scholars. It highlights the importance of communication and the recognition of the unique experiences that impact how health information and health care are understood through diverse racial and cultural perspectives.

Each chapter advances various divergent health issues and disparities pertinent to Black, Latino/a/x, and AI/AN communities, so that the powerful aspect of the human condition to know and be known as it relates to the negotiation of health and communication can be clearly understood. Contributions to this volume unabashedly call for more equitable, community-centric, tribally centered, and transparent scholarship on topics of health disparities, health care, marginality, medical mistrust, social justice, and media and new technology as it relates to people of color. The authors in this book are committed to research areas that invigorate and reimagine conversations among clinicians, public health professionals, classroom environments, and communities.

This insightful volume seeks to shift the dominant culture paradigms and locate authors of color and their research experiences and scholarship as central to their work. It provides a space to amplify the voices of our collective lived experiences through the vehicle of rigorous engaged scholarship. This book was originally published as a special issue of *Health Communication*.

Angela Cooke-Jackson's expertise is in Health Communication and Behavioral Science. She uses community-based participatory research and health literacy to help communities curate and design innovative, practical applications for sustainable change. She is also the co-director of the Intimate Communication Lab (www.intimatecommlab.org). She envisions her research at the nexus of culture, health disparities, and marginalized populations.

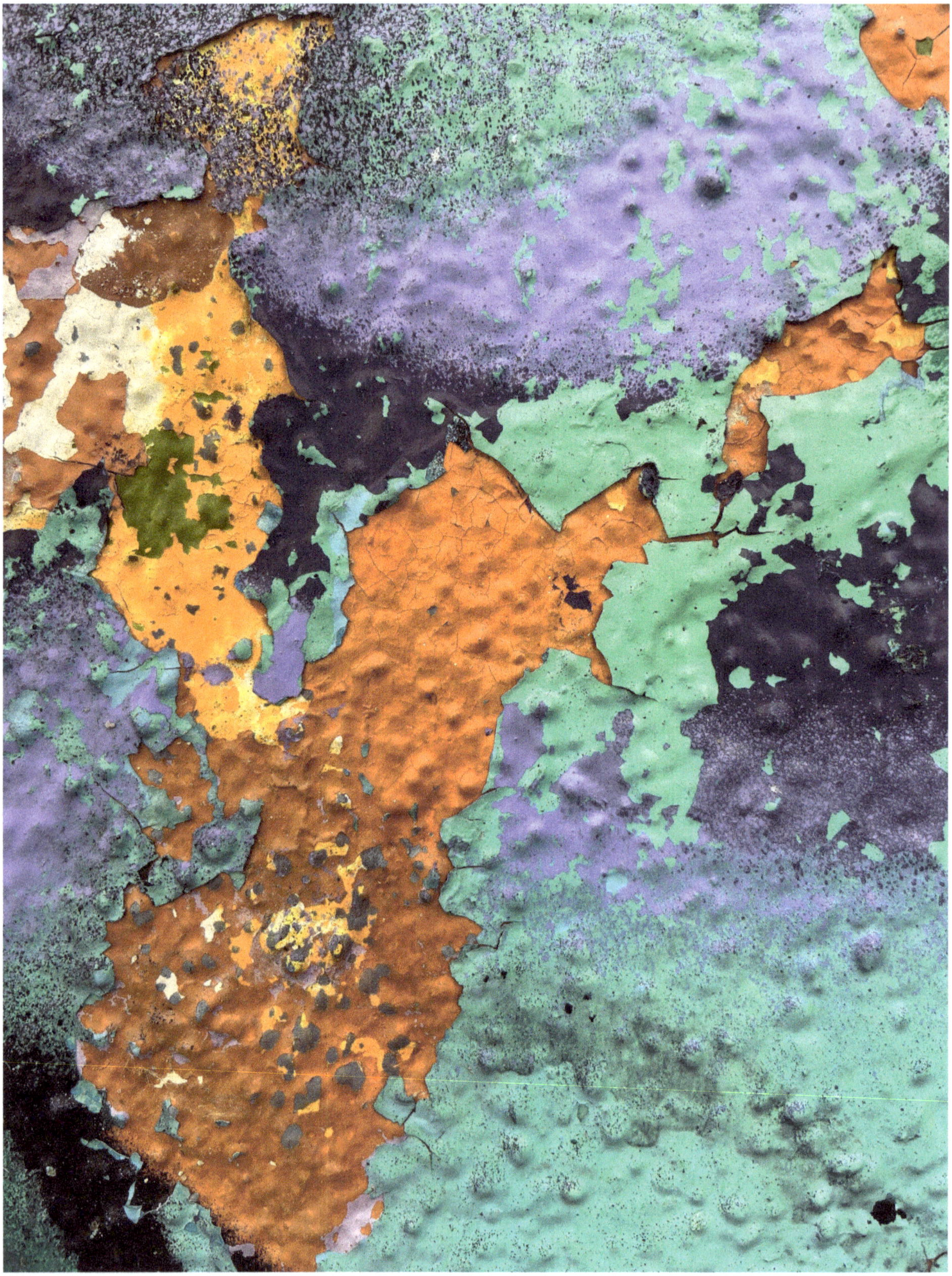

Emergent Health Communication Scholarship from and about African American, Latino/a/x, and American Indian/ Alaskan Native Peoples

Edited by
Angela Cooke-Jackson

Routledge
Taylor & Francis Group
NEW YORK AND LONDON

First published 2024
by Routledge
605 Third Avenue, New York, NY 10158

and by Routledge
4 Park Square, Milton Park, Abingdon, Oxon, OX14 4RN

Routledge is an imprint of the Taylor & Francis Group, an informa business

British Library Cataloguing-in-Publication Data
A catalogue record for this book is available from the British Library

ISBN13: 978-1-032-66122-3 (hbk)
ISBN13: 978-1-032-66126-1 (pbk)
ISBN13: 978-1-032-66128-5 (ebk)

DOI: 10.4324/9781032661285

Typeset in Minion Pro
by codeMantra

Publisher's Note
The publisher accepts responsibility for any inconsistencies that may have arisen during the conversion of this book from journal articles to book chapters, namely the inclusion of journal terminology.

Contents

Citation Information

The chapters in this book were originally published in the journal *Health Communication*, volume 37, issue 9 (2022). When citing this material, please use the original page numbering for each article, as follows:

Introduction

Emergent Health Communication Scholarship from and about African American, Latino/a/x, and American Indian/Alaskan Native Peoples
Angela Cooke-Jackson
Health Communication, volume 37, issue 9 (2022) pp. 1057–1060

Chapter 1

Beyond Personal Experiences: Examining Mediated Vicarious Experiences as an Antecedent of Medical Mistrust
Lillie D. Williamson
Health Communication, volume 37, issue 9 (2022) pp. 1061–1074

Chapter 2

Community-Based Participatory Research (CBPR) to Enhance Participation of Racial/Ethnic Minorities in Clinical Trials: A 10-Year Systematic Review
Soroya Julian McFarlane, Aurora Occa, Wei Peng, Oluwatumininu Awonuga, and Susan E. Morgan
Health Communication, volume 37, issue 9 (2022) pp. 1075–1092

Chapter 3

The Effect of an Entertainment-Education Intervention on Reproductive Health of Young Women of Color
Camille J. Saucier, Sapna Suresh, John J. Brooks, Nathan Walter, Aaron Plant, and Jorge A. Montoya
Health Communication, volume 37, issue 9 (2022) pp. 1093–1103

Chapter 4

A Theoretically Based Analysis of Twitter Conversations about Trauma and Mental Health: Examining Responses to Storylines on the Television Show Queen Sugar
Diane B. Francis and LeChrista Finn
Health Communication, volume 37, issue 9 (2022) pp. 1104–1112

Chapter 5

"After Philando, I Had to Take a Sick Day to Recover": Psychological Distress, Trauma and Police Brutality in the Black Community
Deion S. Hawkins
Health Communication, volume 37, issue 9 (2022) pp. 1113–1122

Chapter 6

A Subjective Culture Approach to Cancer Prevention: Rural Black and White Adults' Perceptions of Using Virtual Health Assistants to Promote Colorectal Cancer Screening

Melissa J. Vilaro, Danyell S. Wilson-Howard, Jordan M. Neil, Fatemeh Tavassoli, Mohan S. Zalake, Benjamin C. Lok, François P. Modave, Thomas J. George, Folakemi T. Odedina, Peter J. Carek, Aubrey M. Mys, and Janice L. Krieger
Health Communication, volume 37, issue 9 (2022) pp. 1123–1134

Chapter 7
African American Women's Maternal Healthcare Experiences: A Critical Race Theory Perspective
Comfort Tosin Adebayo, Erin Sahlstein Parcell, Lucy Mkandawire-Valhmu, and Oluwatoyin Olukotun
Health Communication, volume 37, issue 9 (2022) pp. 1135–1146

Chapter 8
Individually Tailoring Messages to Promote African American Men's Health
Derek M. Griffith, Emily Cornish Jaeger, Andrea R. Semlow, Jennifer M. Ellison, Erin M. Bergner, and Elizabeth C. Stewart
Health Communication, volume 37, issue 9 (2022) pp. 1147–1156

Chapter 9
The Influence of Memorable Message Receipt on Dietary and Exercise Behavior among Self-Identified Black Women
Natasha R. Brown and La'Marcus T. Wingate
Health Communication, volume 37, issue 9 (2022) pp. 1157–1166

Chapter 10
Count Me Out: Perceptions of Black Patients Who are on Dialysis but Who are Not on a Transplant Waitlist
Charles R. Senteio and Matthew K. Ackerman
Health Communication, volume 37, issue 9 (2022) pp. 1167–1179

Chapter 11
In Our Sacred Voice – An Exploration of Tribal and Community Leader Perceptions as Health Communicators of Disease Prevention among American Indians in the Plains
Crystal Y. Lumpkins, Ryan Goeckner, Jason Hale, Charley Lewis, Jordyn Gunville, River Gunville, Chris M. Daley, and Sean M. Daley
Health Communication, volume 37, issue 9 (2022) pp. 1180–1191

Chapter 12
A Comparative Analysis of Health News in Indigenous and Mainstream Media
Victoria L. LaPoe, Candi S. Carter Olson, Cristina L. Azocar, Benjamin R. LaPoe, Bharbi Hazarika, and Parul Jain
Health Communication, volume 37, issue 9 (2022) pp. 1192–1203

Chapter 13
Family Connections and the Latino Health Paradox: Exploring the Mediating Role of Loneliness in the Relationships Between the Latina/o Cultural Value of Familism and Health
Monica L. Gallegos and Chris Segrin
Health Communication, volume 37, issue 9 (2022) pp. 1204–1214

Chapter 14
A Pilot Study of Latinx Lesbian, Gay, and Bisexual Adolescent Patients' Goal Prioritizations in Patient-Provider Sexual Orientation and Health Disclosures
Suzanne Burdick and Sarah Nicholus
Health Communication, volume 37, issue 9 (2022) pp. 1215–1228

Chapter 15

When Engagement Leads to Action: Understanding the Impact of Cancer (Mis)information among Latino/a Facebook Users
Yonaira M. Rivera, Meghan B. Moran, Johannes Thrul, Corinne Joshu, and Katherine C. Smith
Health Communication, volume 37, issue 9 (2022) pp. 1229–1241

Chapter 16

Construyendo Conexiones Para Los Niños: Environmental Justice, Reproductive Feminicidio, and Coalitional Possibility in the Borderlands
Sarah De Los Santos Upton, Carlos A. Tarin, and Leandra H. Hernández
Health Communication, volume 37, issue 9 (2022) pp. 1242–1252

Notes on Contributors

Matthew K. Ackerman, School of Communication and Information, Rutgers University, USA.

Comfort Tosin Adebayo, Department of Communication Studies, Towson University, USA.

Oluwatumininu Awonuga, Department of Communication Studies, University of Georgia, Athens, USA.

Cristina L. Azocar, Journalism, San Francisco State University, USA.

Erin M. Bergner, Center for Research on Men's Health, Vanderbilt University, Nashville, USA.

John J. Brooks, School of Communication, Northwestern University, Evanston, USA.

Natasha R. Brown, Department of Communication, Indiana University Northwest, Gary, USA.

Suzanne Burdick, Department of Communication Studies, University of Texas at Austin, USA.

Peter J. Carek, Community Health & Family Medicine, University of Florida, USA.

Candi S. Carter Olson, Journalism, Utah State University, USA.

Angela Cooke-Jackson, California State University, Los Angeles, USA.

Chris M. Daley, Lehigh College of Health, Institute for Indigenous Studies, USA.

Sean M. Daley, Lehigh College of Health, Institute for Indigenous Studies, USA.

Sarah De Los Santos Upton, Department of Communication, The University of Texas at El Paso, USA.

Jennifer M. Ellison, Center for Research on Men's Health, Vanderbilt University, Nashville, USA.

LeChrista Finn, College of Agriculture, Communities, and the Sciences, Kentucky State University, Frankfort, USA.

Diane B. Francis, Department of Communication, University of Kentucky, Lexington, USA.

Monica L. Gallegos, Department of Communication Studies, California State University, USA.

Thomas J. George, Hematology & Oncology, University of Florida, USA.

Ryan Goeckner, Department of Anthropology, Ohio State University, Columbus, USA.

Derek M. Griffith, Center for Research on Men's Health, Vanderbilt University; Department of Medicine Health & Society, Vanderbilt University, Nashville, USA.

Jordyn Gunville, Lehigh College of Health, Institute for Indigenous Studies, USA.

River Gunville, Lehigh College of Health, Institute for Indigenous Studies, USA.

Jason Hale, Lehigh College of Health, Institute for Indigenous Studies, USA.

Deion S. Hawkins, Department of Communication Studies, Emerson College, USA.

Bharbi Hazarika, Scripps School of Journalism, Ohio University, Athens, USA.

Leandra H. Hernández, Department of Communication, Utah Valley University, Orem, USA.

Emily Cornish Jaeger, Center for Research on Men's Health, Vanderbilt University, Nashville, USA.

Parul Jain, Scripps School of Journalism, Ohio University, Athens, USA.

Corinne Joshu, Department of Epidemiology, Johns Hopkins School of Public Health, USA.

Janice L. Krieger, STEM Translational Communication Center, University of Florida, USA.

Benjamin R. LaPoe, Communication Studies, Ohio University, Athens, USA.

Victoria L. LaPoe, Scripps School of Journalism, Ohio University, Athens, USA.

Charley Lewis, Lehigh College of Health, Institute for Indigenous Studies, USA.

Benjamin C. Lok, Computer & Information Science & Engineering, University of Florida, USA.

Crystal Y. Lumpkins, Department of Family Medicine and Community Health, University of Kansas Medical Center; William Allen White School of Journalism and Mass Communications, University of Kansas-Lawrence, USA.

Soroya Julian McFarlane, Department of Communication Studies, University of Georgia, Athens, USA.

Lucy Mkandawire-Valhmu, College of Nursing, University of Wisconsin-Milwaukee, USA.

François P. Modave, Health Outcomes & Biomedical Informatics, University of Florida, USA.

Jorge A. Montoya, Department of Communication Studies, Sentient Research, USA.

Meghan B. Moran, Department of Health, Behavior & Society, Johns Hopkins School of Public Health, USA.

Susan E. Morgan, School of Communication, University of Miami, Coral Gables, USA.

Aubrey M. Mys, STEM Translational Communication Center, University of Florida, USA.

Jordan M. Neil, Health Policy Research Center, Department of Medicine, Harvard Medical School, USA.

Sarah Nicholus, Women's, Gender, and Sexuality Studies, University of Texas at Austin, USA.

Aurora Occa, Department of Communication, University of Kentucky, Lexington, USA.

Folakemi T. Odedina, Pharmacotherapy & Translational Research, University of Florida, USA.

Oluwatoyin Olukotun, School of Nursing, University of Portland, USA.

Erin Sahlstein Parcell, Department of Communication, University of Wisconsin-Milwaukee, USA.

Wei Peng, Murrow College of Communication, Washington State University, USA.

Aaron Plant, Department of Communication Studies, Sentient Research, USA.

Yonaira M. Rivera, Department of Communication, School of Communication & Information, Rutgers University, USA.

Camille J. Saucier, School of Communication, Northwestern University, Evanston, USA.

Chris Segrin, Department of Communication, University of Arizona, USA.

Andrea R. Semlow, Center for Research on Men's Health, Vanderbilt University, Nashville, USA.

Charles R. Senteio, School of Communication and Information, Rutgers University, USA.

Katherine C. Smith, Department of Health, Behavior & Society, Johns Hopkins School of Public Health, USA.

Elizabeth C. Stewart, Department of Surgery, Meharry Medical College, USA.

Sapna Suresh, School of Communication, Northwestern University, Evanston, USA.

Carlos A. Tarin, Department of Communication, The University of Texas at El Paso, USA.

Fatemeh Tavassoli, Computer & Information Science & Engineering, University of Florida, USA.

Johannes Thrul, Department of Mental Health, Johns Hopkins School of Public Health, USA.

Melissa J. Vilaro, STEM Translational Communication Center, University of Florida, USA.

Nathan Walter, School of Communication, Northwestern University, Evanston, USA.

Lillie D. Williamson, Department of Communication Arts, University of Wisconsin-Madison, USA.

Danyell S. Wilson-Howard, Chemistry, Bethune-Cookman University, USA.

La'Marcus T. Wingate, College of Pharmacy, Department of Clinical & Administrative Pharmacy Sciences, Howard University, Washington, D.C., USA.

Mohan S. Zalake, Computer & Information Science & Engineering, University of Florida, USA.

INTRODUCTION

Emergent Health Communication Scholarship from and about African American, Latino/a/x, and American Indian/Alaskan Native Peoples

Angela Cooke-Jackson

ABSTRACT

It is a privilege and honor to welcome you to this special issue of Health Communication which is based on scholarship that advances various divergent health issues pertinent to African American, Latino/a/x, and American Indian/Alaskan Native (AI/AN) peoples. The vision for this special issue which is a microcosm of the impactful research literature emerging from our field by Black, Latino/a/x, and American Indian peoples was to call attention to and acknowledge the breath of theoretically grounded and methodologically appropriate research in health communication. The 16 original articles featured in this issue reflect a robust compilation of topics from medical mistrust to tribal and elder leaders as health communicators and health promoters. The vision for the issue is that these articles serve as a platform that starts a meaningful and needed dialog within the field of health communication about the need for accessible and diverse scholarship from often-absent voices and/or narratives.

> *The process of developing a worldview that differs from the dominant worldview requires active intellectual work on the part of the knower, because schools, society, and the structure and production of knowledge are designed to create individuals who internalize the dominant worldview and knowledge production and acquisition processes.* (Ladson-Billings, 2021, p. 158)

The field of health communication has experienced an emergence of scholarship by African American, Latino/a/x, and American Indian/Alaskan Native (AI/AN) communication scholars over the past decade. These scholars are ambitious and passionate and have a clear vision of how the field could better encompass the experiences of Black, Brown, and Indigenous folks of color.

As a senior scholar, I am transfixed by their ability to vocalize through their respective research endeavors the importance and need for more transparent and immersive scholarship. Scholarship that locates our lived experiences and narratives as central to shift the dominant culture paradigms is deeply valuable.

These scholars are committed to their own specific research areas to invigorate and reimagine conversations among clinicians, public health professionals, classroom environments, and communities. They are unabashedly calling for more equitable, community-centric, tribally centered, and transparent scholarship on topics of health disparities, health care, marginality, medical mistrust, social justice, and media and new technology as it relates to people of color. Their work advances various divergent health issues pertinent to Black, Latino/a/x, and AI/AN groups so that we clearly understand the powerful aspect of the human condition to know and be known as it relates to the negotiation of health and communication (Ladson-Billings, 2000). Invariably, this research provides a space to amplify the voices of our collective lived experiences through the vehicle of rigorous engaged scholarship.

It is a privilege to welcome you to the manifestation of this special issue. This is a compilation which I have envisioned for the past two decades. One does not always have the privilege to bring to fruition a compilation of this magnitude. For that reason, I am deeply appreciative of the receptiveness, support, and mentorship of the editor, Dr Teri Thompson. When I requested in a simple e-mail to Dr Thompson that the journal *Health Communication* provides a space for Black, Latino/a/x, and American Indian/Alaskan Native health communication scholars to advance innovative scholarship, she without hesitation said yes. The call went out in October 2019. There were 50 plus abstract submissions from which 25 went through the blind-review process. Sixteen were accepted for publication. Over the course of the months, in the midst of the COVID-19 pandemic, these scholars excelled. Thank you to the team of folks who etched out time in their busy lives to read through the first round of abstracts – Dr Kristina Ruiz-Mesa, Dr John Youngblood, Dr Lorenda Belone, and Dr Diane Francis. Thank you to the blind review scholars – a collection of experienced expert professors and practitioners – who understood the challenge and goal to not simply read the 16 manuscripts but provide detailed recommendations to each author with the intent to mentor them through the publication process and understand the importance of their research. The outcome is a profoundly rich compilation of scholarship which is a testament to the agility and dedication of people to work collectively to complete something greater than themselves. I hope each scholar can pause to see themselves in the issue, but more importantly, the worth of their voices and health and health-care research scripted into this special issue and into the field. Representation does matter.

The histories of Black, Brown, and Indigenous people in the U.S. are steeped in high rates of infectious diseases, chronic illnesses, mental health illnesses, low birth rates, infant mortality rates, and high maternal mortality that stem from centuries of racism, invisibility, inequality, and marginalization. The current cultural and political climate marks a point in which our experiences, stories, and truths are being mindfully and intentionally studied and shared. Shifting the paradigm continues to take time, but we must thoughtfully and strategically pursue this end, understanding that our field is enriched when we incorporate communication perspectives from health scholars of the African American, Latino/a/x, and American Indian/Alaskan Native diaspora. The 16 peer-reviewed articles featured in this special issue address these critical intersections.

This issue begins with Lillie Williamson's article on the topic of medical mistrust. She notes that African Americans consistently report higher levels of medical mistrust than their White counterparts. She observes that even though most studies call for more research on medical mistrust, they neglect the vicarious experiences that transpire among Black people. Her detailed recruitment strategies used snowball sampling to garner participation from underserved populations in her online survey. Medical mistrust was measured with the Medical Mistrust Index (MMI) and her analytic procedure applied structural equation modeling to the hypothesis that racial discrimination leads to less trust in health care. Dr Williamson's findings provide a wealth of insights, among which is that health-care providers must recognize the impact of the media environment and ways they represent and remind people of structural barriers and oppressive systems especially during the COVID-19 pandemic. Dually important, she notes, is the extension of research that investigates medical mistrust among Latino/a/x and Indigenous populations.

Next, Soroya Julian McFarlane and colleagues dive into the topic of community-based participatory research (CBPR) as a method that "centers on effective dialogue between research and community stakeholders with the goal of creating an equitable partnership for health and social change" (2021, p. 2). The authors provide a comprehensive 10-year systematic review of the status of empirical research on elements of CBPR that have been used to improve the rate of accrual of members of racial and ethnic minority communities for clinical trials. Their review notes a large increase in CBPR and a positive outcome in community participation. Findings address the value of more transparency about the extent of community participation and more accurate, thorough descriptions about the nature of partnership with minority communities with the intent of building on the literature on community-engaged methods.

Camille Saucier and colleagues explore the rates of unplanned pregnancies among Black and Latina teens using an entertainment-education video intervention – "Plan A." The video intervention, which was developed in close collaboration with Black and Latina women aged 18–19, sought to ensure that the content was relevant, engaging, and motivational. The sample included Black, Latina, and non-Latina White women, with younger and White women included for comparison purposes. The authors found that exposure to "Plan A" significantly improved attitudes toward long-acting reversible contraceptives (LARCs) among all age groups and specifically among young Black and Latina women. They state that their findings may be explained by participant's identification with the Black and Latina lead characters, both of whom model positive reproductive health behaviors. One of the most valuable conclusions from this study is the realization that collaborative approaches with intended audiences (Black and Latina women) can result in more dynamic entertainment-education interventions.

Moving from entertainment-education videos to entertainment programming, Diane Francis and LeChrista Finn used a culture-centric approach to investigate the role of television storylines in facilitating health-related conversations on the social media site Twitter. The authors examined Twitter conversations on the fictional television drama "Queen Sugar" to investigate sexual and police-involved trauma. Using a culture-centric model of narratives in health promotion, they classified 1671 tweets into four main thematic categories (identification, social proliferation, emotions, and intention). Although the authors note some limitations with the use of their hashtag #QueenSugarTalks and an inability to examine demographic data, they contend that Twitter may be an important vehicle for engaging difficult conversations, specifically for mental health communication with Black Americans.

As we consider the theme of police brutality and mental health among Black communities, Deion Hawkins' article introduces us to another important juxtaposition of scholarship. Drawing on Critical Race Theory (CRT), he addresses the too frequent incidents of police brutality. His article takes a phenomenological approach as he analyzes 27 semi-structured interviews with African Americans on topics of psychological distress, trauma, and police brutality in the Black community. His findings acknowledge the importance and usefulness of creating trauma-based communication models that frame brutality as a health communication issue as well as blueprints that advance police–community relationships in Black communities.

Although Critical Race Theory has been a debated framework, it is an imperative theoretical approach for understanding inequity. As such, the next article by Melissa J. Vilaro and colleagues provides a comprehensive overview of race and the usefulness of CRT for the development of culturally tailored approaches to reduce cancer inequities, specifically colorectal cancer (CRC). The authors investigate the use of virtual health assistants (VHA) to promote colorectal cancer screening among rural Black and White study participants. Their analysis with 28 focus groups (Black = 85, White = 69) tested the VHA intervention on mobile phones. Not only did Black focus group members prefer receiving information about colorectal cancer risk from VHA, they also expressed the value of sharing the intervention and colorectal cancer screening messages with younger members of their network. Among other recommendations, the authors observe the value of Critical Race Theory, health communication, and technology as a bridge for inclusive colorectal cancer messages.

Comfort Tosin Adebayo and colleagues also propose Critical Race Theory as a means to understand Black women's experiences of pregnancy-related complications. The authors note the intersections of race, maternal health, marginality, and the structural barriers to pregnancy that are specific to how Black women are impacted by maternal health care. The study recruited 31 African American women to engage in interviews that took place in Milwaukee County, Wisconsin. The authors' findings ask health-care administrators to be more vigilant in addressing the needs of African American women and other minority populations. This includes trainings that address racism and health inequities that might manifest knowingly and unknowingly in institutional practices. They also encourage active collaborations among individuals and organizations that care for women of color.

Derek Griffith and colleagues center the theoretical framework of African American Manhood to address the importance of scholarship that is population-specific and uses individualized messages to address minority health and achieve health equity. Their scholarship articulates the value of synergistically weaving manhood, tailored health messages for African American men, and intersectionality together. Their use of illustrations of African American men provides a powerful depiction of how distinct messaging can address societal factors like racism, gendered norms, values, and social expectations of Black men across a lifespan. The scholarship has a dynamic extension to other racial/ethnic groups and is valuable toward a better understanding of screening hesitancy, particularly of people of color, as well as distinct health intervention messages and educational materials for Black men.

Natasha R. Brown and La'Marcus T. Wingate introduce readers to health-related memorable messages and self-reports of diet and exercise behavior among Black women. Additionally, the authors use Control Theory to explain behavioral responses to memorable messages. Their cross-sectional survey was used to understand the relationship between receipt of memorable messages and dietary and exercise behaviors in Black women. Findings from this study suggest that receiving memorable messages not only impacts dietary choices but also acts to motivate greater frequency of exercise among Black women. Although the authors address the limitations of their work, they note that their research expands the literature on memorable messages and how Black women might enact holistic health-promoting behaviors through diet and exercise behaviors.

Charles R. Senteio and Matthew K. Ackerman tackle the critical topic of Black patients, dialysis, and awareness of transplantation and being on the transplant list. They present the implication of this racial disparity using Uncertainty Management Theory (UMT) to understand African American barriers and to getting on the transplant list and remaining there. Twenty-four Black end-stage renal disease (ESRD) patients participated in semi-structured interviews sharing their dialysis experiences and their understanding of transplants. The authors found that uncertainty is multilayered and social support can both dissuade the patients from getting on the transplant list and decrease uncertainty, especially when individuals wanted to be on the transplant list so they could be with family. The authors call for improved patient education surrounding treatment options and better communication of relevant transplant health information.

One observation that I have noted from this special topic issue is that we have a long way to go in the field of health communication toward advancing literature from and about American Indians. The article from Crystal Y. Lumpkins and colleagues is a relevant and necessary contribution. The authors delve into the topic of tribal and elder leaders as health communicators and health promoters within the Central Plains communities (Kansas, Iowa, Missouri, and South Dakota). Thirty-nine in-depth interviews were conducted by members of the Center for American Indian Community Health. The interviewees were all members of federally recognized tribes living in reservation and urban tribal communities across the region. The results from this compelling study indicate that these elders and tribal leaders do not necessarily see themselves as "authority" health communicators or health promoters within their tribe or community. However, the elders did feel that social and cultural authority using tailored and targeted messages from trusted sources could bolster health communication programs and have a positive impact on health outcomes among American Indian populations. The article ends by encouraging those who partner with Indigenous communities to communicate with community members to better understand if they feel health communication via trusted leaders would be useful.

A second distinct contribution to American Indian scholarship comes from Victoria LaPoe and colleagues. The authors use mediatization theory to understand US media coverage and Indigenous US media coverage of COVID-19. The goal was to observe its potential to impact policy decision and thus address the importance of evaluating health coverage of Indigenous communities by both Indigenous and non-Indigenous news sources. The authors used a qualitative textual analysis of the Indigenous and mainstream digital new sources, collecting 326 news stories for analysis. The findings from this study are deeply profound, providing a robust and important contribution to health communication scholarship. One primary take away is that mainstream news sources must produce stories about Indigenous health issues that are free from stereotypes which have "inculcated enduring schemas about Indigenous people" (2021, p. 10). Additional findings note that for diverse coverage, newsrooms must have reporters who are connected to Indigenous communities and that these reporters should have space to tell specific stories and need other critical opportunities for covering health in Indian country.

Latino/a/x scholarship was another important contribution included in this special issue. First, we hear from Monica Gallegos and Chris Segrin, who investigate the relationship between Latina/o cultural values of *familism* and health. The Latino Health Paradox, which is the central component of their scholarship, is investigated in combination with the theoretical model of loneliness and health. This study included 139 Latina/o and 116 non-Latina/o White participants who were from a parent study that documented the Latino health paradox in the sample. The authors' findings suggest that *familism* may be a psychological resource in the Latina/o community and thus makes sense of lower loneliness and indirectly greater health. One valuable insight from the authors is understanding how cultural values, especially those based on interpersonal connections, can protect outcomes related to health and wellbeing.

Next, Suzanne Burdick and Sarah Nicholus provide a pilot study on a dually important topic, Latinx lesbian, gay, and bisexual (LGB) adolescent patients' disclosure of personal sexual orientation and health to health-care providers. Their article highlights the layers of marginalization that reside between Latinx LGB patients' cultural identity, sexual orientation, and sexual health. The authors used a participatory action research paradigm to conduct one-on-one interviews with participants that identified as Latinx. They found that Latinx LGB individuals have different reasons and motivations for disclosing information to health-care providers. One important call to action is to encourage health-care providers and systems to engage in diversity, equity, and inclusion training to mitigate unconscious bias and inadvertent microaggressions.

Yonaira M. Rivera and colleagues shed light on social media platforms, specifically one of the largest – Facebook – as a means to engage with and empower Latinos/as to participate in cancer control and prevention. Their mixed-methods study explores how Latinos/as engage with and act on cancer prevention screening information (CPSI) on Facebook. Findings from this study suggest that cultural values and other aspects of cultural connection influence how Latinos/as engage with, interpret, and act on cancer prevention screening information on Facebook. This work, which is the first to explore these phenomena, offers a valuable perspective on how to leverage social media, using it to curtail the effects of health misinformation as well as to create cancer education interventions and communication campaigns that have culturally tailored content.

To round out this special issue, we hear from authors Sarah De Los Santos Upton, Carlos A. Tarin, and Leandra H. Hernandez, whose scholarship is creating a powerful research space on environmental and reproductive justice, the U.S.–Mexico border, and health communication. In their article, they use *reproductive feminicidio* to explore the public advocacy efforts of Familias Unidas as a case study on gender violence against women on the reproductive spectrum. Their work identifies three rhetorical strategies – *familia, comunidad*, and *(in)justicia* – employed by Familias Unidas to shape their public argument(s). The most generative analysis this article brings forward is the reality that organizing efforts can highlight how "issues affecting marginalized communities are frequently obfuscated in health communication literature" (2021, p. 9).

In closing, the articles published in this special issue *Emergent Health Communication Scholarship from and about African American, Latino/a/x, and Native American/First Peoples* each highlight the importance of synergy and collective voices while they envelop the importance of representation – particularly at this time in our history. Each article speaks to the depth and breadth of talent, diversity of methodology, and the locations of health behaviors, perspectives, and health communication topics. They offer theoretical and practical approaches and applications to consider when engaging in research in partnership with and/or on African American, Latino/a/x, and Alaskan Indian/Native American peoples. The vision for this undertaking is to make sure Black, Latino/a/x, and American Indian researchers have a seat at the table of scholarship that is transpiring in the field of health communication. The publication process has its own set of challenges, but I hope we see a growth in theoretically grounded and methodologically appropriate scholarship from a breadth of racially, gendered diverse folks. I especially hope that scholars see the field of health communication and this journal as a safe and accessible space for their often-absent voices and/or narratives.

Disclosure statement

No potential conflict of interest was reported by the author.

Funding

The author reported that there is no funding associated with the work featured in this article.

References

De Los Santos Upton, S., Tarin, C. A., & Hernández, L. H. (2021). Construyendo conexiones para los niños: Environmental justice, reproductive feminicidio, and coalitional possibility in the borderlands. *Health Communication*, 1–11. Advance online publication. https://doi.org/10.1080/10410236.2021.1911386

Ladson-Billings, G. (2000). Racialized discourses and ethnic epistemologies. In N. Denzin & Y. Lincoln (Eds.), *Handbook of qualitative research* (2nd ed., pp. 257–277). Sage.

Ladson-Billings, G. (Ed.). (2021). *Critical race theory in education: A scholar's journey*. Teachers College Press.

LaPoe, V. L., Carter Olson, C. S., Azocar, C. L., LaPoe, B. R., Hazarika, B., & Jain, P. (2021). A comparative analysis of health news in Indigenous and mainstream media. *Health Communication*, 1–12. Advance online publication. https://doi.org/10.1080/10410236.2021.1945179

McFarlane, S. J., Occa, A., Peng, W., Awonuga, O., & Morgan, S. E. (2021). Community-based participatory research (CBPR) to enhance participation of racial/ethnic minorities in clinical trials: A 10-year systematic review. *Health Communication*, 1–18. Advance online publication. https://doi.org/10.1080/10410236.2021.1943978

Beyond Personal Experiences: Examining Mediated Vicarious Experiences as an Antecedent of Medical Mistrust

Lillie D. Williamson

ABSTRACT

African Americans consistently report higher levels of medical mistrust than their White counterparts. As a result, medical mistrust is considered to be a contributor to racial health disparities. Despite calls to address medical mistrust, few studies have explicitly examined it as a phenomenon of interest; those that have, tended to focus on personal experiences while neglecting vicarious experiences. The current study a) explicitly tests the effects of two types of news story content on reported levels of medical mistrust within an African American adult sample and b) examines two widely used medical mistrust measures. Participants ($N = 410$) were randomly assigned to view a news story based on a 2 (health care, non-health care) x 2 (racial discrimination, nonracial discrimination) experimental design. Results indicated that individually, both health care content and racial discrimination content increased race-based medical mistrust, but had no effect on general medical mistrust. However, when all four conditions were examined, exposure to health-related racial discrimination stories resulted in higher levels of race-based and general medical mistrust than non-health, nonracial discrimination stories. Findings are discussed in terms of the theoretical and practical implications for health communication scholars.

African Americans[1] consistently report higher levels of medical mistrust than their White counterparts. This distrust in the motives of medical personnel and institutions is associated with decreased likelihood of engagement in several health behaviors including routine health checkups (Hammond et al., 2010), cancer screenings (Shelton et al., 2010), treatment adherence (Kalichman et al., 2016), and registering as an organ donor (Morgan, 2004). As a result, medical mistrust is considered a contributor to racial health disparities, making this distrust in medical personnel and institutions crucial for health scholars to understand and address. Medical mistrust has long been recognized, but takes on renewed concern in the midst of public health crises, like COVID-19 (Jaiswal et al., 2020), which disproportionately affect African American communities (Centers for Disease Control and Prevention, 2020).

Despite calls to address medical mistrust, few studies have explicitly investigated it as a phenomenon of interest. As a result, there is little known about the antecedents of medical mistrust (Benkert et al., 2019). The work that has been done has heavily focused on the Tuskegee Syphilis Study (for discussion, see Jaiswal & Halkitis, 2019) and primarily centered personal experiences, neglecting the role of vicarious experiences. Mediated vicarious experiences, in particular, as suggested by Bandura (2009), have been largely absent from work on medical mistrust. Recent scholarship, such as Williamson, Smith et al. (2019), has begun to highlight the impact of news content on medical mistrust; however, this work examined the framing of a single type of news content, only examined one type of medical mistrust (race-based), and was conducted with a college student sample.

The current study begins to fill these gaps by experimentally testing the effects of health care content and racial discrimination content in news stories on medical mistrust. In doing so, the study moves the literature forward in two important ways. First, it expands the examination of vicarious experiences via mediated communication (i.e., news stories) as an antecedent of medical mistrust within an African American adult sample by specifically testing types of news content. Second, this study investigates the potential differential effects of content on both general and race-based medical mistrust, two widely used measures of medical mistrust. Below, the need to understand medical mistrust antecedents, the importance of mediated vicarious experiences, and the nuances of medical mistrust measures are discussed.

The need to understand medical mistrust antecedents beyond tuskegee

Medical mistrust – distrust in the motives of medical personnel and organizations (Omodei & McLennan, 2000) – represents a widespread barrier for health communication scholars to address. There has been a great deal of work on medical mistrust (Benkert et al., 2019), much of which has focused on the relationship between medical mistrust and health outcomes. As a result, there is an abundance of knowledge surrounding the various health outcomes influenced by medical mistrust (for a review of health contexts, see Williamson & Bigman, 2018); however, much less is known about what precedes and contributes to medical mistrust. In recognition of this, scholars have recently called for more work on medical mistrust antecedents (Benkert et al., 2019)

While there has been work conducted on antecedents of medical trust or skepticism (e.g., Jensen et al., 2011; Tian & Yoo, 2020), there is little work that examines medical mistrust specifically. Although similar, trust and mistrust are distinct concepts. Trust refers to the ability to feel vulnerable and know that one's needs will be met (Hall et al., 2001), whereas mistrust refers to perceptions of negative motives on the part of medical personnel and institutions (Thompson et al., 2004). In other words, individuals can believe healthcare providers will not meet their needs without being mistrustful. For example, believing a provider does not have enough experience to correctly diagnosis an issue does not mean an individual believes the provider is working against their best interests. Thus, medical mistrust is, as Jaiswal and Halkitis (2019) define it, "not merely the opposite of trust" and more than "simply the absence of trust" but instead "the belief that the entity that is the object of mistrust is acting against one's best interest or well-being" (p. 80).

When medical mistrust among African Americans is considered, the focus is often on the lingering effects of the Tuskegee Syphilis Study (Tuskegee), in which the US Public Health Service told African American men they were being treated for "bad blood" but instead withheld treatment for syphilis, even after penicillin was a known cure. Incidents of mistreatment and abuse began well before Tuskegee and continued long after (for a review, see Washington, 2006). Although Tuskegee is a well-known, salient example of the earned distrust of medical institutions, the enduring focus on Tuskegee may conceal the other historical and present-day examples of mistreatment and abuse of African American communities (Jaiswal & Halkitis, 2019). Thus, in answering Benkert et al.'s (2019) call for needed work on medical mistrust antecedents, scholars must also look beyond Tuskegee and knowledge of that incident. Instead, Tuskegee should be thought of as a notable example representing broader issues (i.e., negative health care experiences, racial discrimination).

The role of mediated vicarious experiences

Some scholarship has branched out beyond Tuskegee and explicitly examined other medical mistrust antecedents. Much of this work, however, has predominantly focused on personal experiences. For instance, Hammond (2010) examined, and found evidence for, the relationships between both healthcare experiences and racial discrimination experiences and medical mistrust. Hammond (2010), however, conceptualized these experiences as participants' own personal experiences. Work in social cognitive theory (SCT; Bandura, 2009) suggests that not only personal experiences, but also vicarious experiences influence medical mistrust. SCT asserts that through the actions of others individuals are able to learn about the world, including the consequences of actions, without directly experiencing events.

There has gradually begun to be work producing empirical support for the effects of vicarious experiences. For instance, work conducted by Bogart et al. (2016) suggested that hearing about others' HIV conspiracy beliefs (i.e., medical mistrust) was associated with decreased antiretroviral therapy adherence. While this particular work demonstrates a potential turn toward vicarious experiences, it only acknowledges those that would result from interpersonal communication (i.e., interpersonal vicarious experiences). A recent review of medical mistrust alluded to the role of vicarious experiences by mentioning vicarious interpersonal experiences (e.g., intergenerational transmission of experiences; Benkert et al., 2019). There was, however, no mention of mediated vicarious experiences, defined in the current study as vicarious experiences that occur as a result of mediated communication. As noted by Bandura (2009), media is one way in which these vicarious processes occur; thus, examining mediated vicarious experiences in considerations of medical mistrust is necessary.

Vicarious experiences via media

Mediated vicarious experiences serve as a way to learn about the world without direct experiential knowledge (Bandura, 2009), including judging risk. Scholars have contended that vicarious experiences result in individuals realizing they themselves are vulnerable to the effects of racism and discrimination (Truong et al., 2016); exposure to news media is one way this might occur. News coverage of racial inequalities often depicts Black disadvantage (Gandy & Li, 2005), which can influence perceptions of inequality (Gandy, 2009) and health risk perceptions (Bigman, 2014). This news coverage may also act as a means of vicariously experiencing the world, affecting perceived likelihood of facing events oneself.

Recently, Williamson, Bigman et al. (2019) found that African American participants specifically pointed to news stories as having influenced their organ donation-related medical mistrust beliefs. For these participants, having seen these news stories allowed them to gain knowledge vicariously about what happened when racial/ethnic minorities engaged with the organ donation, and medical, system, thus influencing their medical mistrust beliefs; they believed these news stories were indicative of what would happen to them. A subsequent experimental study conducted by Williamson, Smith et al. (2019) found evidence that news stories depicting racial discrimination experiences influenced medical mistrust, suggesting that mediated vicarious experiences in the form of news stories can, in fact, influence medical mistrust. This study, however, only examined racial discrimination content, which is unlikely to be the only type of news content that influences medical mistrust; racial discrimination may not be the only vicarious experience related to medical mistrust. Thus, there remains a need to understand the types of news content that influences medical mistrust.

News content

The question then becomes what types of news content might influence medical mistrust. Based on SCT, the realms in which personal experiences influence medical mistrust, should be the areas that vicarious experiences would be expected to influence medical mistrust. In other words, the type of incidents that would influence medical mistrust for individuals if personally experienced, should be the type of incidents that influence medical mistrust when experienced vicariously via depictions in news stories. Previous work suggests that this would occur in the domains of racial discrimination experiences (Hammond, 2010; Williamson, Smith et al., 2019), as well as health care experiences (Hammond, 2010).

Considering the mental representation of medical mistrust provides additional theoretical rationale for expecting depictions of both racial discrimination and negative health care experiences to influence medical mistrust. Medical mistrust is an attitude; as such, part of its mental representation is an attitudinal schema (Pratkanis, 1989). This attitudinal schema is comprised of knowledge about an object (i.e., healthcare providers) and its associated attributes. Given the history of mistreatment of Black patients, it is reasonable to think that there may be a link between health care providers (i.e., the object) and discrimination (i.e., an attribute). This linkage would be activated not only when individuals encounter information about the healthcare system, but also when the associated node is activated. As a result, exposure to racial discrimination content in news stories may prime thoughts of racial discrimination more broadly, including in the health care system, resulting in increased medical mistrust.

H1: Exposure to racial discrimination content in news stories will result in higher levels of medical mistrust than exposure to nonracial discrimination news stories.

The attitudinal schema for medical mistrust is likely to be comprised of a myriad of other attributes for the healthcare system. It may be the case that exposure to healthcare content, regardless of its attachment to discrimination, may prime associations and result in medical mistrust, particularly if this healthcare content depicts an undesirable encounter with a healthcare provider. Exposure to this type of content may prime other negative attributes associated with healthcare providers. For instance, if individuals believe providers care more about profit than their patients (Jacobs et al., 2006), exposure to content depicting unsatisfactory healthcare experiences may prime attributes, like greed, and result in medical mistrust.

H2: Exposure to health care content in news stories will result in higher levels of medical mistrust than exposure to non-health care news stories.

It is also possible to consider how these two types of message content may interact to influence medical mistrust. Messages that do not contain either of these types of content should produce the lowest reported medical mistrust, whereas messages that contain both types of content should result in the highest levels of medical mistrust. There is, however, no current indication of how other combinations of health care and racial discrimination content in messages may influence medical mistrust. Thus,

H3: Exposure to health care, discrimination news stories will result in higher reported medical mistrust than exposure to all other news story types.

H4: Exposure to non-health care, nondiscrimination news stories will result in lower reported medical mistrust than exposure to all other news story types.

RQ1: Does exposure to health care, nondiscrimination news stories result in different levels of medical mistrust than exposure to non-health care, racial discrimination news stories?

General versus race-based medical mistrust

The current study also presents an opportunity to examine the potential differential impact of news stories on general and race-based medical mistrust. Examining the relationship between news content and both types of medical mistrust may help disentangle the nuances of these types of medical mistrust (e.g., whether exposure influences general mistrust, mistrust that stems from marginalization and social positioning, or both). As documented by Williamson and Bigman (2018), these widely used measures of medical mistrust rely on different referents (general: people should be mistrustful versus race-based: people who belong to my race/ethnicity). In light of historical relationships between Africans Americans and the medical system, asking about whether, "Patients have sometimes been deceived or misled by healthcare providers" (LaVeist et al., 2009, p. 2100) is very different than asking items about whether individuals believe their group is more likely to be misled (e.g., "Healthcare providers sometimes hide information from people of my race/ethnicity;" Thompson et al., 2004, p. 213). The latter directly calls upon African Americans' social positioning. Recent work has suggested these types of medical mistrust can have consequential differences in their relation to other variables (Pellowski et al., 2017); however, most studies only examine one type of medical mistrust (Williamson & Bigman, 2018). Given the lack of work examining differences between general and race-based medical mistrust:

RQ2: Do health care content and racial discrimination content impact both general and race-based medical mistrust?

Method

Participants and recruitment

Participants (N = 462) were recruited through a Qualtrics survey panel in July 2019. All participants were adults over the age of 18 who self-identified as African American. Fifty-two participants were removed from the data set for providing irrelevant responses to open-ended items (e.g., "Avenger end game because I want a scam webs they all game ... ") or for streamlining answers (i.e., answering "3" for every Likert-scale item) resulting in a final sample of 410 participants. Participants were primarily women (73.8%) and reported being heterosexual (83.7%). They ranged in age from 18 to 75 with a mean age of 36.04 (SD = 15.67). Most participants reported being from the South (59%). Finally, a majority of participants did not hold a bachelor's degree (70.7%) and reported making less than 50,000 USD (63.7%).

Procedure

Following approval from the Institutional Review Board at the University of Illinois at Urbana-Champaign (Protocol # 19737)

participants completed an online experimental survey. Participants were told they were taking part in two short, unrelated surveys: a "news study" and a "health study" to address the concern that letting participants assume exposure and subsequent items were related could be problematic. Without this precaution, individuals exposed to non-health care, racial discrimination news stories would have been exposed to a discrimination news story and then subsequently presented with health items without any explanation or justification.

In the "news study," participants were asked a few questions about their news media habits (e.g., how credible they perceive news stories to be). They were then exposed to a message that corresponded to the condition they were randomized into (e.g., non-health care, racial discrimination). After exposure to the message, participants were asked to engage in a thought-listing exercise about their thoughts while reading the study, as well as asked whether and where they had previously read a similar article (not discussed here). As a precaution, story credibility was also assessed.[2] In the "health study," participants were asked items about their current health and medical mistrust. As two types of medical mistrust were presented (i.e., general medical mistrust and race-based medical mistrust), the order of presentation for these two measures was counterbalanced. At the end, participants were debriefed and informed of the true relationship between the two "studies."

Stimuli

A 2 (health care, non-health care) x 2 (racial discrimination, nonracial discrimination) design was employed creating four types of news stories: health care, racial discrimination; health care, nonracial discrimination; non-health care, racial discrimination; and non-health care, nonracial discrimination. Two stories were created for each message type. Health care content for this study depicted an inability to access either an oncologist or a therapist (i.e., negative health care experiences). For the non-health care news stories, lack of access to home internet and to ride-sharing services (e.g., Lyft) were used. News stories depicting racial discrimination utilized racialized geographic regions and mentioned the difficulty Black residents had procuring the discussed service. For nonracial discrimination content new stories, the differences were ascribed to geographic region (i.e., residents of small rural towns had difficulty accessing services). These topics were chosen as they could be used for both racial discrimination and issues of region and had appeared in recent news stories (e.g., Krull, 2019).

Messages were created to resemble news stories individuals may encounter in everyday life. Each was presented as a short news report on the findings of a recent study or institutional report; this included a quote from a researcher involved in the study explaining the report and its recommendations. Messages were made as consistent as possible in terms of content and length. Sentiment analysis conducted in ConTEXT (Diesner et al., 2015) revealed that the stories did not vary in tone. The resulting messages represent probabilistic social comparison frames (Bigman, 2014; Gandy & Li, 2005). Example stimuli are presented in Appendix A.

Measures

Medical mistrust

General medical mistrust. General medical mistrust was assessed using a modified version of the Medical Mistrust Index (MMI; LaVeist et al., 2009). The original index asks participants how much they agree with statements about health-care organizations; the measure was modified to refer to healthcare providers (e.g., "Patients have sometimes been deceived or misled by healthcare providers"). Participants were asked to respond from 1 (strongly disagree) to 5 (strongly agree). The MMI has been found to be a reliable scale among Black populations (e.g., Brandon et al., 2005). For the current study, the items formed a reliable scale (α =.86).

Race-based medical mistrust. Race-based medical mistrust was assessed using the Group-Based Medical Mistrust Scale (GBMMS; Thompson et al., 2004). The GBMMS asks participants whether individuals of their race/ethnicity should be distrustful of medical personnel; in other words, the referent group for items is participants' own race/ethnic group. The 12-item scale contains items such as "People of my race/ethnicity should be suspicious of modern medicine." For the current study, as all participants were African American, "people of my race/ethnicity" was replaced with "African Americans." Participants rated their level of agreement from 1 (strongly disagree) to 5 (strongly agree). Previous work has found the scale to be reliable for Black populations (e.g., Greer et al., 2014). Although all items formed a reliable scale in the current study (α = .88), analyses indicated removal of reverse coded items; the remaining eight items also formed a reliable scale (α = .89).

Demographics

Demographic information on sex, age, socioeconomic status, and sexual orientation were also collected. Scholarship has suggested that variables such as biological sex (Greer et al., 2014), age (Hammond, 2010), and socioeconomic status (Maly et al., 2008) are associated with medical mistrust; thus, these were included as possible covariates.

Analysis

Structural equation modeling procedures were utilized using Mplus Version 8 (Muthén & Muthén, 2017). In all models, both general and race-based medical mistrust were treated as latent variables. Based on the bivariate correlations, general and race-based medical mistrust were entered into the same model; they were not so highly correlated as to suggest multicollinearity (r = .47, p < .001). A confirmatory factor analysis (CFA) was conducted for the general medical mistrust and race-based medical mistrust variables. After the CFA, a structural model was tested in which health care content and racial discrimination content were dummy coded and entered as exogenous variables in the model. Based on recommendations by Kline (2016), the comparative fit index (CFI), root mean square error of approximation (RMSEA), and standardized root mean squared residual (SRMR) are reported alongside the chi-square statistic. A CFI greater than .90, a RMSEA below .08, and a SRMR below .09 served as indicators of adequate fit.

Structural equation modeling is not optimally suited to ascertain differences among all conditions (e.g., differences in medical mistrust for those exposed to health care, nonracial discrimination news stories versus those exposed to non-health care, racial discrimination news stories). Thus, ANOVAs were conducted in SPSS Version 25; separate analyses were run for general medical mistrust and race-based medical mistrust. As two outcomes were examined for the purposes of later examining the comparatives effects on outcomes, the *p*-value was adjusted to provide a conservative estimate; thus, the *p*-value was set to .025 (i.e., .05/2).

Results

Manipulation check

A manipulation check was conducted to ensure that participants perceived differences between message conditions. To examine the effects of the health care manipulation, independent samples t-tests were conducted for health care versus non-health care conditions. Participants were asked two questions related to the health content of the article: "The story I read was about health" and "The story I read was about an individual with a health issue." There were significantly higher levels of agreement that the story was about health for those in the health care condition ($M = 4.14$, $SD = 1.05$) than in the non-health care condition ($M = 2.34$, $SD = 1.36$), $t(381.26) = 14.94$, $p < .001$. Similarly, there were higher levels of agreement that the individual had a health issue for those in the health care condition ($M = 3.72$, $SD = 1.21$) than those in the non-health care condition ($M = 2.28$, $SD = 1.31$), $t(407.26) = 11.65$, $p < .001$.

To examine the effects of the racial discrimination manipulation, independent samples t-tests were conducted for racial discrimination versus nonracial discrimination conditions. Participants were asked two questions related to racial discrimination content of the article: "The story I read mentioned racial discrimination" and "The story I read was about an individual who experienced racial discrimination." There were significantly higher levels of agreement that the story mentioned racial discrimination for those in the racial discrimination condition ($M = 3.88$, $SD = 1.22$) than in the nonracial discrimination condition ($M = 2.56$, $SD = 1.27$), $t(410) = 10.75$, $p < .001$. Similarly, there were higher levels of agreement that the individual in the story experienced racial discrimination for those in the racial discrimination condition ($M = 3.72$, $SD = 1.18$) than those in the nonracial discrimination condition ($M = 2.47$, $SD = 1.26$), $t(410) = 10.38$, $p < .001$.

Main analysis

Structural equation model

Confirmatory factor analysis. The initial model did not fit the data, $\chi^2(151, N = 410) = 1147.89$, $p < .001$, $CFI = .72$, $RMSEA = .13$ (90% CI: .120, .134), $SRMR = .10$. An examination of item loadings revealed that four items for race-based medical mistrust loaded below a threshold of .40 (Matsunaga, 2010). These items were also the reverse coded items in the scale. Given concerns about reverse coded items (Weems & Onwuegbuzie, 2001) and their loadings (e.g., Zhang et al., 2016), these items were removed. The removal of these items bettered fit, but still produced an ill-fitting model, $\chi^2(89, N = 410) = 337.71$, $p < .001$, $CFI = .91$, $RMSEA = .08$ (90% CI: .073, .092), $SRMR = .05$. Correlating error terms for one pair of general medical mistrust items and two pairs of race-based medical mistrust items produced an adequately fitting model, $\chi^2(86, N = 410) = 222.29$, $p < .001$, $CFI = .95$, $RMSEA = .06$ (90% CI: .052, .072), $SRMR = .04$.

Structural model. H1 and H2 posited that exposure to racial discrimination content (H1) and health care content (H2) would result in higher levels of medical mistrust. Given the nature of the analyses, this would be represented as a positive relationship between content and medical mistrust. Demographic variables were not related to medical mistrust and thus, were not included in models as covariates.[3] This model provided adequate fit, $\chi^2(112, N = 410) = 249.22$, $p < .001$, $CFI = .95$, $RMSEA = .06$ (90% CI: .046, .064), $SRMR = .04$. The unstandardized path coefficients (UPC) and standardized path coefficients (SPC) are presented.

There was no significant relationship between racial discrimination content and general medical mistrust (UPC = .11, SPC = .10, $p = .06$). Nor was there a significant relationship between negative health care content and general medical mistrust (UPC = .09, SPC = .08, $p = .15$). There was, however, a positive relationship between racial discrimination content and race-based medical mistrust (UPC = .21, SPC = .11, $p = .03$), as well as between health care content and race-based medical mistrust (UPC = .22, SPC = .12, $p = .03$). This would suggest that there is no effect of these types of content on general medical mistrust, but there is an effect on race-based medical mistrust. Thus, H1 and H2 were supported for race-based medical mistrust, but not general medical mistrust. The final structural model is shown in Figure 1.

Analysis of variance

H3 posited that health care-related racial discrimination news stories would result in higher reported medical mistrust than all other news story types. H4 posited that news stories that are not about health care or racial discrimination (i.e., non-health care, nonracial discrimination news stories) would result in

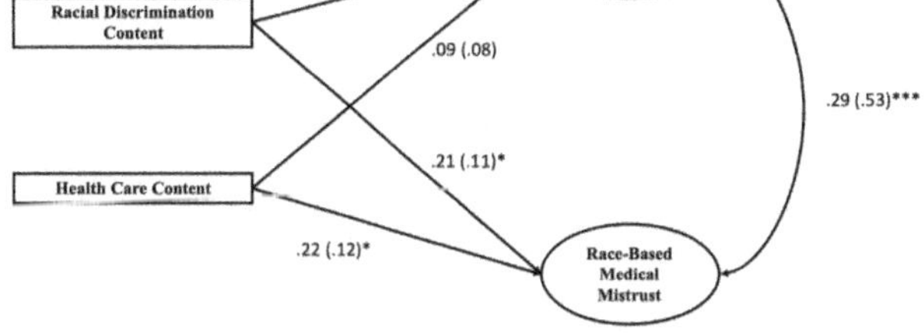

Figure 1. Structural model of associations between exposure to content type and medical mistrust. Unstandardized estimates are listed first, followed by standardized estimates in parentheses. *p <.05, ***p <.001

lower reported medical mistrust than all other message types. Finally, RQ1 asked whether there was a difference in reported medical mistrust between only health care-related (i.e., health care, nonracial discrimination) news stories and only racial discrimination-related (i.e., non-health care, racial discrimination) news stories.

Planned contrasts revealed that there was only a marginal difference in general medical mistrust for those exposed to health care-related, racial discrimination news stories ($M = 3.70$, $SD = .76$) in comparison to those who were exposed to non-health care, nonracial discrimination news stories ($M = 3.46$, $SD = .78$), $F(1, 406) = 4.99$, $p = .03$, $\eta^2 = .01$. However, for race-based medical mistrust, exposure to health care-related, racial discrimination news stories resulted in higher levels of mistrust ($M = 3.00$, $SD = 1.05$) than exposure to non-health care, nonracial discrimination news stories ($M = 2.62$, $SD = .81$), $F(1, 406) = 9.05$, $p = .003$, $\eta^2 = .02$. There were no other significant differences in medical mistrust among conditions. Thus, there was only partial support for H3 and H4. Furthermore, there was no significant difference between reported levels of medical mistrust for those exposed to health care, nonracial discrimination news stories in comparison to those exposed to non-health care, racial discrimination news stories. Full ANOVA results can be found Table 1.

Post-hoc analysis

Given the pattern of results found from the SEM and ANOVA analyses, a subsequent post-hoc analysis was conducted. The SEM model tested found significant relationships for exposure to both negative health care content and racial discrimination content for race-based medical mistrust. Based on the ANOVA analyses, it seemed that the health care-related, racial discrimination news studies may be driving these differences. As

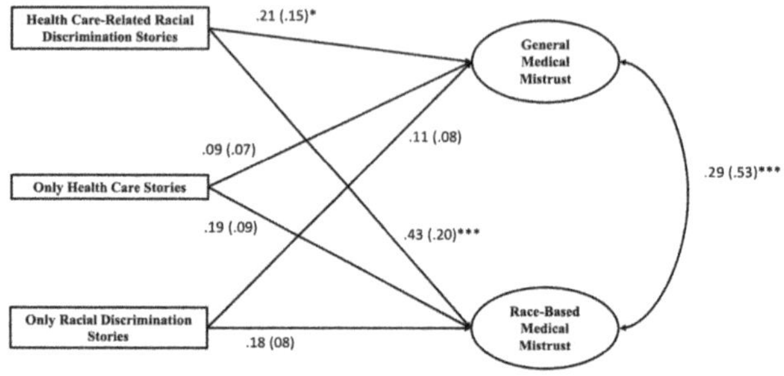

Figure 2. Structural model of associations between news story type and medical mistrust. Unstandardized estimates are listed first, followed by standardized estimates in parentheses. The model shows each news story type in comparison to non-health care, nonracial discrimination news stories. *p <.05, ***p <.001

a result, an additional SEM model was run with conditions dummy coded so that each was compared to the non-health care, nonracial discrimination condition, allowing for the effects of exposure to health care-related discrimination stories versus non-health care, nonracial discrimination stories to be examined while accounting for each type of medical mistrust. This model provided good fit, $\chi^2(125, N = 410) = 258.32$, $p < .001$, $CFI = .95$, $RMSEA = .05$ (90% CI: .042, .060), $SRMR = .04$ and revealed significant relationships for both general (UPC = .21, SPC = .15, $p = .02$) and race-based medical mistrust (UPC = .43, SPC = .20, $p = .001$). The full model is depicted in Figure 2.

Furthermore, while demographic variables were not associated with medical mistrust when examined as covariates, it still remained possible that these variables could be acting as moderators. To begin to investigate this possibility, age was tested as a moderator. The model provided good fit, $\chi^2(177, N = 410) = 323.45$, $p < .001$, $CFI = .95$, $RMSEA = .05$ (90% CI: .037, .053), $SRMR = .04$; however, there was no evidence of age moderating these effects; see Table 2 for results. The distribution of data did not allow for other demographic variables to be tested.

Table 1. Planned contrasts examining differences in medical mistrust by condition.

Conditions Compared		General Medical Mistrust F	p	η^2	Race-Based Medical Mistrust F	p	η^2
H/D	H/ND	1.46	0.23	0.004	2.53	0.11	0.01
H/D	NH/D	0.87	0.35	0.002	2.00	0.16	0.01
H/D	NH/ND	4.99	0.03	0.01	9.05	0.003	0.02
H/ND	NH/ND	1.03	0.31	0.003	1.99	0.16	0.01
NH/D	NH/ND	1.56	0.21	0.004	2.34	0.13	0.01
H/ND	NH/D	0.06	0.80	0.00	0.02	0.88	0.00

H/D = Health Care, Racial Discrimination, H/ND = Health Care, Nonracial Discrimination, NH/D = Non-Health Care, Racial Discrimination, NH/ND = Non-Health Care, Nonracial Discrimination. As these are planned contrasts, df = 1 for all tests.

Discussion

Medical mistrust is a recurrent barrier to engagement of likelihood of engaging in health behaviors. To date, the focus on Tuskegee's role in medical mistrust has contributed to a dearth of work considering other factors influencing medical mistrust among African Americans. Additionally, when antecedents of medical mistrust have been considered, the work has largely neglected the possible role of vicarious experiences. The

Table 2. Parameter estimates of moderated model.

	General Medical Mistrust b	B	SE	p	95% CI	Race Based Medical Mistrust b	B	SE	p	95% CI
H/D	0.19	0.14	0.09	0.03	[.02,.36]	0.44	0.2	0.14	0.002	[.17,.71]
H/ND	0.07	0.05	0.09	0.43	[−.11,.25]	0.19	0.09	0.13	0.15	[−.07,.44]
NH/D	0.1	0.07	0.09	0.26	[−.07,.26]	0.2	0.09	0.13	0.14	[−.07,.45]
Age	0.01	0.2	0.004	0.05	[.00,.02]	0.001	0.01	0.01	0.91	[−.01,.01]
H/D x Age	−0.01	−0.07	0.01	0.35	[−.02,.01]	−0.01	−0.07	0.01	0.34	[−.03,.01]
H/ND x Age	0.001	0.01	0.01	0.9	[−.01,.01]	0.004	0.03	0.01	0.62	[−.01,.02]
NH/D x Age	−0.01	−0.11	0.01	0.16	[−.02,.003]	−0.01	−0.09	0.01	0.19	[−.03,.01]

H/D = Health Care, Racial Discrimination, H/ND = Health Care, Nonracial Discrimination, NH/D = Non-Health Care, Racial Discrimination, NH/ND = Non-Health Care, Nonracial Discrimination.

current study utilized an experimental method to examine mediated vicarious experiences by testing the effects of exposure to health care content and racial discrimination content in news stories on two types of medical mistrust.

It was posited that negative health care content and racial discrimination content in news stories would be positively related with medical mistrust. Considered individually, both negative health care content and racial discrimination content in news stories were positively related to race-based medical mistrust, but not general medical mistrust. This suggests that these types of content in news stories result in medical mistrust that centers social positioning (i.e., race-based) but not general mistrust. Such a conclusion, however, may be premature given the pattern of findings for the four individual conditions.

When examining the four individual conditions, health care-related racial discrimination news stories resulted in higher levels of race-based medical mistrust than non-health, nonracial discrimination news stories. There was a marginal difference in general medical mistrust between those exposed to these two types of news stories. Additionally, there was no significant differences in medical mistrust for those exposed to health care, nonracial discrimination news stories versus those exposed to non-health care, racial discrimination stories. The subsequent model examining the effects of health-care related, racial discrimination stories (in comparison to non-health care, nonracial discrimination news stories) on both types of medical mistrust simultaneously found that exposure to health-care related, racial discrimination stories resulted in higher levels of both general and race-based medical mistrust than non-health care, nonracial discrimination stories. Thus, the effects of exposure to both types of content on race-based medical mistrust may be driven by the effect of exposure to health care-related, racial discrimination stories. It is possible that the combination of negative health care content and racial discrimination content approximate perceived racism in health care, thus contributing to medical mistrust (Hammond, 2010). Future work should investigate the role of mediators, like perceived racism, in the impact of news stories exposure on medical mistrust.

While there was evidence of an impact of health care-related racial discrimination news stories, there was no evidence that non-health care, racial discrimination stories influenced medical mistrust. This is consistent with previous work that found no differences in race-based medical mistrust for explicit racial discrimination news stories (Williamson, Smith et al., 2019). Given the pervasiveness of racial discrimination in the U.S. (Reskin, 2012), African Americans may reasonably assume that the default is racism. This would explain the lack of differences between exposure the explicit racial discrimination frame and control both in the current study and in Williamson, Smith et al. (2019). A closer examination of manipulation check items in the current study revealed that although racial discrimination was not *mentioned* (and participants realized this), they still reported higher agreement that the individual had *experienced* racial discrimination when exposed to the health care, nonracial discrimination stories as compared to the non-health care, nonracial discrimination news stories. This would suggest that participants assumed racial discrimination was still at play, even when it was not explicitly mentioned. If this is the case, an additional layer may be required to trigger medical mistrust, above and beyond the baseline. This may be the health care context, as seen in the current study, or when it is seen as hiding the racism, which could be an interpretation of the implicit frame used in Williamson, Smith et al. (2019). These two studies appear to begin to outline the conditions under which explicit racial discrimination in news stories increases medical mistrust.

Additionally, there was no effect of health care, nonracial discrimination stories on medical mistrust. Operationalizing health care content as lack of access to services may not prime attributes that are a part of the knowledge structure for medical mistrust. Alternatively, given continued issues surrounding access to health care (United States Department of Health and Human Services, 2020), this manipulation of negative health care experiences content (i.e., lack of access to resources) may seem like the norm and not a novel or egregious enough offense to heighten medical mistrust. Future work should examine other operationalizations of health care content. The possibility that the effect sizes for the impact health care content and racial discrimination content are much smaller than anticipated should also be noted. If this is the case, the current sample size may not have been large enough to detect these differences.

Finally, a research question was also asked regarding differential effects on general and race-based medical mistrust. An initial examination suggested that the particular types of news story content had an impact on race-based medical mistrust, but not general medical mistrust. Further investigation revealed, however, that when accounting for both types of medical mistrust, exposure to health care-related racial discrimination news stories influenced both race-based and general medical mistrust. Based on the standardized estimates of these relationships, there appears to be slightly larger impact for race-based medical mistrust than general medical mistrust. This is unsurprising as race-based medical mistrust directly calls upon the political and social position of being African American. It remains notable, however, that the effects were present for both general and race-based medical mistrust.

Theoretical implications

The current investigation builds upon previous work by examining the effect of news stories (i.e., mediated vicarious experiences) on medical mistrust in a sample of African American adults. The findings indicate that investigations into medical mistrust may be missing part of the picture by not accounting for exposure to mediated vicarious racial discrimination and health experiences. As scholars answer recent calls to further examine the antecedents of medical mistrust and use more sophisticated techniques (Benkert et al., 2019), theorizing about medical mistrust must include mediated vicarious experiences. Although previous work has examined discrimination as an antecedent to medical mistrust (e.g., Durant et al., 2011; Hammond, 2010), these studies focused on individuals' own experiences of discrimination. The current study suggests that as communication scholarship is used to more carefully examine medical mistrust, theories, such as social cognitive theory, that are designed to account for vicarious experiences, including through media, may be fruitful avenues for theoretically grounding these studies.

Additionally, as the stories utilized in this study represent probabilistic social comparison frames, specifically disparity frames, the current findings also suggest that theses frames might influence medical mistrust and have implications for communication about health inequalities. Previous work on these frames has examined medical mistrust as a moderator of the effects of these frames (Nicholson et al., 2008), but to my knowledge, no studies have directly examined the effects of these frames directly on medical mistrust. It will be beneficial for future work to examine this phenomenon in conjunction with other health-risk frames (e.g., impact frames), as well as other potentially associated constructs (e.g., linked fate).

The current work supports the idea that despite being related constructs, there are differences in general and race-based medical mistrust. The bivariate relationships and the structural model indicated that these two types of medical mistrust are, in fact, related. Additionally, the relationship between health care-related discrimination news stories (versus non-health care, nonracial discrimination news stories) and general medical mistrust was revealed when race-based medical mistrust was accounted for within the model. Scholars so far have primarily chosen *either* the general medical mistrust or race-based medical mistrust scale (Williamson & Bigman, 2018). To fully understand the relationship between general medical mistrust and race-based medical mistrust future work must include both measures; this may illuminate how they operate similarly or differently with other constructs of interest. Additionally, as general and race-based medical mistrust appear to be related but not overlapping constructs, it will be beneficial to know whether general medical mistrust is a precursor to race-based medical mistrust or race-based medical mistrust feeds into general medical mistrust. It is also possible that general medical mistrust moderates the relationship between news stories and race-based medical mistrust. Thus, subsequent studies may want to assess general medical mistrust prior to message exposure.

Practical implications

News stories have the potential to influence medical mistrust, and in turn, impact a wide range of health behaviors. The current study provides evidence that news stories discussing discrimination using social comparison frames influence medical mistrust, particularly in the context of health care. Some may argue that this is inconsequential as content analyses suggest this type of news story may be infrequent (Gandy & Li, 2005; Nagler et al., 2016). However, given the increased exposure to news via social media (Matsa & Shearer, 2018) and that Black Americans report being exposed to race-related content more often (Anderson & Hitlin, 2016) and are more likely to share news stories showing disparate racial impact (Bigman et al., 2019), exposure to health care-related racial discrimination stories is still possible.

Thus, the current investigation serves as a reminder of the importance of understanding the other messages that may be present in the information environment (Randolph & Viswanath, 2004). In promoting behaviors (e.g., routine check-ups, cancer screenings, etc.), health scholars must recognize and be mindful of the effect exposure to these stories (e.g., reports chronicling the difficulty African American women face during childbirth or Virginia's Governor Northam black-face medical school yearbook picture) would have on medical mistrust, and in turn, a variety of health behaviors. More recently, in light of the recent COVID-19 pandemic, we must keep in mind the impact news stories about Black Americans' difficulties seeking care and getting tested for COVID-19 (e.g., Mitropoulos & Moseley, 2020) could have on medical mistrust and willingness to seek care if experiencing symptoms. Moving forward, it may also impact behaviors related to COVID-19 vaccination.

Additionally, the findings of this study speak to the way in which healthcare providers may deal with the role of negative healthcare experiences and racial discrimination experiences by keeping this in mind during interactions with patients. There have been calls for structural competency in medical training and practice, which differs from cultural competency (Metzl & Hansen, 2014). Cultural competency refers to the ability to identify expressions of illness and health across cultures, whereas structural competency advocates for a recognition of the institutions and social conditions that impact health. Metzl and Hansen (2014) discuss this as thinking about how "such variables as race, class, gender, and ethnicity are shaped both by the interactions of the two persons in a room, but by the larger structural contexts in which their interactions take place" (p. 3). Thus, health-care providers might consider that patients' hesitancy to come in for appointments, or perhaps see a new doctor, could be fueled by current news stories and societal events.

More broadly, the current study, taken with Williamson, Smith et al. (2019), illuminates the need to take care in how medical mistrust is discussed and addressed. Medical mistrust is associated with exposure to individuals' experiences of racial discrimination both in the context of the health care (the current study) and when it is being "hidden" (i.e., mentioned implicitly) in a variety of contexts (Williamson, Smith et al., 2019). This would point toward medical mistrust being tied to the myriad of inequities, discrimination, and racism that exists in systems in the U.S. Medical mistrust should not be framed as something that needs to be changed within individuals. African Americans' medical mistrust is considered to be a specific type of cultural mistrust (Thompson et al., 2004), which has previously been framed in ways that might be interpreted as being located within the individual (e.g., pertinent to paranoia as a clinical diagnosis; Whaley, 2001). The current study should not be taken to mean that decreasing exposure to these stories or convincing individuals that racial discrimination does not exist within the health care system is the answer. Instead of locating the solution within individuals, the solution should be properly placed on systems. While some individual measures may mitigate medical mistrust and get individuals necessary care, addressing medical mistrust should ultimately involve advocacy that deals with racism and, in turn, begin to decrease the frequency of these types of experiences.

Limitations

The findings of this study must be considered in the context of its limitations. Financial constraints tied to recruiting through Qualtrics limited survey length and the number conditions. Subsequent work should include a no-exposure control and items that would help verify that vicarious processes are taking place. Furthermore, participants were exposed to a single news story. In everyday life, participants are inundated with messages, sometimes within a short period of time (e.g., scrolling through social media). Although steps were taken to ensure the stories looked like those they might have encountered, participants knew they were taking part of a study and were presented with a stand-alone article. Future work should consider testing the impact of these stories in a more ecologically valid presentation of the news stories that would provide a closer approximation of how individuals encounter these news stories in the world. For instance, participants could be presented with a mock news feed with multiple stories as in Bigman et al. (2019). Finally, the current study was unable to fully investigate whether demographic variables played a role in the relationship between news stories and medical mistrust. Subsequent studies should strive to have enough representation and variation in their samples to be able to investigate these nuances. Despite these limitations, the current study provides a window into the impact of these messages.

Conclusion

In addressing medical mistrust, both in the context of the current pandemic, as well as the legacy of health disparities, health scholars must consider the message environment outside of the doctor's office. Furthermore, viewing African Americans' medical mistrust as solely the result of personal experiences is too narrow; mediated vicarious experiences must also be considered. The results of the present study indicate a need to be attuned to the impact of racial discrimination news stories, particularly those that are health-related, could have on African Americans' medical mistrust. Given our focus on these types of messages, health communication scholars are poised to undertake the work that pushes medical mistrust scholarship beyond Tuskegee and personal experiences to mediated vicarious experiences.

Notes

1. African American is used in this piece to specifically reference this particular group. Black Americans is used in certain places to denote the use in a specific body of literature or story in which Black Americans would include African Americans, as well as other individuals of African descent (i.e., Afro-Caribbean).
2. Story credibility did not vary by condition, $F(3, 406) = 2.46, p = .06$.
3. News credibility, measured using Flanagin and Metzger (2000) information credibility scale, was also evaluated as a potential covariate. It was ultimately unrelated to medical mistrust and subsequently removed from analyses.

Acknowledgments

The author thanks Cabral A. Bigman and two anonymous reviewers for their valuable comments on earlier drafts of this manuscript.

Disclosure of potential conflict of interest

This article is based on the dissertation completed by Williamson (2019).

ORCID

Lillie D. Williamson http://orcid.org/0000-0001-5735-1416

References

Anderson, M., & Hitlin, P. (2016). *Social media conversations about race: How social media users see, share and discuss race and the rise of hashtags like #BlackLivesMatter*. Pew Research Center. http://www.pewinternet.org/wp-content/uploads/sites/9/2016/08/PI_2016.08.15_Race-and-Social-Media_FINAL.pdf

Bandura, A. (2009). Social cognitive theory of mass communication. In J. O. Bryant & M. B. Oliver (Eds.), *Media effects: Advances in theory and research* (3rd ed., pp. 94–124). Routledge.

Benkert, R., Cuevas, A., Thompson, H. S., Dove-Meadows, E., & Knuckles, D. (2019). Ubiquitous yet unclear: A systematic review of medical mistrust. *Behavioral Medicine*, *45*(2), 86–101. https://doi.org/10.1080/08964289.2019.1588220

Bigman, C. A. (2014). Social comparison framing in health news and its effect on perceptions of group risk. *Health Communication*, *29*(3), 267–280. https://doi.org/10.1080/10410236.2012.745043

Bigman, C. A., Smith, M. A., Williamson, L. D., Planey, A. M., & McNeil Smith, S. (2019). Selective sharing on social media: Examining the effects of disparate racial impact frames on intentions to retransmit news stories among US college students. *New Media & Society*, *21* (11–12), 2691–2709. https://doi.org/10.1177/1461444819856574

Bogart, L. M., Wagner, G. J., Green, H. D., Mutchler, M. G., Klein, D. J., McDavitt, B., Lawrence, S. J., & Hilliard, C. L. (2016). Medical mistrust among social network members may contribute to antiretroviral treatment nonadherence in African Americans living with HIV. *Social Science & Medicine*, *164*, 133–140. https://doi.org/10.1016/j.socscimed.2016.03.028

Brandon, D. T., Isaac, L. A., & LaVeist, T. A. (2005). The legacy of Tuskegee and trust in medical care: Is Tuskegee responsible for race differences in mistrust of medical care? *Journal of the National Medical Association*, *97*(7), 951–956. https://www.ncbi.nlm.nih.gov/pmc/articles/PMC2569322/pdf/jnma00188-0013.pdf

Centers for Disease Control and Prevention. (2020). *COVID-19 in racial and ethnic minority groups*. https://www.cdc.gov/coronavirus/2019-ncov/need-extra-precautions/racial-ethnic-minorities.html

Diesner, J., Aleyasen, A., Chin, C., Mishra, S., Soltani, K., & Tao, L. (2015). *ConTEXT: Network construction from texts* [Computer software]. http://context.ischool.illinois.edu/

Durant, R. W., Legedza, A. T., Marcantonio, E. R., Freeman, M. B., & Landon, B. E. (2011). Different types of distrust in clinical research among whites and African Americans. *Journal of the National Medical Association*, *103*(2), 123–130. https://doi.org/10.1016/S0027-9684(15)30261-3

Flanagin, A. J., & Metzger, M. J. (2000). Perceptions of Internet information credibility. *Journalism & Mass Communication Quarterly*, *77*(3), 515–540. https://doi.org/10.1177/107769900007700304

Gandy, O. H., Jr. (2009). *Coming to terms with chance: Engaging rational discriminationa and cumulative disadvantage*. Ashgate.

Gandy, O. H., Jr., & Li, Z. (2005). Framing comparative risk: A preliminary analyis. *Howard Journal of Communication*, *16*(2), 71–86. https://doi.org/10.1080/10646170590948956

Greer, T. M., Brondolo, E., & Brown, P. (2014). Systemic racism moderates effects of provider racial biases on adherence to hypertension treatment for African Americans. *Health Psychology*, *33*(1), 35–42. https://doi.org/10.1037/a0032777

Hall, M. A., Dugan, E., Zheng, B., & Mishra, A. K. (2001). Trust in physicians and medical institutions: What is it, can it be measured, and does it matter? *Milbank Quarterly*, *79*(4), 613–639. https://doi.org/10.1111/1468-0009.00223

Hammond, W. P. (2010). Psychosocial correlates of medical mistrust among African American men. *American Journal of Community Psychology*, *45*(1–2), 87–106. https://doi.org/10.1007/s10464-009-9280-6

Hammond, W. P., Matthews, D., & Corbie-Smith, G. (2010). Psychosocial factors associated with routine health examination scheduling and receipt among African American men. *Journal of the National Medical Association*, *102*(4), 276–289. https://doi.org/10.1016/S0027-9684(15)30600-3

Jacobs, E. A., Rolle, I., Ferrans, C. E., Whitaker, E. E., & Warnecke, R. B. (2006). Understanding African Americans' views of the trustworthiness of physicians. *Journal of General Internal Medicine*, *21*(6), 642–647. https://doi.org/10.1111/j.1525-1497.2006.00485.x

Jaiswal, J., & Halkitis, P. N. (2019). Towards a more inclusive and dynamic understanding of medical mistrust informed by science. *Behavioral Medicine*, *45*(2), 79–85. https://doi.org/10.1080/08964289.2019.1619511

Jaiswal, J., LoSchiavo, C., & Perlman, D. C. (2020). Disinformation, misinformation and inequality-driven mistrust in the time of COVID-19: Lessons learned from AIDS denialism. *AIDS and Behavior*, *24*(10), 2776–2780. https://doi.org/10.1007/s10461-020-02925-y

Jensen, J. D., Carcioppolo, N., King, A. J., Bernat, J. K., Davis, L., Yale, R., & Smith, J. (2011). Including limitations in news coverage of cancer research: Effects of news hedging on fatalism, medical skepticism, patient trust, and backlash. *Journal of Health Communication*, *16*(5), 486–503. https://doi.org/10.1080/10810730.2010.546491

Kalichman, S. C., Eaton, L., Kalichman, M. O., Grebler, T., Merely, C., & Welles, B. (2016). Race-based medical mistrust, medication beliefs and HIV treatment adherence: Test of a mediation model in people living with HIV/AIDS. *Journal of Behavioral Medicine*, *39*(6), 1056–1064. https://doi.org/10.1007/s10865-016-9767-1

Kline, R. B. (2016). *Principles and practice of structural equation modeling*. Guilford Press.

Krull, R. (2019). In St. Louis' digital divide, North City suffers from poor internet access. *River Front Times*. https://www.riverfronttimes.com/newsblog/2019/02/11/in-st-louis-digital-divide-north-city-suffers-from-poor-internet-access

LaVeist, T. A., Isaac, L. A., & Williams, K. P. (2009). Mistrust of health care organizations is associated with underutilization of health services. *Health Services Research*, *44*(6), 2093–2105. https://doi.org/10.1111/j.1475-6773.2009.01017.x

Maly, R. C., Stein, J. A., Umezawa, Y., Leake, B., & Anglin, M. D. (2008). Racial/ethnic differences in breast cancer outcomes among older patients: Effects of physician communication and patient empowerment. *Health Psychology*, *27*(6), 728–736. https://doi.org/10.1037/0278-6133.27.6.728

Matsa, K. E., & Shearer, E. (2018). *News use across social media platforms 2018*. Pew Research Center. https://www.journalism.org/2018/09/10/newsuse-across-social-media-platforms-2018/

Matsunaga, M. (2010). How to factor-analyze your data right: Do's, don'ts, and how-to's. *International Journal of Psychological Research*, *3*(1), 97–110. http://doi.org/10.21500/20112084.854

Metzl, J. M., & Hansen, H. (2014). Structural competency: Theorizing a new medical engagement with stigma and inequality. *Social Science & Medicine*, *103*, 126–133. https://doi.org/10.1016/j.socscimed.2013.06.032

Mitropoulos, A., & Moseley, M. (2020, April 28). *Beloved Brooklyn teacher, 30, dies of coronovirus after she was twice denied a COVID-19 test*. ABC News. https://abcnews.go.com/Health/beloved-brooklyn-teacher-30-dies-coronavirus-denied-covid/story?id=70376445

Morgan, S. E. (2004). The power of talk: African Americans' communication with family members about organ donation and its impact on the willingness to donate organs. *Journal of Social and Personal Relationships*, *21*(1), 112–124. https://doi.org/10.1177/0265407504039845

Muthén, L. K., & Muthén, B. O. (2017). *Mplus (Version 8). [Computer software]*. Muthen and Muthen. https://www.statmodel.com/

Nagler, R. H., Bigman, C. A., Ramanadhan, S., Ramamurthi, D., & Viswanath, K. (2016). Prevalence and framing of health disparities in local print news: Implications for multilevel interventions to address cancer inequalities. *Cancer Epidemiology, Biomarkers & Prevention*, *25* (4), 603–612. https://doi.org/10.1158/1055-9965.EPI-15-1247

Nicholson, R. A., Kreuter, M. W., Lapka, C., Wellborn, R., Clark, E. M., Sanders-Thompson, V., Jacobsen, H. M., & Casey, C. (2008). Unintended effects of emphasizing disparities in cancer communication to African-Americans. *Cancer Epidemiology, Biomarkers & Prevention*, *17* (11), 2946–2953. https://doi.org/10.1158/1055-9965.EPI-08-0101

Omodei, M. M., & McLennan, J. (2000). Conceptualizing and measuring global interpersonal mistrust-trust. *The Journal of Social Psychology*, *140*(3), 279–294. https://doi.org/10.1080/00224540009600471

Pellowski, J. A., Price, D. M., Allen, A. M., Eaton, L. A., & Kalichman, S. C. (2017). The differences between medical trust and mistrust and their respective influences on medication beliefs and ART adherence among African-Americans living with HIV. *Psychology & Health*, *32*(9), 1127–1139. https://doi.org/10.1080/08870446.2017.1324969

Pratkanis, A. R. (1989). The cognitive representation of attitudes. In A. R. Pratkanis, S. J. Breckler, & A. G. Greenwald (Eds.), *Attitude structure and function* (pp. 71–98). Psychology Press.

Randolph, W., & Viswanath, K. (2004). Lessons learned from public health mass media campaigns: Marketing health in a crowded media world. *Annual Review of Public Health*, *25*(1), 419–437. https://doi.org/10.1146/annurev.publhealth.25.101802.123046

Reskin, B. (2012). The race discrimination system. *Annual Review of Sociology*, *38*(1), 17–35. https://doi.org/10.1146/annurev-soc-071811-145508

Shelton, R. C., Winkel, G., Davis, S. N., Roberts, N., Valdimarsdottir, H., Hall, S. J., & Thompson, H. S. (2010). Validation of the group-based medical mistrust scale among urban Black men. *Journal of General Internal Medicine*, *25*(6), 549–555. https://doi.org/10.1007/s11606-010-1288-y

Thompson, H. S., Valdimarsdottir, H. B., Winkel, G., Jandorf, L., & Redd, W. (2004). The group-based medical mistrust scale: Psychometric properties and association with breast cancer screening. *Preventive Medicine*, *38*(2), 209–218. https://doi.org/10.1016/j.ypmed.2003.09.041

Tian, Y. T., & Yoo, J. H. (2020). Medical drama viewing and medical trust: A moderated mediation approach. *Health Communication*, *35*(1), 46–55. https://doi.org/10.1080/10410236.2018.1536959

Truong, K. A., Museus, S. D., & McGuire, K. M. (2016). Vicarious racism: A qualitative analysis of experiences with secondhand racism in graduate education. *International Journal of Qualitative Studies in Education*, *29*(2), 224–247. https://doi.org/10.1080/09518398.2015.1023234

United States Department of Health and Human Services (2020). *Access to health services*. https://www.healthypeople.gov/2020/topics-objectives/topic/Access-to-Health-Services/national-snapshot

Washington, H. A. (2006). *Medical apartheid: The dark history of medical experimentation on Black Americans from colonial times to the present*. Doubleday Books.

Weems, G. H., & Onwuegbuzie, A. J. (2001). The impact of midpoint responses and reverse coding on survey data. *Measurement and Evaluation in Counseling and Development*, *34*(3), 166–176. https://doi.org/10.1080/07481756.2002.12069033

Whaley, A. (2001). Cultural mistrust: An important psychological construct for diagnosis and testing of African Americans. *Professional Psychology, Research and Practice*, *32*(6), 555–562. https://doi.org/10.1037/0735-7028.32.6.555

Williamson, L. D., & Bigman, C. A. (2018). A systematic review of medical mistrust measures. *Patient Education and Counseling*, *101*(10), 1786–1794. https://doi.org/10.1016/j.pec.2018.05.007

Williamson, L. D., Bigman, C. A., & Quick, B. L. (2019). A qualitative examination of African Americans' organ donation-related medical mistrust beliefs. *Howard Journal of Communications*, *30*(5), 430–445. https://doi.org/10.1080/10646175.2018.1512064

Williamson, L. D., Smith, M. A., & Bigman, C. A. (2019). Does discrimination breed mistrust? Examining the role of mediated and non-mediated discrimination experiences in medical mistrust. *Journal of Health Communication*, *24*(10), 791–799. https://doi.org/10.1080/10810730.2019.1669742

Zhang, X., Noor, R., & Savalei, V. (2016). Examining the effect of reverse worded items on the factor structure of the need for cognition scale. *PloS One*, *11*(6), 1–15. https://doi.org/10.1371/journal.pone.0157795

Appendix. Example Stimuli

Example of stimuli used. Photographs are from Pixabay and used under the terms of their license: https://pixabay.com/service/license.

Stimuli for Therapist Version of the Health Care, Racial Discrimination (H/D) Condition

Baltimore Residents Have Tougher Time Seeing a Therapist

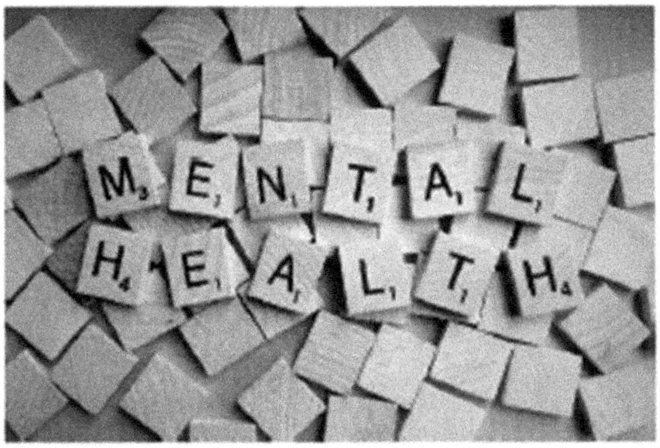

Study findings raise concerns about unequal access to mental health treatment

Black residents in Baltimore, Maryland have a significantly harder time getting an appointment with a therapist than other Maryland residents.

Courtney Wilson, a Black cashier, has struggled to get a therapist in Maryland for the past year. She thought she was alone, but it turns out many other Baltimore residents like Wilson are struggling to get appointments.

A recent Mental Health Association of Maryland report shows that Black residents in Baltimore are less likely to have nearby practices that are accepting new patients. The report finds that they can have a lot of difficulty securing an appointment with a therapist.

The findings are raising concerns about unequal access to mental health treatment for Black residents in cities like Baltimore.

"What we are seeing is that people living in Black areas are still not receiving the same levels of access," said Steve Anderson, a researcher at the Mental Health Association of Maryland and co-author of the report.

The report recommends that the private and public sector work together to find solutions and increase access in historically underserved Black communities.

Stimuli for Therapist Version of Health Care, nonracial Discrimination (H/ND) Condition

Rural Residents Have Tougher Time Seeing a Therapist

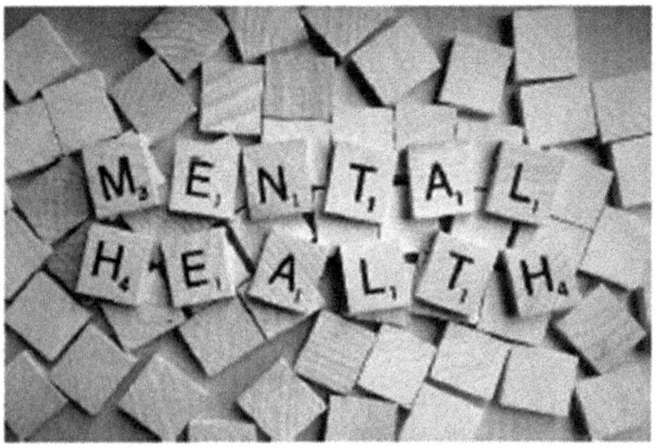

Study findings raise concerns about unequal access to mental health treatment

Residents in rural towns in Maryland have a significantly harder time getting an appointment with a therapist than other Maryland residents.

Courtney Wilson, a White cashier, has struggled to get a therapist in Maryland for the past year. She thought she was alone, but it turns out many other rural residents like Wilson are struggling to get appointments.

A recent Mental Health Association of Maryland report shows that rural residents in Maryland are less likely to have nearby practices that are accepting new patients. The report finds that they can have a lot of difficulty securing an appointment with a therapist.

The findings are raising concerns about unequal access to mental health treatment for residents in rural towns.

"What we are seeing is that people living in rural areas are still not receiving the same levels of access," said Steve Anderson, a researcher at the Mental Health Association of Maryland and co-author of the report.

The report recommends that the private and public sector work together to find solutions and increase access in historically underserved rural communities.

Stimuli for Internet Version of Non-health Care, Racial Discrimination (NH/D) Condition

Ferguson Residents Have Tougher Time Getting Home Internet

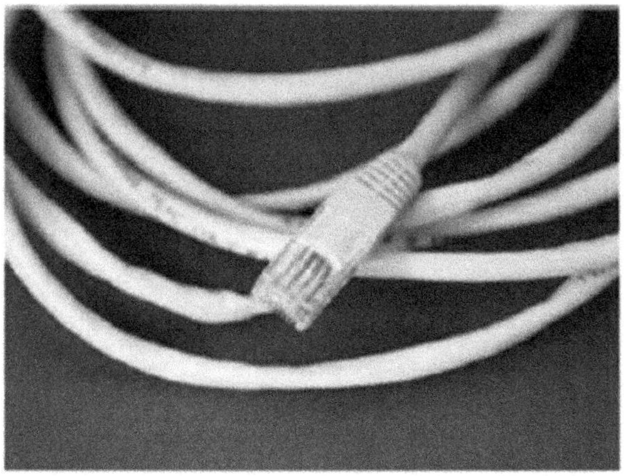

Study findings raise concerns about unequal access to home internet services

Black residents in Ferguson, Missouri have a significantly harder time getting home internet access than other Missouri residents.

Brandon Jones, a Black postal worker, has struggled to get high-speed internet access in his home for the past year. He thought he was alone, but it turns out many other Ferguson residents like Jones are struggling to get home internet access.

A recent Brookings Institute report shows that Black residents in Ferguson are less likely to have internet access in their place of residence. The report finds that they can have a lot of difficulty securing high-speed internet access.

The findings are raising concerns about unequal access to internet services for Black residents in cities like Ferguson.

"What we are seeing is that people living in Black areas are still not receiving the same levels of access," said Steve Anderson, a researcher at the Brookings Institute and co-author of the report.

The report recommends that the private and public sector work together to find solutions and increase access in historically underserved Black communities.

Stimuli for Internet Version of Non-health Care, nonracial Discrimination (NH/ND) Condition

Rural Residents Have Tougher Time Getting Home Internet

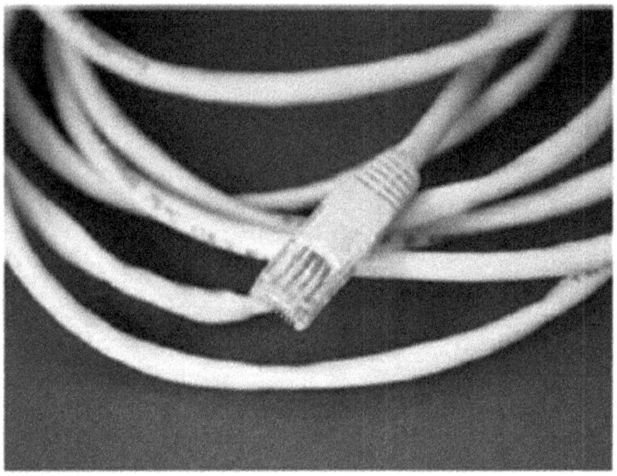

Study findings raise concerns about unequal access to home internet services

Residents in rural towns in Missouri have a significantly harder time getting home internet access than other Missouri residents.

Brandon Jones, a White postal worker, has struggled to get high-speed internet access in his home for the past year. He thought he was alone, but it turns out many other rural residents like Jones are struggling to get home internet access.

A recent Brookings Institute report shows that rural residents in Missouri are less likely to have internet access in their place of residence. The report finds that they can have to a lot of difficulty securing high-speed internet access.

The findings are raising concerns about unequal access to internet services for residents in rural towns.

"What we are seeing is that people living in rural areas are still not receiving the same levels of access," said Steve Anderson, a researcher at the Brookings Institute and co-author of the report.

The report recommends that the private and public sector work together to find solutions and increase access in historically underserved rural communities.

Community-Based Participatory Research (CBPR) to Enhance Participation of Racial/ Ethnic Minorities in Clinical Trials: A 10-Year Systematic Review

Soroya Julian McFarlane, Aurora Occa, Wei Peng, Oluwatumininu Awonuga, and Susan E. Morgan

ABSTRACT

There has not been a significant improvement in the rate of clinical trial accrual in more than 20 years. Worse, the challenge of inadequate representation among racial and ethnic minorities also persists, deepening disparities in health. Community-Based Participatory Research (CBPR) is a participatory communication method that centers on effective dialogue between researchers and community stakeholders with the goal of creating an equitable partnership for health and social change. The objective of the current study was to provide an update since a systematic review in 2012, on the current status of the empirical research, with a particular focus on the elements of CBPR methods used to improve the rate of accrual of members of racial and ethnic minority communities for clinical trials. Our systematic review found a large increase in the number of CBPR related studies and studies related to racial and ethnic representation in research. More than 85% of studies employing CBPR methods saw statistically positive outcomes. Specifically, the elements of CBPR that are associated with these positive outcomes include community partner participation in (1) a study advisory committee, (2) data collection, (3) the development of interventions, and (4) participant recruitment. However, the results of our study indicate that researchers need to be more transparent about the extent of community participation as well as more thoroughly and accurately describe the nature of the partnership with members of minority communities in order to build upon the scientific literature on community-engaged methods.

Recent research has continually emphasized the need to increase public participation in clinical trials, which currently stands at around 3% (Michaels et al., 2012). The importance of including the medically underserved, including members of minority communities, is even more pressing (Laufman, 2009). Vulnerable groups usually present higher risk and prevalence of various disease conditions, yet they are the least likely to participate in clinical trials (Ford et al., 2008). This challenge of improving recruitment practices has been approached from several perspectives, leading to the development of interventions that aim to increase the diversity of participants in clinical trials and research studies. For example, educational interventions have tended to either address gaps in competence and awareness on the side of the medical provider, or the patient, or both. Despite well-documented barriers faced by patients, especially members of minority populations, who might be eligible to participate in clinical trials, (Albrecht et al., 2008; Occa et al., 2018), there is a paucity of research that focuses on interventions to effectively address these barriers.

The process of recruitment for clinical trials necessarily includes communication between patients and health system providers and/or clinical research staff. Approaches to increase community participation in clinical trials by improving communication often focus on adjusting the provider's verbal and nonverbal behavior – from specific wording, to tone, pitch, speech rate, and facial expressions (Krieger, 2014; Morgan et al., 2017). Specific communication-related behaviors of patients and providers that might support the informed consent process during clinical trial recruitment have also been identified (see Albrecht et al., 2008; Krieger, 2014; Morgan, Occa, Mouton et al., 2017; Morgan, Occa, Potter et al., 2017; Occa & Morgan, 2018). Less studied are methods of effectively integrating community members' perspective and worldview, which ultimately influence the success of the encounter between patients and their health care providers and/or clinical research professionals. However, some studies have suggested that improving the participation of members of vulnerable groups requires a meaningful level of community-engagement, motivated by ethics, social justice and inclusive values (Ross et al., 2010; Seifer et al., 2010; Wallerstein & Duran, 2008).

Community-based Participatory Research (CBPR) is widely considered the optimal approach within the Community Engagement Continuum (CENR) for both communities and researchers who share a social change objective (Ross et al., 2010). There continues to be a high degree of support for CBPR approaches, as evidenced by inclusion in funding mechanisms, such as the NIH Trust Initiative and Clinical and Translational Science Award program (Seifer et al., 2010). However, because of the nature of CBPR (explained in the next section) collecting scientific and statistical data on the implementation or outcomes of this approach is difficult, which makes causal inferences from a CBPR intervention on a specific disease outcome challenging (Wallerstein et al., 2008).

Nonetheless, CBPR methodologies have been used as the foundation of the development of a number of strategies and interventions to support the recruitment of members of minority communities in clinical trials and research studies. In 2012, a systematic review of research using CBPR to inform clinical research in racial and ethnic minorities was published, and results indicated that the outcomes associated with the use of this set of methodologies was overwhelmingly positive (De Las Nueces et al., 2012). However, a key finding at the time of the study was that the degree of community "participation," a critical aspect of true CBPR, varied significantly across interventions. Because there has also been a substantial increase in the number of recent peer-reviewed publications that use CBPR in clinical trial research, this suggests that an updated review may support intervention planning, development, and implementation. Therefore, the goal of this current research will be to provide an update on the current status, effectiveness and the extent of participation of racial and ethnic minority communities in clinical trials using CBPR methods, and the role of communication, based on recent literature.

Literature review

Clinical trials are responsible for most advancements in treatments and cures for various illnesses, but without adequate representation across racial, ethnic and cultural backgrounds, findings from clinical trials are of diminished value since they may not be generalizable (Michaels et al., 2015). Previous studies have documented the knowledge and attitudes of members of the general public regarding clinical trial participation (see Krieger, 2014; Krieger et al., 2015; Miller et al., 2011); these studies point to the importance of building awareness of clinical trials, particularly among members of vulnerable groups (Tanner et al., 2015). However, an overemphasis on "raising awareness" as the main route to improving rates of participation may prove short-sighted. Research has already demonstrated that in 2012, 72.9% (up from 67.6% in 2008) of the general population were aware of clinical trials. Awareness has also been increasing in Black/African American and Hispanic minority groups (67.1% and 59.8%, respectively,), which is a faster rate of increase than among Caucasians (Leiter et al., 2015). On the other hand, improving knowledge and perceptions about clinical trials is necessary to increase intentions to participate and ultimately increase accrual rates (Morgan et al., 2020).

Individuals from underrepresented groups face additional barriers that require careful attention. These barriers can be individual- or system-based (Morgan & Mouton, 2015). For example, the financial reimbursement system for health-care providers creates pressure on physicians to limit the time that they spend with each patient, which makes it more challenging for physicians to discuss clinical trials with their patients (Howerton et al., 2007). Other difficulties associated with communicating about clinical trials are aggravated in race-discordant interactions about clinical trials (Eggly et al., 2015). Features of clinical trials themselves also present significant barriers. For example, Lie et al. (2019) discovered that patients cited the length of many clinical trials as a barrier to study participation. Additionally, rigid inclusionary criteria for participation in most clinical trials increase the time required to talk about clinical trials with patients and limits the number of people who are eligible to participate (Morgan & Mouton, 2015).

Some of the barriers faced by individuals from underrepresented groups can be better addressed by using complementary methods for protocol design and study implementation (Ford et al., 2008). Developing protocols and procedures through in-depth discussions with members from the community may help researchers and practitioners anticipate those hidden needs before they become barriers. Therefore, identifying empirically supported best practices to increase motivation and develop shared understanding with patients and community-based stakeholder groups, particularly within minority communities may help to increase participation in clinical trials among members of these groups.

Community-based participatory methods

The goal of interventions related to clinical trial accrual are not to persuade people to join clinical trials but rather to increase informed consent, or informed refusal to participate, through clear and accurate messages (Krieger, 2014). Three recommendations have been suggested for promoting clinical trials in communities by Michaels et al. (2015); these CBPR-grounded recommendations go beyond exhortations to "increase awareness" and instead focus on the importance of helping patients access information about available trials and eventually, to make an informed decision about participation. First, message design must advocate for clinical trials as a social justice issue, address any historical or cultural misunderstanding and include a call for action that holds the community itself accountable for increasing participation (for example, through training community leaders). Second, this work should be a part of a long-term, patient-centered, trust-building plan that acknowledges institutional responsibility. Third, measures of success should include indirect and/or proximal variables to accrual, such as changes in attitudes or increases in community dialogue about the subject rather than simply focusing on the number of minority patients enrolled in a study as the key outcome.

To accomplish these goals, researchers have increasingly employed Community-Based Participatory Methods (CBPR) as a part of their recruitment of participants for clinical trials (Swanson & Ward, 1995). The community-engaged research (CeNR) continuum, developed by National Center for Research Resources (NCRR) at the National Institutes of Health (NIH), identifies approaches to orientations to research, from less- to more-desirable: (a) investigator-driven, (b) community-placed, (c) community-based research, (d) Community-based Participatory Research (CBPR), (e) community-driven research. The ideal of social justice and community engagement, within the confines of an academic research project, therefore, has been embodied by the CBPR approach (Ross et al., 2010). CBPR is a participatory communication method that centers on effective dialogue between community and researcher stakeholders as equal partners in a process of social change (Peterson & Gubrium, 2011). CBPR facilitates community involvement in all areas of leadership and decision-making in the implementation of a research project to improve community health outcomes (Ross et al., 2010).

One of the main challenges to implementation of CBPR methodologies for clinical trials is the mobilization of communities; competing values and worldviews of stakeholders at the individual level present challenges for working together effectively. CBPR is especially effective in targeting underserved or vulnerable groups (Minkler, 2004; Wallerstein et al., 2008) who are, by definition, more at risk of a particular disease or poor health outcomes, and usually have limited ability to deploy resources to adequately intervene (Nyamathi et al., 2007). While women, children, and the elderly, people of color, LGBTQ, immigrants, homeless people, and people living with HIV have all been considered vulnerable populations (Nyamathi et al., 2007), the participation (or lack thereof) of racial and ethnic minorities has been the focus of much of the existing literature addressing disparities in clinical trial accrual in underserved populations (see Heller et al., 2014; Katz et al., 2008; A. Langford et al., 2010). De Las Nueces et al. (2012) suggest that CBPR is becoming more commonly integrated into research that targets racial and ethnic minorities for participation in clinical trials, but there is limited recent evidence to support this claim. We therefore sought to address this with the following research question:

RQ1: Has there been an increase since the 2012 systematic review in the use of CBPR methods to enhance racial and ethnic participation in clinical trials?

When done well, successful CBPR looks like effective dialogue, involving community leaders that are held in high esteem by the community, a flexible Principal Investigator who listens and responds accordingly, resulting in the creation of sustainable relationships built on a foundation of demonstrated dedication, shared values, and an equitable power structure (Wallerstein et al., 2008). The process of establishing this two-way dialogue between researchers and community usually begins with the establishment of a Community Advisory Board (CAB). Working with a CAB is time-consuming and involves various types of activities. Iterative steps employed by researchers and CABs may include strategizing, community engagement, creating recruitment material, ongoing dissemination of findings via presentations and discussions, and follow-up at the community, program and policy levels (McDavitt et al., 2016). These activities require consistent communication and the details reveal the true nature of these partnerships.

Effective communication between community and research stakeholders, while time-intensive, predicts better outcomes from CBPR projects (Wallerstein et al., 2008). However, communication processes are not necessarily straightforward or easy. Researchers must be wary of CPBR elements that can potentially reinforce existing power structures in communities. For example, community representation on the CAB may not be as democratic as CBPR ideals promote. In a project described by Horowitz et al. (2009), community leaders were in charge of regular updates and enforced strict schedules and procedures. An overly dogmatic CAB approach may actually be incongruous with the values of CBPR, which can be summarized as the "need to better understand the non-project nature of people's lives, the complex livelihood inter-linkages that make an impact in one area likely to be felt in others and the potential for unintended consequences" (Cleaver, 1999, p. 599). Very restricted timelines have been associated with investigator-driven goals and success indicators, and with instrumental goals of governmental funding (e.g., NIH), which have been suggested to be incompatible with transformative CBPR methods (Peterson & Gubrium, 2011). CBPR methodologies may need to be thought of as advancing a long-term program of research and the development of a set of sustained relationships between members of a research institution and the communities with which it collaborates in order to generate meaningful and generalizable research that is consistent with values on social justice.

Regardless of the degree to which researchers faithfully implement all principles of CBPR, 89% of studies found the method to be effective, according to the 2012 systematic review (De Las Nueces et al., 2012). Only one study suggested that CBPR might be less effective; UyBico et al. (2007) found that only 13% of studies that used community-engaged strategies were effective to aid recruitment. However, it was suggested that the heterogeneity of the populations included and other factors related to the methodology of the study may have resulted in this anomalous finding. Balcázar et al. (2010) also reported mixed findings: while both the treatment and intervention groups saw significant and positive changes because of the CPBR-based intervention, there was no significant difference between the two groups on several outcomes. In spite of the growing use of CBPR methodologies and their importance to achieving more equitable health outcomes, there has not been a follow-up systematic review of the efficacy of CBPR for clinical trial recruitment in racial and ethnic minority groups since the 2012 publication. Therefore, our second research question aimed to understand the recent evidence for the efficacy of CBPR for increasing participation of racial and ethnic minorities in clinical trials, and the role of communication strategies to achieving these outcomes:

RQ2a: What is the current evidence of the effectiveness of CBPR in improving participation of racial and ethnic minorities in clinical trials?

RQ2b: What communication strategies are employed in some of the studies associated with successful CBPR implementation?

While Neuces's systematic review (De Las Nueces et al., 2012) is the starting point for our work, an important caveat to the early study's findings is that many of the projects reviewed in 2012 did not technically meet the definition of CBPR; rather, a number of the included studies used community-engaged research methods. In other words, the degree of community "participation," a critical aspect of CBPR, varied significantly across the projects under review. For example, while Balcázar et al. (2010), described the integration of community health workers into a randomized control trial (RCT) with the help of a community advisory council, the article does not provide details as to the extent of the community participation and autonomy in managing the project. True community participation means that intergroup communication between community and researchers effectively validates and navigates identity, perspectives and experiences of both parties – researchers and community representatives (Wallerstein et al., 2008). This experience is typically evidenced by the engagement of a Community Advisory Board (CAB) as well as community involvement in all (not some) of these areas: identifying research questions, development of intervention, recruitment of subjects, delivery of intervention, data collection, quantitative and qualitative data analysis, and dissemination of findings (Israel et al., 2012). We would therefore like to document evidence of community participation in clinical trials utilizing CBPR methods in recent years, and understand if there has been improvement in the implementation of true, participatory CBPR.

RQ3a: Which elements of CBPR processes are associated with improved research participation by members of minority communities (and other positive study outcomes)?

RQ3b: Has the rigor of the application of CBPR in clinical trial research improved since 2012?

Herein, we share the methods and results of our findings on the effectiveness of CBPR for increasing participation of racial and ethnic minorities in clinical trials, based on a systematic review of the literature over the past 10 years.

Methods

Data sources and search strategy

A comprehensive literature search was performed of peer-reviewed articles using PubMed, Medline, Web of Science, and CINAHL using the PRISMA approach (Moher et al., 2010) to guide our search strategy. The search was limited to the articles published in English from January 2010 to December 2020 (De Las Nueces et al., 2012 systematic review publication covered up to May 2010). Several keywords were used to retrieve the articles, including ("Community-Based Participatory Research"[Mesh] OR "community-based participatory research" OR "community-based participatory action research" OR "participatory action research" OR "participatory research"))) AND ("Patient Selection"[Mesh] OR participant* OR recruit*))) AND (((("clinical trial*" OR "intervention study")) OR clinical trial as topic [MeSH Terms] OR "randomized controlled"))).

To be included in the current systematic review, articles had to (1) describe the process to recruit participants for clinical trials, had to (2) adopt a community-based participatory research process, and had to (3) target racial and ethnic minority groups (study demographic included more than 90% nonwhite population). Articles were excluded if they: (1) were not US-based (2) did not claim to be CBPR or related (e.g., community-engagement, action research etc.), (3) were not a clinical trial (as defined by the NIH), (4) did not target members of one or more racial/ethnic minority groups, (5) did not report results, or were only descriptive case studies or lessons learnt, (7) were systematic review articles, and (8) if the intervention described did not directly target the community (for example, interventions that targeted medical providers were excluded). While the 2012 systematic review aimed to understand the effectiveness of CBPR strategies for racial and ethnic groups, the search still included many studies not specifically targeting racial and ethnic minorities. In order to understand CBPR effectiveness among racial and ethnic minorities to enhance participation in clinical trials, we found it important to focus only on studies that specifically targeted racial and ethnic minorities. Duplicate articles were excluded from the sample. This process led to a final sample of 104 articles.

Data collection process

After receiving an initial training, four coders independently coded a portion of the retrieved articles. Reviewers' agreement was measured for each of the variables (kappa = 0.74). Given the agreement was satisfactory, the coders coded the remaining articles independently. Figure 1 shows a diagram detailing the study selection process.

The variables coded included the presence of differences between control and study groups; the types of outcomes under study; the type of trial and type of randomization used; the number of participants eligible, enrolled, and retained in the studies. We also coded the presence (or absence) of an advisory committee and the level and type of involvement of the advisory committee.

Analysis

Below we describe the data included in the studies identified through this systematic review. Data were retrieved and synthesized into tables. Where studies did not report levels of community participation in the planning or implementation of the CBPR projects,[1] we combined "No" or "Not reported" into "No/Not reported" for the purpose of data analysis. We conducted chi-square analyses to understand relationships between variables (e.g., study outcomes and CBPR rigor). As in the previously published systematic review (De Las Nueces et al., 2012), it was not possible to complete a meta-analysis because the studies were too heterogeneous. However, we identified and reported frequencies and means.

Results

Characteristics of the articles

Excluding one article that did not clearly indicate the type of study design, 80 of these articles (76.9%) were randomized control trials. Another 14 articles (13.5%) employed randomized control design with delayed intervention. Of the articles using cluster randomization, 38 (36.5%) randomized participants by recruitment sites and another 20 (19.2%) randomized by their communities. Nine studies (8.7%) used cluster randomization by schools. The vast majority of the studies reported the details of baseline (n = 93, 89.4%) and outcome measures (n = 97, 93.3%). When evaluating the effects of the interventions, 46 studies (44.2%) adjusted the differences in the analysis.

We found that Black or African Americans were recruited as the only participants in 32 studies. Nineteen studies recruited Asians or Pacific Islanders as the only participants and another 19 studies had Latino or Hispanic participants as the sole participants. American Indian, Alaska Native, and Indigenous people were recruited as the only participants in 12 articles. About 22 studies recruited mixed or unspecified demographic groups (e.g., Black and Latino) as the participants.[2] Thus, the majority of studies recruited members

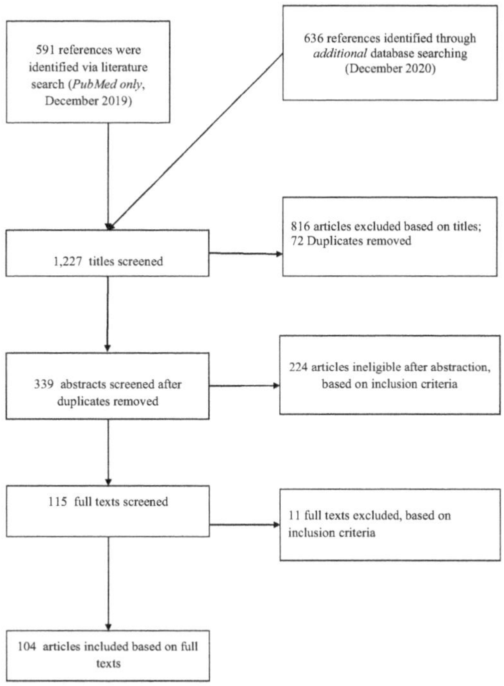

Figure 1. PRISMA flow diagram detailing study selection.

of a single minority ethnic population. The mean number of participants enrolled in 100 studies which reported the data was 390 (range = 23– 1,834). The mean number of participants retained in follow-up studies was 311 (range = 12– 1630).

RQ1: increase in use of CBPR methods

The first RQ aimed to determine if there has been an increase since the 2012 systematic review in the use of CBPR methods to enhance racial and ethnic participation in clinical trials. Our systematic review covered 104 articles published between 2010 and 2020, compared to only 19 eligible studies in the 2012 systematic review by De Las Nueces and colleagues. This represents a substantial increase in published studies claiming CBPR methods since the 2012 review. Notably, the areas of focus in the articles of the present review have significantly expanded than those included in the 2012 review. A variety of health-related topics have been addressed by CBPR-based intervention. Table 1 has provided the list of topics and the percentages of each topic in the sample.

Table 1. Quantity and percentages of health-related topics in the sampled articles of CBPR interventions.

Health Topics	n	%
Diet, weight, and lifestyle	23	22.1
Non-cancer chronic diseases	20	19.2
Cancer	13	12.5
Alcohol and substance use	13	12.5
Infectious diseases	13	12.5
Healthcare service and research	9	8.7
Mental health	7	6.7
Family and parenting	3	2.9
Acute diseases	2	1.9
Other	1	1.0
Total	104	100.0

RQ2: effectiveness of CBPR and the role of communication

Effectiveness of CBPR

RQ2a aimed to determine the effectiveness of CBPR in recruitment of racial and ethnic minorities for clinical trials. The majority of the studies (n = 88, 84.6%) have successfully achieved their primary outcome. Table 2 presents detailed information about the study results.

Behavioral outcomes were most commonly examined as found in 77 (74%) articles of this review. Typical behavioral outcomes were used to measure the effects of CBPR-based interventions on actual behaviors of the participants, such as smoking cessation (Apata et al., 2019) and physical exercise (Saunders et al., 2014). Another 30 studies (28.9%) reported clinical results. Examples of clinical outcomes include BMI (Wright et al., 2013) and reduction in HbA1c (McElfish et al., 2020). Only 12 studies (11.5%) reported process outcomes related to the development of a treatment or intervention program, such as intervention planning and training or service use costs (Chung et al., 2018). A total of 13 studies reported both behavioral and clinical outcomes. Two studies reported both process and clinical outcomes.

Role of communication

RQ2b aimed to understand what communication strategies are employed in some of the studies associated with successful CBPR implementation. In projects that implemented 6 or more of the elements of CBPR, the following communication strategies were noted. First, regular and transparent communication between researchers and community leaders was key to shared decision making and mutual understanding (Aisenberg et al., 2012; Kaufman et al., 2014; Lowe et al., 2012; Tingen et al., 2013). For example, Tingen et al. (2013) reported that there was consistent feedback from the

Table 2. Presentation of results – CBPR for clinical trial participation.

Primary Author	Significant baseline differences adjusted for in results*	Types of Outcomes under study	Baseline measures reported	Outcome measures reported	Primary Outcomes of Study	Health Topic Categories	Study successful in achieving primary outcome	Funding Source
Aisenberg et al. (2012)	No	Process (Recruitment; Other)	Yes	Yes	Patient & Healthcare provider response; intervention adaptation; ongoing partnership and partnership development	Healthcare service and research	Yes	NIH/Gov
Allen et al. (2016)	Yes		Yes	Yes	Behavior (number of EBS offered)	Cancer	Yes	NIH/Gov
Andreae et al. (2012)	No	Process (Recruitment; Other)	Yes	N/A	Strategies that created community, partnerships and facilitated recruitment	Non-cancer chronic disease	Yes	Private/ NGO
Andrews et al. (2016)	No	Behavioral	Yes	Yes	Smoking, abstinence	Alcohol and substance use	Yes	NIH/Gov
Apata et al. (2019)	Yes	Behavioral	Yes	Yes	Smoking cessation	Alcohol and substance use	No	NIH/Gov
Baker et al. (2016)	Yes	Behavioral,Clinical	Yes	Yes	Hypertension, BMI, and self-reported behavior change	Non-cancer chronic disease	Yes	NIH/Gov
Balcázar et al. (2010)	Yes	Behavioral	Yes	Yes	Awareness, self-efficacy, and improved dietary habits.	Diet, weight, and lifestyle	Yes	NIH/Gov
Berkley-Patton et al. (2016)	No	Behavioral	Yes	Yes	HIV testing.	Infectious diseases	Yes	NIH/Gov
Berns et al. (2017)	No	Behavioral	Yes	Yes	Weight status, acceptability of intervention	Diet, weight, and lifestyle	Yes	NIH/Gov
Bird Jernigan et al. (2019)	No	Behavioral	Yes	Yes	Perceived healthy stores; healthy shopping frequency	Healthcare service and research	Yes	NIH/Gov
Blakeney et al. (2015)	No	Process (Recruitment; Other)	N/A	N/A	Training material appropriateness	Non-cancer chronic disease	Yes	NIH/Gov
Blumenthal et al. (2010)	Yes	Behavioral	Yes	Yes	Knowledge, screening	Cancer	Yes	NIH/Gov
Boden-Albala et al. (2014)	No	Behavioral	Yes	Yes	Knowledge	Acute Diseases	Yes	NIH/Gov
Brown and Moyer (2010)	No	Process (Recruitment; Other)	No	No	Recruitment	Healthcare service and research	Yes	NIH/Gov
Calderón et al. (2014)	No	Behavioral	Yes	Yes	Health literacy (STOFHLA/DHLS)	Non-cancer chronic disease	Yes	NIH/Gov
Celano et al. (2012)	No	Behavioral	Yes	Yes	Asthma management and family functioning, caregiver stress	Non-cancer chronic disease	Yes	NIH/Gov
Cené et al. (2013)	No	Behavioral	Yes	Yes	Feasibility of an educational program	Non-cancer chronic disease	Yes	NIH/Gov
Chan et al. (2011)	No	Behavioral	Yes	Yes	Informed decision making (IDM), intention to screen	Cancer	Yes	NIH/Gov
Chung et al. (2018)	No	Process (Recruitment; Other)	Yes	Yes	Intervention planning and training, service use costs	Mental Health	No	NIH/Gov
Clifasefi and Collins (2020)	Yes	Behavioral	Yes	Yes	Self-reported alcohol and quality of life outcomes	Alcohol and substance use	Yes	NIH/Gov
Corrigan et al. (2017)	Yes	Behavioral	Yes	Yes	General health status, psychological experience of physical health, recovery, quality of life, reduction in homelessness, increase in insurance coverage	Mental Health	Yes	NIH/Gov
Cukor et al. (2018)	No	Behavioral	Yes	Yes	Adherence to treatment following intervention	Non-cancer chronic disease	Yes	NIH/Gov
Daley et al. (2018)	No	Behavioral	Yes	Yes	Tobacco use, nicotine dependence, motivation and confidence	Alcohol and substance use	Yes	NIH/Gov
DeHaven et al., (2011)	No	Behavioral	Yes	Yes	Dietary changes, level of physical activity	Diet, weight, and lifestyle	Yes	NIH/Gov NIH/ Gov
Depue et al. (2013)	No	Process (Recruitment; Other)	Yes	Yes	Dose, cost, content of the intervention, patient safety, fidelity	Non-cancer chronic disease	Yes	

(*Continued*)

Table 2. (Continued).

Primary Author	Significant baseline differences adjusted for in results*	Types of Outcomes under study	Baseline measures reported	Outcome measures reported	Primary Outcomes of Study	Health Topic Categories	Study successful in achieving primary outcome	Funding Source
Derose et al. (2019)	No	Behavioral	N/A	Yes	Weight loss, healthy eating, BP, physical activity minutes	Non-cancer chronic disease	Yes	NIH/Gov
Fang et al. (2017)	No	Behavioral	Yes	Yes	Screening rate	Cancer	Yes	Multiple
Flores et al. (2017)	Yes	Behavioral,Process (Recruitment;Other)	No	Yes	Intervention implementation and evaluation	Healthcare service and research	Yes	NIH/Gov
Fung et al. (2018)	Yes	Clinical	Yes	Yes	Cancer Prevention knowledge	Cancer	Yes	NIH/Gov
Gao et al. (2014)	No	Behavioral	Yes	Yes	HBV Knowledge & participation in biospecimen research	Infectious diseases	Yes	NIH/Gov
Gesell et al. (2015)	No	Behavioral	Yes	Yes	Weight gained during pregnancy	Diet, weight, and lifestyle	Yes	Multiple
Green et al. (2015)	No	Clinical	Yes	Yes	Knowledge and attitude toward cancer clinical trials	Cancer	Yes	NIH/Gov
Halbert et al. (2014)	No	Behavioral	No	Yes	Intervention Completion Rate	Diet, weight, and lifestyle	No	NIH/Gov
Harmon et al. (2014)	Yes	Behavioral	Yes	Yes	Increase fruit and vegetable intake; lower fat intake	Diet, weight, and lifestyle	Yes	Academic
Hawk (2013)	No	Behavioral	Yes	Yes	Increase in HIV Testing and risk reduction	Infectious diseases	Yes	Multiple
Heisler et al. (2014)	No	Behavioral	Yes	Yes	Knowledge, satisfaction, descional conflict	Non-cancer chronic disease	Yes	NIH/Gov
Inouye et al. (2014)	No	Behavioral	Yes	Yes	Recruitment and retention feasibility, changes in self-efficacy for diet and exercise, and weight and fasting insulin level change	Diet, weight, and lifestyle	Yes	Unclear
Islam et al. (2013)	No	Yes	Yes	Yes	Diabetes Prevention, improved healthy behaviors, and clinical measurements	Non-cancer chronic disease	Yes	NIH/Gov
Izquierdo et al. (2018)	No	N/A	Yes	Yes	Depressive symptoms, mental health- related quality of life	Mental Health	Yes	Unclear
Kaholokula et al. (2017)	Yes	Yes	Yes	Yes	Weight regain prevention	Diet, weight, and lifestyle	Yes	NIH/Gov
Kataoka et al. (2011)	No	Yes	Yes	Yes	Academic Outcome	Mental Health	Yes	NIH/Gov
Kaufman et al. (2014)	No	Yes	Yes	Yes	Sexual activity & HIV knowledge	Infectious diseases	Yes	NIH/Gov
Kegler et al. (2017)	No	Yes	Yes	Yes	Reducing energy intake and improving home environment	Diet, weight, and lifestyle	Yes	NIH/Gov
Kelly et al. (2010)	No	Yes	Yes	Yes	Reduction in violence-related attitudes	Other	Yes	NIH/Gov
Kieffer et al. (2013)	Yes	Yes	Yes	Yes	Reduction in depressive symptoms	Mental Health	Yes	Multiple
Kim et al. (2014)	No	Yes	Yes	Yes	Improvement in heart health	Non-cancer chronic disease	Yes	NIH/Gov
Komro et al. (2017)	Yes	Yes	Yes	Yes	Underage alcohol use prevention	Alcohol and substance use	Yes	NIH/Gov
Kulis et al. (2016)	Yes	Yes	Yes	Yes	Parenting skills and family functioning	Family and Parenting	Yes	NIH/Gov
Kulis et al. (2017)	No	Yes	Yes	Yes	Substance Use prevention	Family and Parenting	Yes	NIH/Gov
A. T. Langford et al. (2015)	Yes	Yes	Yes	Yes	Enrollment in clinical trials	Healthcare service and research	Yes	NIH/Gov
Leake et al. (2012)	No	Yes	No	No	Attendance, class size, program evaluation	Non-cancer chronic disease	Yes	NIH/Gov
Lee et al. (2018)	No	Yes,N/A	No	No	"phase Yes: knowledge, attitude, and HPV vaccination intention; phase No:	Cancer.	Yes	Academic
Lowe et al. (2012)	Yes	Yes,N/A	Yes	Yes	HPV vaccination uptake and intention."	Alcohol and substance use	Yes	NIH/Gov
Ma et al. (2012)	Yes	Yes,N/A	Yes	Yes	Global Assessment of Individual Needs (overall health problems)	Infectious diseases	Yes	NIH/Gov
Ma et al. (2014)	Yes	N/A	Yes	Yes	Knowledge, screening, utilization of clinic	Healthcare service and research	Yes	NIH/Gov
Ma et al. (2018)	Yes	Yes,N/A	Yes	Yes	Knowledge	Infectious diseases	Yes	NIH/Gov
Martin et al. (2015)		Yes	Yes	Yes	HBV Screening rate, HBV vaccination completion rate	Non-cancer chronic disease	No	NIH/Gov

(*Continued*)

Table 2. (Continued).

Primary Author	Significant baseline differences adjusted for in results*	Types of Outcomes under study	Baseline measures reported	Outcome measures reported	Primary Outcomes of Study	Health Topic Categories	Study successful in achieving primary outcome	Funding Source
Mayer et al. (2019)	Yes	Yes,Multiple	Yes	Yes				NIH/Gov
McDonnell et al. (2011)	No	N/A	Yes	Yes	Adherence to ICS and decrease home asthma triggers	Alcohol and substance use	No	NIH/Gov
McElfish et al. (2020)	Yes	N/A	Yes	Yes	Losing weight	Non-cancer chronic disease	Yes	Multiple
Menkin et al. (2019)	Yes	N/A	Yes	Yes	"quit smoking for at least	Acute diseases	Yes	NIH/Gov
Mendel et al. (2020)	Yes	No	Yes	Yes	N/A0 days at the end of the study"	Mental Health	Yes	NIH/Gov
Miller III et al. (2016)	Yes	Yes	Yes	Yes	Reduction in HbAYesc	Diet, weight, and lifestyle	No	NIH/Gov
Morgan et al. (2010)	No	Yes,N/A	Yes	Yes	Pedometer-measured change in steps	Cancer	Yes	NIH/Gov
Morrison et al. (2017)	No	Yes	Yes	Yes	Type of services and interactions	Diet, weight, and lifestyle	No	NIH/Gov
Moskowitz et al., (2016)	Yes	Yes	Yes	Yes	Blood pressure change	Alcohol and substance use	Yes	NIH/Gov
Napoles et al. (2015)	Yes	N/A	Yes	Yes	Breast cancer-specific quality of life and distress, general symptoms of distress.	Cancer	Yes	Multiple
Napoles et al. (2020)	Yes	N/A	Yes	Yes	Breast cancer-specific Quality of life	Cancer	No	Multiple
Nassar et al. (2014)	No	N/A	No	Yes	HYesNYes immunization	Infectious Diseases	No	NIH/Gov
					Mental health, socioeconomic factors, and service use			NIH/Gov
Ngo et al. (2016)	Yes	Yes,N/A	Yes	Yes	Health research information-seeking behavior	Mental health	Yes	NIH/Gov
Nickell et al. (2019)	Yes	Yes,N/A	Yes	Yes	Weight change from baseline to YesNo months	Cancer	No	Private/ NGO
Paskett et al. (2018)	Yes	N/A	Yes	Yes	Self-efficacy with health insurance navigation	Cancer	No	NIH/Gov
Patel et al. (2019)	Yes	Yes	Yes	Yes	Tobacco abstinence	Healthcare service and research	Yes	NIH/Gov
Patten (2012)	No	Yes	No	No	Change in facility-level transplant referral for patients aged less than 70 years from baseline to YesNo months	Alcohol and substance use	No	NIH/Gov
Patzer et al. (2017)	Yes	No	Yes	Yes	Acceptability, and Quiz Scores of IRB module training	Healthcare service and research	Yes	Multiple
Pearson et al. (2014)	No	No,N/A	No	Yes	Change in cancer clinical trial knowledge and attitudes,	Healthcare service and research	Yes	Academic
Pelto et al. (2016)	Yes	N/A	Yes	Yes	Condom use and HIV test	Cancer	Yes	NIH/Gov
Rhodes et al. (2011)	Yes	N/A	Yes	Yes	Consistent condom use	Infectious Diseases	Yes	NIH/Gov
Rhodes et al. (2017)	Yes	Yes	Yes	Yes	HIV testing, condom use	Infectious Diseases	Yes	NIH/Gov
Rhodes et al. (2020)	Yes	Yes	Yes	Yes	Physical activity, fruit and vegetable consumption	Infectious Diseases	Yes	NIH/Gov
Saunders et al. (2014)	Yes	Yes	Yes	Yes	Healthy eating and physical activity; breast and cervical cancer screening.	Diet, weight, and lifestyle	Yes	NIH/Gov
Scarinci et al. (2014)	Yes	Yes,N/A	Yes	Yes	Physical activity; cardiovascular health indicators	Diet, weight, and lifestyle	Yes	NIH/Gov
Schulz et al. (2015)	No	Yes	Yes	Yes	Vegetable, Fiber, Added Sugar, Total Fat	Diet, weight, and lifestyle	Yes	NIH/Gov
Shah et al. (2015)	No	Yes	Yes	Yes	Parent & Youth outcomes	Diet, weight, and lifestyle	Yes	Multiple
Sieving et al. (2017)	Yes	Yes	Yes	Yes	Systolic or diastolic blood pressure; intervention feasibility	Family and Parenting	Yes	NIH/Gov
Skolarus et al. (2018)	No	No,N/A	Yes	Yes	Hemoglobin AYesc (HbAYesc) level	Non-cancer chronic disease	No	Multiple
Spencer et al. (2011)	Yes	N/A	Yes	Yes	Breast cancer-specific quality of life and distress, general symptoms of distress.	Non-cancer chronic disease	Yes	Multiple
Tingen et al. (2013)	No	Yes	Yes	Yes	Recruitment strategy	Alcohol and Substance Use	Yes	NIH/Gov

(*Continued*)

Table 2. (Continued).

Primary Author	Significant baseline differences adjusted for in results*	Types of Outcomes under study	Baseline measures reported	Outcome measures reported	Primary Outcomes of Study	Health Topic Categories	Study successful in achieving primary outcome	Funding Source
Tingey et al. (2015)	Yes	Yes	Yes	Yes	Self-efficacy, response efficacy, response cost, intrinsic reward, extrinsic reward, severity, and vulnerability)	Infectious Diseases	Yes	NIH/Gov
Tomayko et al. (2016)	No	N/A	Yes	Yes	BMI, nutrition & activity behaviors	Diet, weight, and lifestyle	No	NIH/Gov
Tong et al. (2018)	No	Yes	Yes	Yes	Knowledge, attitudes, smoker behavior	Alcohol and Substance Use	No	Multiple
Tovar et al. (2013)	No	Yes	Yes	Yes	Feeding styles; obesity	Diet, weight, and lifestyle	Yes	NIH/Gov
Tucker et al. (2017)	No	Yes,N/A	Yes	Yes	Healthy eating, physical activity, weight	Diet, weight, and lifestyle	Yes	Private
Ursua et al. (2018)	No	Yes	Yes	Yes	BP control, changes in SBP and DBP, and changes in appointment keeping	Non-cancer chronic disease	Yes	NIH/Gov
Wagner et al. (2016)	No	Yes	Yes	Yes	Smoking cessation	Smoking cessation	No	NIH/Gov
Wieland et al. (2018)	No	Yes	Yes	Yes	Healthy eating and Physical activity	Alcohol and Substance Use	Yes	NIH/Gov
Wilcox et al., (2013)	Yes	Yes	Yes	Yes	Physical activity and healthy eating	Diet, weight, and lifestyle	Yes	NIH/Gov
Williams et al. (2016)	Yes	Yes	Yes	Yes	Alcohol & cigarette use	Alcohol and Substance Use	Yes	NIH/Gov
Wilson et al. (2019)	Yes	Yes	Yes	Yes	HIV risk reduction skills	Infectious Diseases	Yes	NIH/Gov
Wingood et al. (2011)	No	Yes	Yes	Yes	HIV Prevention (condom use, gender role perceptions, self-efficacy, HIV knowledge)	Infectious Diseases	Yes	NIH/Gov
Woods et al. (2013)	No	Yes,N/A	Yes	Yes	Diet, nutrition and physical activity	Diet, weight, and lifestyle	Yes	NIH/Gov
Wright et al. (2013)	No	Yes,N/A	Yes	Yes	BMI, physical activity	Diet, weight, and lifestyle	Yes	Multiple
Yeh et al. (2016)	Yes	Yes,N/A	Yes	Yes	Diabetes prevention	Non-cancer chronic disease	Yes	NIH/Gov
Zoellner et al. (2011)	No	Yes,N/A	Yes	Yes	Blood Pressure	Non-cancer chronic disease	Yes	NIH/Gov

*Studies coded as 'no' include those studies that did, and did not, have significant differences in their target populations at baseline.

researchers to school representatives throughout the project as well as efforts to show appreciation, either financially or with special tokens of appreciation. Second, ensuring clarity in communication by validating and adapting messages based on literacy levels, before dissemination, (Tingen et al., 2013) and/or as a part of interventions (Kim et al., 2014), was also important. Tools like animation were also used to translate technical information to be suitable for lower literacy audiences (Calderón et al., 2014).

Third, surface and deep level cultural targeting of messages and materials (as defined by Resnicow et al., 1999), informed through community engagement, were important components of successful CBPR projects. Examples of surface level targeting included: adapting foods (Islam et al., 2013; Tingen et al., 2013) and religious symbols and rituals (A. T. Langford et al., 2015; Tingen et al., 2013), using the preferred language of participants (Derose et al., 2019; Islam et al., 2013), creating ethnic concordance between researchers/staff and members of the target group, e.g., in vignette characters or peer navigators (Aisenberg et al., 2012; A. T. Langford et al., 2015; Tingen et al., 2013; Zoellner et al., 2011). Examples of deep level cultural targeting included: ensuring integration of study protocols and prospective participants' values such as family (Aisenberg et al., 2012; Islam et al., 2013), acknowledgment of the population's sociohistorical context (Leake et al., 2012), and addressing misconceptions and myths in messages (Islam et al., 2013), adapting or developing training programs for community capacity building (Blakeney et al., 2015; Kelly et al., 2010), developing culturally grounded curricula according to community beliefs (Gao et al., 2014; Kieffer et al., 2013; Lowe et al., 2012) or lifestyle preferences (Inouye et al., 2014; Leake et al., 2012).

RQ3: rigor of CBPR application

Minority populations and CBPR rigor

RQ3a sought to understand which elements of CBPR processes are associated with improved research participation by members of minority communities (and other positive study outcomes). Most of the studies reviewed achieved community involvement in several ways, including: an advisory committee (n = 67, 64.4%), data collection (n = 72, 69.2%), development of interventions (n = 87, 83.7%), and participant recruitment (n = 77, 74.0%), and delivery of the intervention (n = 78, 75.0%). In contrast, 35 (33.7%) and 44 (42.3%) of the studies had community partners work together to disseminate results and identify research questions, respectively. Twenty-five (24.0%) and 23 (22.1%) studies had community partners participating in qualitative or quantitative interpretations of research findings.

About 63.2% of the studies (n = 12) with Asian or Pacific Islander participants had community partners on the advisory committee, followed by 62.5% of the studies with Black or African American participants, 58.3% with Native or Indigenous participants, 57.9% with Latinx or Hispanic participants. About 77.3% of the studies that focused on the population of two or more races or unspecified race had community members at advisory committees, the highest percentage.

We did not observe notable differences in qualitative and quantitative interpretations of the results among the studies with different population races. Fewer than one-third of the studies corresponding to each population had community partners support interpretation of their findings. In contrast, a significantly greater number of studies involved community partners in data collection. Despite no significant difference across different racial/ethnic populations, community partners supported data collection in about two-thirds of the studies.

We further found that community partners involved in the dissemination of results were found more commonly among the studies focusing on Asians or Pacific Islanders (47.4%) as well as Native or Indigenous (41.4%) communities. By contrast, only approximately 30% or less of the studies focusing on other races had community partners in result dissemination. Importantly, when evaluating the CBPR principle of involving community partners in developing and delivering intervention as well as recruiting participants, we found that the percentages of the studies implementing these three principles were lowest among those focusing on the Native or Indigenous population (58.3%, 66.7%, and 58.3%, respectively). Lastly, only 31.8% of the studies with more than one or unspecified race populations had support from community partners to identify study questions, compared with more than 40% of the studies in other race populations.

Study outcomes and CBPR rigor

We conducted a series of additional analyses to understand the relationship between greater fidelity and more successful outcomes. First, our analysis showed that the number of CBPR principles implemented by the studies achieving their primary outcomes was not significantly different from those not achieving such goals ($t = -.96$, $df = 102$, $p = 34$). Second, the number of CBPR principles implemented was not related to either the number of participants enrolled ($r = .07$, $p = .51$) or the number of participants retained ($r = .10$, $p = .35$). The results suggest that although implementing more CBPR principles might slightly increase participants enrolled and retained, such effects were not statistically significant. Third, we further conducted chi-square analyses to test whether achieving the primary outcome was a function of the implementation of each individual CBPR principle (e.g., presence of advisory board). None of the analyses supported such an association that the inclusion of one particular CBPR principle would result in achieving the primary research outcome.

Funding

Our review showed that most of the studies were funded by the federal or national government (n = 80, 76.9%), followed by studies funded by multiple sources (n = 13, 12.5%). Very few studies were funded by academic (n = 3), private (n = 1), non-governmental organizations (n = 4), or multiple sources (n = 13). Additionally, we did not find significant differences in the implementation of CBPR principles between studies of different funding sources [$F(5, 98) = 1.29$, $p = .28$].

CBPR rigor and Improvement since 2012 review

RQ3b aimed to determine if the rigor of the application of CBPR in clinical trial research has improved since 2012. A comparison of the percentages from the 2012 systematic review, indicates that there may be lower community participation in several of the present 2020 study categories, specifically in identifying study questions (63% in 2012 vs. 42.3% in 2020), recruitment of subjects (84% in 2012 vs. 74.0% in 2020), delivery of intervention (84% in 2012 vs. 75.0% in 2020), qualitative interpretation of findings (37% in 2012 vs. 24.0% in 2020), dissemination of results (47% in 2012 vs. 33.7% in 2020). Our analysis did not show a significant change in the presence of an advisory committee (63.2% in 2012 vs. 64.4% in 2020) and quantitative interpretation of findings (21.1% in 2012 vs. 22.1% in 2020). In only two categories do communities appear to be more involved in the 2020 compared to the 2012 study: development of the intervention (74% in 2012 vs. 83.7% in 2020) and data collection (68% in 2012 vs. 69.2% in 2020).

Discussion

The current research presents an update on the use of CBPR methods to enhance participation of racial and ethnic minorities in clinical trial research in the United States. We summarized the literature published since 2012 to meet several objectives. First, we wanted to understand whether there has been an increase in the application of CBPR. Second, we were interested in examining the effectiveness of this methodology to enhance participation of underrepresented individuals in clinical research, including the role played by communication. Third, we wanted to assess the rigor with which the CBPR methodology was applied, and to this purpose we included an analysis of specific dimensions not considered in the systematic review published in 2012 (De Las Nueces et al., 2012).

Adoption of CBPR methods

We noted a significant increase in the number of CBPR interventions being published across a variety of journals. Despite more restrictive inclusion criteria in our study (i.e. we focused on studies that targeted racial and ethnic minorities only), we found more than 4 times the number of eligible studies compared to the 2012 De Las Nueces review. This represents significant progress since a 2004 report of the Agency of Healthcare Research and Quality (AHRQ) which found only 30 interventional studies utilizing CBPR methods in a 28-year period (Viswanathan et al., 2004) and the 2012 De Las Nueces systematic review which found 19 clinical trials in 7 years. There may be several reasons behind this increase in the number of studies adopting a CBPR methodology. Lack of diversity in clinical trials is now considered a scientific and ethical issue (Caplan & Friesen, 2017). Interest in CBPR methodologies has also been fueled by an increased recognition of the importance of engaging participants from traditionally underrepresented groups to ensure the generalizability of clinical research results (Nazha et al., 2019). In response, government agencies have developed grant mechanisms specifically dedicated to fund CBPR research (NIH, 2018), thus providing more opportunities to conduct CBPR-driven projects and also demonstrating a greater commitment to address inequalities. The important role of agency support is apparent from the results of this systematic review. It is also possible that this increase in the number of CBPR related publications reflects the growth of health-related published research observed in the past years (Asmundson & Asmundson, 2018; Sweileh et al., 2017).

Engagement of underrepresented individuals

In the current review, CBPR was integrated into projects targeting diverse racial and ethnic groups, including Black/African Americans, Asians or Pacific Islanders, Hispanic, American Indian/Alaska Native and mixed racial and ethnic minority groups. Data showed a significant improvement in representation compared to the 2012 review in which at least 6 out of the 19 studies reviewed focused on non-Hispanic White populations or did not report participants' race; the other 13 studies in that review did not exclusively target racial/ethnic minorities. This suggests that researchers increasingly believe this method may offer powerful advantages over other methodologies designed to recruit ethnic minority populations participants for clinical trials. The increase in racial and ethnic representation in clinical trial enrollment may be a function of the capacity of CBPR-based recruitment processes to affirm and accommodate diverse identities and backgrounds (Scholl et al., 2011).

The importance of internal communication processes in the (assumed equal) partnership between researchers and communities was often understated in many of these outcome-focused articles. At best, regular meetings and updates were highlighted as examples of transparency and shared decision-making. However, details on the reflexive exercises, conversations and events that aimed to shift balance of power, increase esteem and cultural understanding as aspects of successful CBPR (Wallerstein et al., 2008) were not generally divulged. On the other hand, external communication, such as cultural targeting of messages and interventions developed in partnership with the CAB, appeared to play a role in the success of CBPR projects. In combination with the general positive outcomes of these projects, the existence of these partnerships is encouraging, indicating that CBPR may be a starting point to achieving a truly person-centered approach to an important issue of social justice – inclusive and representative clinical trial participation.

Rigor of the application of CBPR methods

An improvement was also notable in the general scientific rigor of the studies; in the current review spanning over 9 years, 76 of the interventional studies utilizing CBPR methods were randomized control trials, compared to 13 in the 2012 systematic review. However, we found that there were no remarkable differences between the 2012 review and the current one in community participation in CBPR projects: presence of an advisory board, or community involvement in determining research questions, data collection, qualitative and quantitative data analysis and dissemination of findings. Paradoxically, there appeared to be less community participation more recently in certain areas, like the selection of study questions, recruitment of subjects, delivery of intervention, qualitative interpretation of findings and dissemination of results. The relative presence of advisory boards did not increase in recent projects, but stayed the same. Even where we observed increases in community participation, studies provided limited information about the quality of the community engagement including, for example, the number of meetings and power over the decision-making process. This, in addition to the numerous articles that focused on cultural tailoring rather than cultural centering (Peterson & Gubrium, 2011), suggests that many of these community engaged projects have a "top down" (Cyril et al., 2015), instrumental approach. These projects may not be considered "transformative CBPR" which is emblematic of leadership and autonomy of communities as experts of their own health (Peterson & Gubrium, 2011).

Finally, in terms of the efficacy of CBPR, the results from the current review were consistent and comparable to the 2012 review; 85% (current study) and 89% (2012 review) of the studies successfully achieved their primary outcome. These results continue to support greater integration of CBPR methods into clinical trial recruitment processes in racial and ethnic minority communities. However, scaling up delivery of interventions, without compromising community participation is a challenge, as noted by Andrews et al. (2016); this study reported reduced efficacy when the intervention was scaled up which the authors attribute to less time spent in communities building relationships in Phase 2 of their project. Projects that report a lack of sustainability may have suffered because the community did not have adequate ownership of the project (Peterson & Gubrium, 2011) Therefore, sustainability of projects may be an important way to assess the effectiveness of CBPR in future studies.

Practical implications to improve the reporting of CBPR

We suggest that future studies that make claim to the use of CBPR methods should report standardized information about their community engagement process in their write-up (examples of paragraphs summarizing the project's CBPR process can be found in Skolarus et al., 2018; Tingen et al., 2013). Descriptions of community participation in the process of data analysis appeared to be particularly underutilized in the articles reviewed in our study. A good example of how to report this information can be found in Tomayko et al. (2016). Alternatively, given page limitations in peer reviewed journals, we suggest that at a minimum, authors may state that the community was involved as an equal partner in every aspect of research, from conceptualization to dissemination and report additional details online on a journal's website.

There are also some solutions that journal outlets may offer to support careful reporting of CBPR studies. For example, journals may provide a detailed checklist (with definitions provided for each category) encouraging authors to convey this information in a systematic manner or in an appendix. This strategy would also help to raise awareness among researchers of the standards for rigor for the use of CBPR methodologies.

Limitations and future research

*There were some limitations in carrying out the current systematic review. As with the 2012 systematic review and other reviews of CBPR methods (see Cook, 2008), we limited our search to peer reviewed literature in the USA, which limits the international generalizability of our findings. However, we believe that health disparities are striking in the United States, particularly as they affect racial/ethnic minorities (LaVeist, 2005), and that this justifies a focus on understanding CBPR as an approach to reducing these disparities in this country's context.

We also cannot claim any causal inference that links CBPR methodology to specific outcomes; although the clinical trials in our review included comparison and/or control groups, the vast majority did not compare methods. In other words, CBPR was simply integrated as a part of these projects and, as such, the results of our review can only suggest that this method may enhance recruitment of racial and ethnic minorities. Future research should continue to test this through randomized control trials comparing CBPR with other methods of recruitment of specific populations. In addition, future research may also explore the efficacy of CBPR for other vulnerable or underserved populations (representation beyond racial minority communities, such as the LBGT+ community). Ultimately, given the encouraging effects of targeted messages, future research should further evaluate messaging strategies and message development methods to more actively represent diverse voices within marginalized and under resourced communities.

Conclusion

This systematic review answers a question that is as relevant today as it was in 2012: Are CBPR methods effective in enhancing the participation of racial and ethnic minorities in clinical trials? In 2012, De Las Nueces and colleagues found that the vast majority of studies that integrated CBPR methods saw statistically positive outcomes. In 2021, our systematic review found similar results, suggesting that CBPR is still a promising avenue to increase the diversity of racial representation in clinical trials, although the rigor of application of these methodologies should be improved. Community-engaged research continues to represent an important move toward social justice and equity in clinical research by facilitating the development of long-term community-academic partnerships based on mutual trust and respect.

Notes

1. Table with details of CBPR elements available from the corresponding author.
2. Characteristics table and complete citations of all included studies are available from the corresponding author.

Acknowledgments

The authors would like to thank the referenced researchers, community leaders and other study participants for leading impressive community-engaged research projects with underserved communities, and for the opportunity to understand the accomplishments and challenges through this systematic review.

ORCID

Soroya Julian McFarlane http://orcid.org/0000-0002-2826-0926
Aurora Occa http://orcid.org/0000-0001-5311-144X
Wei Peng http://orcid.org/0000-0002-2229-4682
Susan E. Morgan http://orcid.org/0000-0002-8403-9484

References

Aisenberg, E., Dwight-Johnson, M., O'Brien, M., Ludman, E. J., & Golinelli, D. (2012). Building a community-academic partnership: Implementing a community-based trial of telephone cognitive behavioral therapy for rural Latinos. *Depression Research and Treatment, 2012*, Article ID 257858. https://doi.org/10.1155/2012/257858

Albrecht, T. L., Eggly, S. S., Gleason, M. E. J., Harper, F. W. K., Foster, T. S., Peterson, A. M., Orom, H., Penner, L. A., & Ruckdeschel, J. C. (2008). Influence of clinical communication on patients' decision making on participation in clinical trials. *Journal of Clinical Oncology: Official Journal of the American Society of Clinical Oncology, 26*(16), 2666–2673. https://doi.org/10.1200/JCO.2007.14.8114

Allen, J. D., Torres, M. I., Tom, L. S., Leyva, B., Galeas, A. V., & Ospino, H. (2016). Dissemination of evidence-based cancer control interventions among Catholic faith-based organizations: Results from the CRUZA randomized trial. *Implementation Science: IS, 11*(1), 74. https://doi.org/10.1186/s13012-016-0430-6

Andreae, S. J., Halanych, J. H., Cherrington, A., & Safford, M. M. (2012). Recruitment of a rural, southern, predominantly African-American population into a diabetes self-management trial. *Contemporary Clinical Trials, 33*(3), 499–506. https://doi.org/10.1016/j.cct.2012.02.005

Andrews, J. O., Mueller, M., Dooley, M., Newman, S. D., Magwood, G. S., & Tingen, M. S. (2016). Effect of a smoking cessation intervention for women in subsidized neighborhoods: A randomized controlled trial. *Preventive Medicine, 90*, 170–176. https://doi.org/10.1016/j.ypmed.2016.07.008

Apata, J., Sheikhattari, P., Bleich, L., Kamangar, F., O'Keefe, A. M., & Wagner, F. A. (2019). Addressing tobacco use in underserved communities through a peer-facilitated smoking cessation program. *Journal of Community Health, 44*(5), 921–931. https://dx.doi.org/10.1007%2Fs10900-019-00635-8

Asmundson, G. J. G., & Asmundson, A. J. N. (2018). Are anxiety disorders publications continuing on a trajectory of growth? A look at Boschen's (2008) predictions and beyond. *Journal of Anxiety Disorders, 56*, 1–4. https://doi.org/10.1016/j.janxdis.2018.05.003

Balcázar, H. G., de Heer, H., Rosenthal, L., Aguirre, M., Flores, L., Puentes, F. A., Cardenas, V. M., Duarte, M. O., Ortiz, M., & Schulz, L. O. (2010). A promotores de salud intervention to reduce cardiovascular disease risk in a high-risk Hispanic border population, 2005-2008. *Preventing Chronic Disease, 7*(2), A28. https://protect-us.mimecast.com/s/9FY7CwpEkBHvVvwyLtX0hv2?domain=cdc.gov

Baker, E. A., Barnidge, E. K., Schootman, M., Sawicki, M., & Motton-Kershaw, F. L. (2016). Adaptation of a modified DASH diet to a rural African American community setting. *American Journal of Preventive Medicine, 51*(6), 967–974.

Berkley-Patton, J., Thompson, C. B., Moore, E., Hawes, S., Simon, S., Goggin, K., Martinez, D., Berman, M., & Booker, A. (2016). An HIV testing intervention in African American churches: Pilot study findings. *Annals of Behavioral Medicine, 50*(3), 480–485. https://doi.org/10.1007/s12160-015-9758-4

Berns, R. M., Tomayko, E. J., Cronin, K. A., Prince, R. J., Parker, T., & Adams, A. K. (2017). Development of a culturally informed child safety curriculum for American Indian families. *The Journal of Primary Prevention, 38*(1–2), 195–205. https://doi.org/10.1007/s10935-012-0275-y

Bird Jernigan, V. B., Salvatore, A. L., Williams, M., Wetherill, M., Taniguchi, T., Jacob, T., Cannady, T., Grammar, M., Standridge, J., Fox, J., Tingle Owens, J., Spiegel, J., Love, C., Teague, T., & Noonan, C. (2019). A healthy retail intervention in Native American convenience stores: The THRIVE community-based participatory research study. American Journal of Public Health, *109*(1), 132–139. https://doi.org/10.2105/AJPH.2018.3047492

Blumenthal, D. S., Smith, S. A., Majett, C. D., & Alema-Mensah, E. (2010). A trial of 3 interventions to promote colorectal cancer screening in African Americans. *Cancer, 116*(4), 922–929. https://doi.org/10.1002/cncr.24842

Blakeney, N., Michaels, M., Green, M., Richmond, A., Long, D., Robinson, W. S., Spicer, C., Elliott-Bynum, S., & Corbie-Smith, G. (2015). Collaborative development of clinical trials education programs for African-American community-based organizations. *Journal of Cancer Education: The Official Journal of the American Association for Cancer Education, 30*(2), 400–406. https://doi.org/10.1007/s13187-014-0673-3

Boden-Albala, B., Edwards, D. F., St Clair, S., Wing, J. J., Fernandez, S., Gibbons, M. C., Hsia, A. W., Morgenstern, L. B., & Kidwell, C. S. (2014). Methodology for a community-based stroke preparedness intervention: The acute stroke program of interventions addressing racial and ethnic disparities study. *Stroke, 45*(7), 2047–2052. https://doi.org/10.1161/STROKEAHA.113.003502

Brown, M., & Moyer, A. (2010). Predictors of awareness of clinical trials and feelings about the use of medical information for research in a nationally representative US sample. *Ethnicity & Health, 15*(3), 223–236. https://doi.org/10.1080/13557851003624281

Calderón, J. L., Shaheen, M., Hays, R. D., Fleming, E. S., Norris, K. C., & Baker, R. S. (2014). Improving diabetes health literacy by animation. *The Diabetes Educator, 40*(3), 361–372. https://doi.org/10.1177/0145721714527518

Caplan, A., & Friesen, P. (2017). Health disparities and clinical trial recruitment: Is there a duty to tweet? *PLoS Biology, 15*(3), e2002040. https://doi.org/10.1371/journal.pbio.2002040

Celano, M. P., Holsey, C. N., & Kobrynski, L. J. (2012). Home-based family intervention for low-income children with asthma: A randomized controlled pilot study. *Journal of Family Psychology: JFP: Journal of the Division of Family Psychology of the American Psychological Association, 26*(2) 171–178. https://doi.org/10.1037/a0027218

Cené, C. W., Haymore, L. B., Ellis, D., Whitaker, S., Henderson, S., Lin, F.-C., & Corbie-Smith, G. (2013). Implementation of the power to prevent diabetes prevention educational curriculum into rural African American communities: A feasibility study. *The Diabetes Educator, 39*(6), 776–785. https://doi.org/10.1177/0145721713507114

Chan, E. C. Y., McFall, S. L., Byrd, T. L., Mullen, P. D., Volk, R. J., Ureda, J., Calderon-Mora, J., Morales, P., Valdes, A., & Kay Bartholomew, L. (2011). A community-based intervention to promote informed decision making for prostate cancer screening among Hispanic American men changed knowledge and role preferences: A cluster RCT. *Patient Education and Counseling, 84*(2), e44–e51. https://doi.org/10.1016/j.pec.2010.07.033

Chung, B., Ong, M., Ettner, S. L., Mccreary, M., Jones, F., Gilmore, J., Ngo, V. K., Sherbourne, C., Tang, L., Dixon, E., Koegel, P., Miranda, J., & Wells, K. B. (2018). 12-month cost outcomes of community engagement versus technical assistance for depression quality improvement: A partnered, cluster randomized, comparative-effectiveness trial. *Ethnicity & Disease, 28*(2), 349–356. https://doi.org/10.18865/ed.28.S2.349

Cleaver, F. (1999). Paradoxes of participation: Questioning participatory approaches to development. *Journal of International Development, 11*(4), 597–612. https://doi.org/10.1002/(SICI)1099-1328(199906)11:4<597::AID-JID610>3.0.CO;2-Q"3.0.CO;2-Q"https://doi.org/10.1002/(SICI)1099-1328(199906)11:4<597::AID-JID610>3.0.CO;2-Q

Clifasefi, S. L., Collins, S. E., & LEAP Advisory Board. (2020). The life-enhancing alcohol-management program: Results from a 6-month nonrandomized controlled pilot study assessing a community based participatory research program in housing first. *Journal of Community Psychology, 48*(3), 763–776. https://doi.org/10.1002/jcop.22291

Cook, W. K. (2008). Integrating research and action: A systematic review of community-based participatory research to address health disparities in environmental and occupational health in the USA. *Journal of Epidemiology and Community Health, 62*(8), 668–676. https://doi.org/10.1136/jech.2007.067645

Corrigan, P. W., Kraus, D. J., Pickett, S. A., Schmidt, A., Stellon, E., Hantke, E., & Lara, J. L. (2017). Using peer navigators to address the integrated health care needs of homeless African Americans with serious mental illness. *Psychiatric Services*, *68*(3), 264–270. https://doi.org/10.1176/appi.ps.201600134

Cukor, D., Pencille, M., Ver Halen, N., Primus, N., Gordon-Peters, V., Fraser, M., & Salifu, M. (2018). An RCT comparing remotely delivered adherence promotion for sleep apnea assessment against an information control in a Black community sample. *Sleep Health*, *4*(4), 369–376. https://doi.org/10.1016/j.sleh.2018.05.001

Cyril, S., Smith, B. J., Possamai-Inesedy, A., & Renzaho, A. M. N. (2015). Exploring the role of community engagement in improving the health of disadvantaged populations: A systematic review. *Global Health Action*, *8*(1), 29842. https://doi.org/10.3402/gha.v8.29842

De las Nueces, D., Hacker, K., DiGirolamo, A., & Hicks, L. S. (2012). A systematic review of community-based participatory research to enhance clinical trials in racial and ethnic minority groups. *Health Services Research*, *47*(3pt2), 1363–1386. https://doi.org/10.1111/j.1475-6773.2012.01386.x

Derose, K. P., Williams, M. V., Flórez, K. R., Griffin, B. A., Payán, D. D., Seelam, R., Branch, C. A., Hawes-Dawson, J., Mata, M. A., Whitley, M. D., & Wong, E. C. (2019). Eat, pray, move: A pilot cluster randomized controlled trial of a multilevel church-based intervention to address obesity among African Americans and Latinos. *American Journal of Health Promotion: AJHP*, *33*(4), 586–596. https://doi.org/10.1177/0890117118813333

Daley, C. M., Daley, S. M., Pacheco, C. M., Smith, T. E., Talawyma, M., McCloskey, C., Choi, W. S., Nazir, N., Filippi, M. K., McKinney, D., Gunville, J., & Greiner, K. A. (2018). Feasibility of implementing the All Nations Breath of Life culturally tailored smoking cessation program for American Indians in multi-tribal urban communities. *Nicotine & Tobacco Research: Official Journal of the Society for Research on Nicotine and Tobacco*, *20*(5), 552–560. https://doi.org/10.1093/ntr/ntx030

DeHaven, M. J., Ramos-Roman, M. A., Gimpel, N., Carson, J., DeLemos, J., Pickens, S., Simmons, C., Powell-Wiley, T., Banks-Richard, K., Shuval, K., Duvahl, J., Tong, L., Hsieh, N., & Lee, J. J. (2011). The GoodNEWS (Genes, Nutrition, Exercise, Wellness, and Spiritual Growth) trial: A community-based participatory research (CBPR) trial with African-American church congregations for reducing cardiovascular disease risk factors–recruitment, measurement, and randomization. *Contemporary Clinical Trials*, *32*(5), 630–640. https://doi.org/10.1016/j.cct.2011.05.017

DePue, J. D., Rosen, R. K., Seiden, A., Bereolos, N., Chima, M. L., Goldstein, M. G., Nu'usolia, O., Tuitele, J., & McGarvey, S. T. (2013). Implementation of a culturally tailored diabetes intervention with community health workers in American Samoa. *The Diabetes Educator*, *39*(6), 761–771. https://doi.org/10.1177/0145721713504630

Eggly, S., Barton, E., Winckles, A., Penner, L. A., & Albrecht, T. L. (2015). A disparity of words: Racial differences in oncologist-patient communication about clinical trials. *Health Expectations: An International Journal of Public Participation in Health Care and Health Policy*, *18*(5), 1316–1326. https://doi.org/10.1111/hex.12108

Fang, C. Y., Ma, G. X., Handorf, E. A., Feng, Z., Tan, Y., Rhee, J., Miller, S. M., Kim, C., & Koh, H. S. (2017). Addressing multilevel barriers to cervical cancer screening in Korean American women: A randomized trial of a community-based intervention. *Cancer*, *123*(6), 1018–1026. https://doi.org/10.1002/cncr.30391

Flores, G., Walker, C., Lin, H., Lee, M., Fierro, M., Henry, M., Portillo, A., & Massey, K. (2017). An innovative methodological approach to building successful community partnerships for improving insurance coverage, health, and health care in high-risk communities. *Progress in Community Health Partnerships: Research, Education, and Action*, *11*(2), 203–213. https://doi.org/10.1353/cpr.2017.0025

Ford, J. G., Howerton, M. W., Lai, G. Y., Gary, T. L., Bolen, S., Gibbons, M. C., Tilburt, J., Baffi, C., Tanpitukpongse, T. P., Wilson, R. F., Powe, N. R., & Bass, E. B. (2008). Barriers to recruiting underrepresented populations to cancer clinical trials: A systematic review. *Cancer*, *112*(2), 228–242. https://doi.org/10.1002/cncr.23157

Fung, L. C., Nguyen, K. H., Stewart, S. L., Chen, M. S., & Tong, E. K. (2018). Impact of a cancer education seminar on knowledge and screening intent among Chinese Americans: Results from a randomized, controlled, community-based trial. *Cancer*, *124*(S7), 1622–1630. https://doi.org/10.1002/cncr.31111

Gao, W., Ma, G. X., Tan, Y., Fang, C., Weaver, J., Jin, M., Lai, P., & Godwin, A. K. (2014). Culturally appropriate education intervention on biospecimen research participation among Chinese Americans. *Cancer Epidemiology, Biomarkers & Prevention: A Publication of the American Association for Cancer Research, Cosponsored by the American Society of Preventive Oncology*, *23*(3), 383–391. https://doi.org/10.1158/1055-9965.EPI-13-0742

Gesell, S. B., Katula, J. A., Strickland, C., & Vitolins, M. Z. (2015). Feasibility and initial efficacy evaluation of a community-based cognitive-behavioral lifestyle intervention to prevent excessive weight gain during pregnancy in Latina women. *Maternal and Child Health Journal*, *19*(8), 1942–1852. https://doi.org/10.1007/s10995-015-1698-x

Green, M. A., Michaels, M., Blakeney, N., Odulana, A. A., Isler, M. R., Richmond, A., Long, D. G., Robinson, W. S., Taylor, Y. J., & Corbie-Smith, G. (2015). Evaluating a community-partnered cancer clinical trials pilot intervention with African American communities. *Journal of Cancer Education: The Official Journal of the American Association for Cancer Education*, *30*(1), 158–166. https://doi.org/10.1007/s13187-014-0764-1

Heller, C., Balls-Berry, J. E., Nery, J. D., Erwin, P. J., Littleton, D., Kim, M., & Kuo, W. P. (2014). Strategies addressing barriers to clinical trial enrollment of underrepresented populations: A systematic review. *Contemporary Clinical Trials*, *39*(2), 169–182. https://doi.org/10.1016/j.cct.2014.08.004

Horowitz, C. R., Brenner, B. L., Lachapelle, S., Amara, D. A., & Arniella, G. (2009). Effective recruitment of minority populations through community-led strategies. *American Journal of Preventive Medicine*, *37*(6 Suppl 1), S195–S200. https://doi.org/10.1016/j.amepre.2009.08.006

Howerton, M. W., Gibbons, M. C., Baffi, C. R., Gary, T. L., Lai, G. Y., Bolen, S., Tilburt, J., Tanpitukpongse, T. P., Wilson, R. F., Powe, N. R., Bass, E. B., & Ford, J. G. (2007). Provider roles in the recruitment of underrepresented populations to cancer clinical trials. *Cancer*, *109*(3), 465–476. http://dx.doi.org/10.4236/health.2010.27113

Halbert, C. H., Bellamy, S., Briggs, V., Bowman, M., Delmoor, E., Johnson, J. C., Kumanyika, S., Melvin, C., Purnell, J., Rogers, R., & Weathers, B. (2014). Intervention completion rates among African Americans in a randomized effectiveness trial for diet and physical activity changes. *Cancer Epidemiology, Biomarkers & Prevention*, *23*(7), 1306–1313. https://doi.org/10.1158/1055-9965.EPI-13-1064

Harmon, B. E., Adams, S. A., Scott, D., Gladman, Y. S., Ezell, B., & Hebert, J. R. (2014). Dash of faith: A faith-based participatory research pilot study. *Journal of Religion and Health*, *53*(3), 747–759. https://doi.org/10.1007/s10943-012-9664-z

Hawk, M. (2013). The girlfriends project: Results of a pilot study assessing feasibility of an HIV testing and risk reduction intervention developed, implemented, and evaluated in community settings. *AIDS Education and Prevention*, *25*(6), 519–534. http://dx.doi.org/10.1521/aeap.2013.25.6.519

Heisler, M., Choi, H., Palmisano, G., Mase, R., Richardson, C., Fagerlin, A., Montori, V. M., Spencer, M., & An, L. C. (2014). Comparison of community health worker-led diabetes medication decision-making support for low-income Latino and African American adults with diabetes using e-health tools versus print materials: A randomized, controlled trial. *Annals of Internal Medicine*, *161*(10), S13–S22. https://doi.org/10.7326/M13-3012

Inouye, J., Matsuura, C., Li, D., Castro, R., & Leake, A. (2014). Lifestyle intervention for Filipino Americans at risk for diabetes. *Journal of Community Health Nursing*, *31*(4), 225–237. https://doi.org/10.1080/07370016.2014.926674

Islam, N. S., Zanowiak, J. M., Wyatt, L. C., Chun, K., Lee, L., Kwon, S. C., & Trinh-Shevrin, C. (2013). A randomized-controlled, pilot intervention on diabetes prevention and healthy lifestyles in the New York City Korean community. *Journal of Community Health*, *38*(6), 1030–1041. https://doi.org/10.1007/s10900-013-9711-z

Israel, B. A., Eng, E., Schulz, A. J., & Parker, E. A. (Eds.). (2012). *Methods for community-based participatory research for health*. John Wiley & Sons.

Izquierdo, A., Ong, M., Pulido, E., Wells, K. B., Berkman, M., Linski, B., Sauer, V., & Miranda, J. (2018). Community partners in care: 6- and 12-month outcomes of community engagement versus technical assistance to implement depression collaborative care among depressed older adults. *Ethnicity & Disease 28*(2), 339–348. http://dx.doi.org/10.18865/ed.28.s2.339

Katz, R. V., Wang, M. Q., Green, B. L., Kressin, N. R., Claudio, C., Russell, S. L., & Sommervil, C. (2008). Participation in biomedical research studies and cancer screenings: Perceptions of risks to minorities compared with Whites. *Cancer Control: Journal of the Moffitt Cancer Center, 15*(4), 344–351. https://doi.org/10.1177/107327480801500409

Kaufman, C. E., Whitesell, N. R., Keane, E. M., Desserich, J. A., Giago, C., Sam, A., & Mitchell, C. M. (2014). Effectiveness of Circle of Life, an HIV-preventive intervention for American Indian middle school youths: A group randomized trial in a Northern Plains tribe. *American Journal of Public Health, 104*(6), e106–e112. https://doi.org/10.2105/AJPH.2013.301822

Kelly, P. J., Lesser, J., Cheng, A.-L., Oscós-Sánchez, M., Martinez, E., Pineda, D., & Mancha, J. (2010). A prospective randomized controlled trial of an interpersonal violence prevention program with a Mexican American community. *Family & Community Health, 33*(3), 207–215. https://doi.org/10.1097/FCH.0b013e3181e4bc34

Kieffer, E. C., Caldwell, C. H., Welmerink, D. B., Welch, K. B., Sinco, B. R., & Guzmán, J. R. (2013). Effect of the healthy MOMs lifestyle intervention on reducing depressive symptoms among pregnant Latinas. *American Journal of Community Psychology, 51*(1–2), 76–89. http://dx.doi.org/10.1007/s10464-013-9568-4

Kim, K. B., Han, H.-R., Huh, B., Nguyen, T., Lee, H., & Kim, M. T. (2014). The effect of a community-based self-help multimodal behavioral intervention in Korean American seniors with high blood pressure. *American Journal of Hypertension, 27*(9), 1199–1208. https://doi.org/10.1093/ajh/hpu041

Krieger, J. L. (2014). Last resort or roll of the die? Exploring the role of metaphors in cancer clinical trials education among medically underserved populations. *Journal of Health Communication, 19*(10), 1161–1177. https://doi.org/10.1080/10810730.2013.801537

Krieger, J. L., Palmer-Wackerly, A., Dailey, P. M., Krok-Schoen, J. L., Schoenberg, N. E., & Paskett, E. D. (2015). Comprehension of randomization and uncertainty in cancer clinical trials decision making among rural, Appalachian patients. *Journal of Cancer Education: The Official Journal of the American Association for Cancer Education, 30*(4), 743–748. https://doi.org/10.1007/s13187-015-0789-0

Kaholokula, J. K., Look, M., Mabellos, T., Zhang, G., de Silva, M., Yoshimura, S., Solatorio, C., Wills, T., Seto, T. B., & Sinclair, K. A. (2017). Cultural dance program improves hypertension management for native Hawaiians and Pacific Islanders: A pilot randomized trial. *Journal of Racial and Ethnic Health Disparities, 4*(1), 35–46. https://doi.org/10.1007/s40615-015-0198-4

Kataoka, S., Jaycox, L. H., Wong, M., Nadeem, E., Langley, A., Tang, L., & Stein, B. D. (2011). Effects on school outcomes in low-income minority youth: Preliminary findings from a community-partnered study of a school-based trauma intervention. *Ethnicity & Disease, 21*(3 Suppl 1), S1–S71–7.

Kegler, M. C., Haardörfer, R., Alcantara, I., Gazmararian, J. A., Gemma, A., Reynolds, P., & Morris, C. (2017). Home environments, physical activity, and energy expenditure among low-income overweight and obese women. *Women & Health, 57*(8), 990–1006. https://doi.org/10.1080/03630242.2016.1235072

Komro, K. A., Livingston, M. D., Wagenaar, A. C., Kominsky, T. K., Pettigrew, D. W., Garrett, B. A., & Cherokee Nation Prevention Trial Team. (2017). Multilevel prevention trial of alcohol use among American Indian and White high school students in the Cherokee Nation. *American Journal of Public Health, 107*(3), 453–459. https://doi.org/10.2105/AJPH.2016.303603

Kulis, S. S., Ayers, S. L., Harthun, M. L., & Jager, J. (2016). Parenting in 2 worlds: Effects of a culturally adapted intervention for urban American Indians on parenting skills and family functioning. *Prevention Sciences, 17*(6), 721–731. https://doi.org/10.1007/s11121-016-0657-0

Langford, A., Resnicow, K., & An, L. (2010). Clinical trial awareness among racial/ethnic minorities in HINTS 2007: Sociodemographic, attitudinal, and knowledge correlates. *Journal of Health Communication, 15*(3), 92–101. https://doi.org/10.1080/10810730.2010.525296

Langford, A. T., Resnicow, K., & Beasley, D. D. (2015). Outcomes from the Body & Soul clinical trials project: A university-church partnership to improve African American enrollment in a clinical trial registry. *Patient Education and Counseling, 98*(2), 245–250. https://doi.org/10.1016/j.pec.2014.10.018

Laufman, L. (2009). Making the invisible visible: Professional education to eliminate disparities in clinical trials. *Journal of Cancer Education: The Official Journal of the American Association for Cancer Education, 24*(2 Suppl), S56–S59. https://doi.org/10.1007/BF03182315

LaVeist, T. A. (2005). *Minority populations and health: An introduction to health disparities in the United States*. John Wiley & Sons.

Leake, A. R., Bermudo, V. C., Jacob, J., Jacob, M. R., & Inouye, J. (2012). Health is wealth: Methods to improve attendance in a lifestyle intervention for a largely immigrant Filipino-American sample. *Journal of Immigrant and Minority Health/Center for Minority Public Health, 14*(3), 475–480. https://doi.org/10.1007/s10903-011-9487-0

Leiter, A., Diefenbach., M. A., Doucette, J., Oh, W. K., & Galsky, M. D. (2015). Clinical trial awareness: Changes over time and sociodemographic disparities. *Clinical Trials, 12*(3), 215–223. https://doi.org/10.1177/1740774515571917

Lee, H., Kim, M., Cooley, M. E., Kiang, P. N.-C., Kim, D., Tang, S., Shi, L., Thiem, L., Kan, P., Peou, S., Touch, C., Chea, P., & Allison, J. (2018). Using narrative intervention for HPV vaccine behavior change among Khmer mothers and daughters: A pilot RCT to examine feasibility, acceptability, and preliminary effectiveness. *Applied Nursing Research: ANR, 40*(April 2018), 51–60. https://doi.org/10.1016/j.apnr.2017.12.008

Lie, M. L. S., Lecouturier, J., & Harding, C. (2019). Should I stay or should I go? A qualitative study exploring participation in a urology clinical trial. *International Urogynecology Journal, 30*(1), 9–16. https://doi.org/10.1007/s00192-018-3784-2

Lowe, J., Liang, H., Riggs, C., Henson, J., & Elder, T. (2012). Community partnership to affect substance abuse among Native American adolescents. *The American Journal of Drug and Alcohol Abuse, 38*(5), 450–455. https://doi.org/10.3109/00952990.2012.694534

Ma, G. X., Gao, W., Tan, Y., Chae, W. G., & Rhee, J. (2012). A community-based participatory approach to a hepatitis B intervention for Korean Americans. *Progress in Community Health Partnerships: Research, Education, and Action, 6*(1), 7–16. https://doi.org/10.1353/cpr.2012.0002

Ma, G. X., Lee, M. M., Tan, Y., Hanlon, A. L., Feng, Z., Shireman, T. I., Rhee, J., Wei, Z., Wong, F., Koh, H. S., Kim, C., & York, W. (2018). Efficacy of a community-based participatory and multilevel intervention to enhance hepatitis B virus screening and vaccination in underserved Korean Americans. *Cancer, 124*(5), 973–982. https://doi.org/10.1002/cncr.31134

Ma, G. X., Tan, Y., Blakeney, N. C., Seals, B. F., Ma, X. S., Zhai, S., Liu, A., Tai, Y., & Michaels, M. (2014). The impact of a community-based clinical trial educational intervention among underrepresented Chinese Americans. *Cancer Epidemiology, Biomarkers & Prevention, 23*(3), 424–432. https://doi.org/10.1158/1055-9965.EPI-13-0773

Martin, M. A., Mosnaim, G. S., Olson, D., Swider, S., Karavolos, K., & Rothschild, S. (2015). Results from a community-based trial testing a community health worker asthma intervention in Puerto Rican youth in Chicago. *Journal of Asthma 52*(1), 59–70. https://doi.org/10.3109/02770903.2014.950426

Mayer, V. L., Vangeepuram, N., Fei, K., Hanlen-Rosado, E. A., Arniella, G., Negron, R., Fox, A., Lorig, K., & Horowitz, C. R. (2019). Outcomes of a weight loss intervention to prevent diabetes among low-income residents of East Harlem, New York. Health Education & Behavior, 46(6), 1073–1082. https://doi.org/10.1177/1090198119868232

McDavitt, B., Bogart, L. M., Mutchler, M. G., Wagner, G. J., Green, H. D., Jr, Lawrence, S. J., Mutepfa, K. D., & Nogg, K. A. (2016). Dissemination as dialogue: Building trust and sharing research findings through community engagement. *Preventing Chronic Disease, 13*(E38). http://dx.doi.org/10.5888/pcd13.150473

McDonnell, D. D., Kazinets, G., Lee, H.-J., & Moskowitz, J. M. (2011). An internet-based smoking cessation program for Korean Americans: Results from a randomized controlled trial. Nicotine & Tobacco Research, 13(5), 336–343. https://doi.org/10.1093/ntr/ntq260

McElfish, P. A., Long, C. R., Bursac, Z., Scott, A. J., Felix, H. C., Schulz, T. K., Worley, M. A., & Rowland, B. (2020). Diabetes self-management education exposure and glycated haemoglobin levels among Marshallese participants in a randomized controlled study. *Diabetic Medicine: A Journal of the British Diabetic Association, 37*(2), 319–325. https://doi.org/10.1111/dme.14189

Mendel, P., O'Hora, J., Zhang, L., Stockdale, S., Dixon, E. L., Gilmore, J., Jones, F., Jones, A., Williams, P., Sharif, M. Z., &Others. (2020). Engaging community networks to improve depression services: A cluster-randomized trial of a community engagement and planning intervention. Community Mental Health Journal, 57(3), 457–469 https://doi.org/10.1007/s10597-020-00632-5

Menkin, J. A., McCreath, H. E., Song, S. Y., Carrillo, C. A., Reyes, C. E., Trejo, L., Choi, S. E., Willis, P., Jimenez, E., Ma, S., Chang, E., Liu, H., Kwon, I., Kotick, J., & Sarkisian, C. A. (2019). "Worth the walk": Culturally tailored stroke risk factor reduction intervention in community senior centers. Journal of the American Heart Association, 8(6), e011088. https://doi.org/10.1161/JAHA.118.011088

Michaels, M., Blakeney, N., Langford, A. T., & Ford, M. E. (2015). Five principles for effective cancer clinical trial education within the community setting. *Journal of Cancer Education: The Official Journal of the American Association for Cancer Education, 30*(1), 197–203. https://doi.org/10.1007/s13187-014-0699-6

Michaels, M., Weiss, E. S., Guidry, J. A., Blakeney, N., Swords, L., Gibbs, B., Yeun, S., Rytkonen, B., Goodman, R., & Jarama, S. L., & Others. (2012). The promise of community-based advocacy and education efforts for increasing cancer clinical trials accrual. *Journal of Cancer Education: The Official Journal of the American Association for Cancer Education, 27*(1), 67–74. https://doi.org/10.1007/s13187-011-0271-6

Miller, J. D., Kotowski, M. R., Comis, R. L., Smith, S. W., Silk, K. J., Colaizzi, D. D., & Kimmel, L. G. (2011). Measuring cancer clinical trial understanding. *Health Communication, 26*(1), 82–93. https://doi.org/10.1080/10410236.2011.527624

Miller, E. R., Cooper, L. A., Carson, K. A., Wang, N.-Y., Appel, L. J., Gayles, D., Charleston, J., White, K., You, N., Weng, Y., & Others. (2016). A dietary intervention in urban African Americans: Results of the "Five Plus Nuts and Beans" randomized trial. *American Journal of Preventive Medicine, 50*(1), 87–95. https://doi.org/10.1016/j.amepre.2015.06.010

Minkler, M. (2004). Ethical challenges for the "outside" researcher in community-based participatory research. *Health Education & Behavior: The Official Publication of the Society for Public Health Education, 31*(6), 684–697. https://doi.org/10.1177/1090198104269566

Moher, D., Liberati, A., Tetzlaff, J., Altman, D. G., & Group, P. R. I. S. M. A. (2010). Preferred reporting items for systematic reviews and meta-analyses: The PRISMA statement. *International Journal of Surgery, 8*(5), 336–341. https://doi.org/10.1016/j.ijsu.2010.02.007

Morgan, S. E., & Mouton, A. (2015). Improving patient accrual to research studies and clinical trials through communication design interventions. In T. R. Harrison & E. A. Williams (Eds.), *Organizations, communication, and health* (pp. 106–124). Routledge. https://doi.org/10.1186/1745-6215-15-399

Morgan, S. E., Occa, A., Peng, W., & McFarlane, S. J. (2020). Evidence-based communication in clinical, mass media, and social media contexts to enhance informed consent for participation in clinical trials and precision medicine initiatives. In D. O'Hair, M. J. O'Hair, E. B. Hester, & S. Geegan (Eds.), *Handbook of applied communication* (pp. 897–915). John Wiley & Sons, Inc. https://doi.org/10.1002/9781119399926.ch49

Morgan, S. E., Occa, A., Mouton, A., & Potter, J. (2017). The role of nonverbal communication behaviors in clinical trial and research study recruitment. *Health Communication, 32*(4), 461–469. https://doi.org/10.1080/10410236.2016.1140266

Morgan, S. E., Occa, A., Potter, J., Mouton, A., & Peter, M. E. (2017). "You need to be a good listener": Recruiters' use of relational communication behaviors to enhance clinical trial and research study accrual. *Journal of Health Communication, 22*(2), 95–101. https://doi.org/10.1080/10810730.2016.1256356

Morgan, P. D., Fogel, J., Tyler, I.D., & Jones, J.R. (2010). Culturally targeted educational intervention to increase colorectal health awareness among African Americans. *Journal of Health Care for the Poor and Underserved 21*(3), 132–147. https://doi.org/10.1353/hpu.0.0357

Morrison, E. J., Clark, M. M., Wieland, M. L., Weis, J. A., Hanza, M. M. K., Meiers, S. J., Patten, C. A., Sloan, J. A., Novotny, P. J., Sim, L. A., Nigon, J. A., & Sia, I. G. (2017). Relationship between negative mood and health behaviors in an immigrant and refugee population. *Journal of Immigrant and Minority Health / Center for Minority Public Health, 19*(3), 655–664. https://doi.org/10.1007/s10903-016-0506-z

Moskowitz, J. M., McDonnell, D. D., Kazinets, G., & Lee, H.-J. (2016). Online smoking cessation program for Korean Americans: Randomized trial to test effects of incentives for program completion and interim surveys. *Preventive Medicine, 86*(May 2016), 70–76. https://doi.org/10.1016/j.ypmed.2016.01.019

Nazha, B., Mishra, M., Pentz, R., & Owonikoko, T. K. (2019). Enrollment of racial minorities in clinical trials: Old problem assumes new urgency in the age of immunotherapy. *American Society of Clinical Oncology Educational Book. American Society of Clinical Oncology. Annual Meeting, 39*(39), 3–10. https://doi.org/10.1200/EDBK_100021

Ngo, V. K., Sherbourne, C., Chung, B., Tang, L., Wright, A. L., Whittington, Y., Wells, K., & Miranda, J. (2016). Community engagement compared with technical assistance to disseminate depression care among low-income, minority women: A randomized controlled effectiveness study. American Journal of Public Health, 106(10), 1833–1841. https://doi.org/10.2105/AJPH.2016.303304

NIH. (2018). *Community-based participatory research program (CBPR).* https://www.nimhd.nih.gov/programs/extramural/community-based-participatory.html

Nyamathi, A., Koniak-Griffin, D., & Greengold, B. A. (2007). Development of nursing theory and science in vulnerable populations research. *Annual Review of Nursing Research, 25*(1), 3–25. https://doi.org/10.1891/0739-6686.25.1.3

Nápoles, A. M., Ortíz, C., Santoyo-Olsson, J., Stewart, A. L., Gregorich, S., Lee, H. E., Durón, Y., McGuire, P., & Luce, J. (2015). Nuevo Amanecer: Results of a randomized controlled trial of a community-based, peer-delivered stress management intervention to improve quality of life in Latinas with breast cancer. *American Journal of Public Health, 105*(3), e55–e63. https://doi.org/10.2105/AJPH.2015.302598

Nassar, A. F., Alemi, F., Hetmyer, A., Alemi, Y., Randolph, L. A., & Ramey, S. L. (2014). Automated monitoring to detect H1N1 symptoms among urban, Medicaid-eligible, pregnant women: A community-partnered randomized controlled trial. *Journal of Community Health, 39*(1), 159–166. https://doi.org/10.1007/s10900-013-9754-1

Nickell, A., Stewart, S. L., Burke, N. J., Guerra, C., Cohen, E., Lawlor, C., Colen, S., Cheng, J., & Joseph, G. (2019). Engaging limited English proficient and ethnically diverse low-income women in health research: A randomized trial of a patient navigator intervention. *Patient Education and Counseling, 102*(7), 1313–1323. https://doi.org/10.1016/j.pec.2019.02.013

Occa, A., & Morgan, S. E. (2018). Training programs for improving communication about medical research and clinical trials: A systematic review. In M. Prostran (Ed.), *Clinical trials in vulnerable populations* (pp. 199–213). IntechOpen. https://doi.org/10.5772/intechopen.70188

Occa, A., Morgan, S. E., & Potter, J. E. (2018). Underrepresentation of Hispanics and other minorities in clinical trials: Recruiters' perspectives. *Journal of Racial and Ethnic Health Disparities, 5*(2), 322–332. https://doi.org/10.1007/s40615-017-0373-x

Paskett, E. D., Baltic, R. D., Young, G. S., Katz, M. L., Lesko, S. M., Webber, K. H., Roberto, K. A., Lengerich, E. J., Schoenberg, N. E., Kennedy, S. K., Mama, S., Midkiff, C. C., & Dignan, M. B. (2018). A group randomized trial to reduce obesity among Appalachian church members: The walk by faith study. *Cancer Epidemiology, Biomarkers & Prevention, 27*(11), 1289–1297. https://doi.org/10.1158/1055-9965.EPI-17-1085

Patel, M. R., Israel, B. A., Song, P. X. K., Hao, W., TerHaar, L., Tariq, M., & Lichtenstein, R. (2019). Insuring good health: Outcomes and acceptability of a participatory health insurance literacy intervention in diverse urban communities. *Health Education & Behavior, 46*(3), 494–505. https://doi.org/10.1177/1090198119831060

Patten, C. A. (2012). Tobacco cessation intervention during pregnancy among Alaska Native women. *Journal of Cancer Education, 27*(1), S86–S90. https://doi.org/10.1007/s13187-012-0317-4

Patzer, R. E., Paul, S., Plantinga, L., Gander, J., Sauls, L., Krisher, J., Mulloy, L. L., Gibney, E. M., Browne, T., Zayas, C. F., McClellan, W. M., Arriola, K. J., Pastan, S. O., & Southeastern Kidney Transplant Coalition. (2017). A randomized trial to reduce disparities in referral for transplant evaluation. *Journal of the American Society of Nephrology, 28*(3), 935–942. https://doi.org/10.1681/ASN.2016030320

Pearson, C. R., Parker, M., Fisher, C. B., & Moreno, C. (2014). Capacity building from the inside out: Development and evaluation of a CITI ethics certification training module for American Indian and Alaska Native community researchers. *Journal of Empirical Research on Human Research Ethics, 9*(1), 46–57. https://doi.org/10.1525/jer.2014.9.1.46

Pelto, D. J., Sadler, G. R., Njoku, O., Rodriguez, M. C., Villagra, C., Malcarne, V. L., Riley, N. E., Behar, A. I., & Jandorf, L. (2016). Adaptation of a cancer clinical trials education program for African American and Latina/o community members. Health Education & Behavior, 43(4), 381–388. https://doi.org/10.1177/1090198115610555

Peterson, J. C., & Gubrium, A. (2011). Old wine in new bottles? The positioning of participation in 17 NIH-funded CBPR projects. *Health Communication, 26*(8), 724–734. https://doi.org/10.1080/10410236.2011.566828

Resnicow, K., Baranowski, T., Ahluwalia, J. S., & Braithwaite, R. L. (1999). Cultural sensitivity in public health: Defined and demystified. *Ethnicity & Disease, 9*(1), 10–21. http://www.jstor.org/stable/26738293

Ross, L. F., Loup, A., Nelson, R. M., Botkin, J. R., Kost, R., Smith, G. R., Jr, & Gehlert, S. (2010). Human subjects protections in community-engaged research: A research ethics framework. *Journal of Empirical Research on Human Research Ethics: JERHRE, 5*(1), 5–17. https://doi.org/10.1525/jer.2010.5.1.5

Rhodes, S. D., Alonzo, J., Mann, L., Song, E. Y., Tanner, A. E., Arellano, J. E., Rodriguez-Celedon, R., Garcia, M., Freeman, A., Reboussin, B. A., & Painter, T. M. (2017). Small-group randomized controlled trial to increase condom use and HIV testing among Hispanic/Latino gay, bisexual, and other men who have sex with men. *American Journal of Public Health, 107*(6), 969–976. https://doi.org/10.2105/AJPH.2017.303814

Rhodes, S. D., Alonzo, J., Mann-Jackson, L., Song, E. Y., Tanner, A. E., Garcia, M., Smart, B. D., Baker, L. S., Eng, E., & Reboussin, B. A. (2020). A peer navigation intervention to prevent HIV among mixed immigrant status Latinx GBMSM and transgender women in the United States: Outcomes, perspectives and implications for PrEP uptake. *Health Education Research, 35*(3), 165–178. https://doi.org/10.1093/her/cyaa010

Rhodes, S. D., McCoy, T. P., Vissman, A. T., DiClemente, R. J., Duck, S., Hergenrather, K. C., Foley, K. L., Alonzo, J., Bloom, F. R., & Eng, E. (2011). A randomized controlled trial of a culturally congruent intervention to increase condom use and HIV testing among heterosexually active immigrant Latino men. *AIDS and Behavior, 15*(8), 1764–1775. https://doi.org/10.1007/s10461-011-9903-4

Saunders, R. P., Wilcox, S., Baruth, M., & Dowda, M. (2014). Process evaluation methods, implementation fidelity results and relationship to physical activity and healthy eating in the Faith, Activity, and Nutrition (FAN) study. *Evaluation and Program Planning, 43*, 93–102. https://doi.org/10.1016/j.evalprogplan.2013.11.003

Scarinci, I. C., Moore, A., Wynn-Wallace, T., Cherrington, A., Fouad, M., & Li, Y. (2014). A community-based, culturally relevant intervention to promote healthy eating and physical activity among middle-aged African American women in rural Alabama: Findings from a group randomized controlled trial. *Preventive Medicine, 69*, 13–20. https://doi.org/10.1016/j.ypmed.2014.08.016

Scholl, J. C., Wilson, J. B., & Hughes, P. C. (2011). Expression of patients' and providers' identities during the medical interview. *Qualitative Health Research, 21*(8), 1022–1032. https://doi.org/10.1177/1049732310393748

Schulz, A. J., Israel, B. A., Mentz, G. B., Bernal, C., Caver, D., DeMajo, R., Diaz, G., Gamboa, C., Gaines, C., Hoston, B., Opperman, A., Reyes, A. G., Rowe, Z., Sand, S. L., & Woods, S. (2015). Effectiveness of a walking group intervention to promote physical activity and cardiovascular health in predominantly non-Hispanic Black and Hispanic urban neighborhoods: Findings from the walk your heart to health intervention. *Health Education & Behavior, 42*(3), 380–392. https://doi.org/10.1177/1090198114560015

Seifer, S. D., Michaels, M., & Collins, S. (2010). Applying community-based participatory research principles and approaches in clinical trials: Forging a new model for cancer clinical research. *Progress in Community Health Partnerships: Research, Education, and Action, 4*(1), 37–46. https://doi.org/10.1353/cpr.0.0103

Sia, I. G. (2016). Healthy immigrant families: Participatory development and baseline characteristics of a community-based physical activity and nutrition intervention. *Contemporary Clinical Trials, 47*(March 2016), 22–31. https://doi.org/10.1016/j.cct.2015.12.004

Sieving, R. E., Allen, M. L., Galvan, A., Rodriguez-Hager, R., Beckman, K., Castillo, M., Gadea, A., Jimbo-Llapa, F., Porta, C., & Svetaz, M. V. (2017). Encuentro: Feasibility, acceptability, and outcomes of a culturally tailored teen-parent health promotion program. *Health Promotion Practice, 18*(5), 751–762. https://doi.org/10.1177/1524839916654462

Shah, M. K., Kieffer, E. C., Choi, H., Schumann, C., & Heisler, M. (2015). Mediators and Moderators of the Effectiveness of a community health worker Intervention that improved dietary outcomes in pregnant Latino women. Health Education & Behavior, 42(5), 593–603. https://doi.org/10.1177/1090198114568307

Skolarus, L. E., Cowdery, J., Dome, M., Bailey, S., Baek, J., Byrd, J. B., Hartley, S. E., Valley, S. C., Saberi, S., Wheeler, N. C., McDermott, M., Hughes, R., Shanmugasundaram, K., Morgenstern, L. B., & Brown, D. L. (2018). Reach Out Churches: A community-based participatory research pilot trial to assess the feasibility of a mobile health technology intervention to reduce blood pressure among African Americans. *Health Promotion Practice, 19*(4), 495–505. https://doi.org/10.1177/1524839917710893

Spencer, M. S., Rosland, A.-M., Kieffer, E. C., Sinco, B. R., Valerio, M., Palmisano, G., Anderson, M., Guzman, J. R., & Heisler, M. (2011). Effectiveness of a community health worker intervention among African American and Latino adults with type 2 diabetes: A randomized controlled trial. *American Journal of Public Health, 101*(12), 2253–2260. https://doi.org/10.2105/AJPH.2010.300106

Swanson, G. M., & Ward, A. J. (1995). Recruiting minorities into clinical trials toward a participant-friendly system. *Journal of the National Cancer Institute, 87*(23), 1747–1759. https://doi.org/10.1093/jnci/87.23.1747

Sweileh, W. M., Al-Jabi, S. W., AbuTaha, A. S., Zyoud, S. H., Anayah, F. M. A., & Sawalha, A. F. (2017). Bibliometric analysis of worldwide scientific literature in mobile - health: 2006–2016. *BMC Medical Informatics and Decision Making, 17*(1), 72. https://doi.org/10.1186/s12911-017-0476-7

Tanner, A., Kim, S.-H., Friedman, D. B., Foster, C., & Bergeron, C. D. (2015). Barriers to medical research participation as perceived by clinical trial investigators: Communicating with rural and African American communities. *Journal of Health Communication, 20*(1), 88–96. https://doi.org/10.1080/10810730.2014.908985

Tingen, M. S., Andrews, J. O., Heath, J., Turnmire, A. E., Waller, J. L., & Treiber, F. A. (2013). Comparison of enrollment rates of African-American families into a school-based tobacco prevention trial using two recruitment strategies in urban and rural settings. *American Journal of Health Promotion: AJHP, 27*(4), e91–e100. https://doi.org/10.4278/ajhp.110204-QUAN-53

Tomayko, E. J., Prince, R. J., Cronin, K. A., & Adams, A. K. (2016). The Healthy Children, Strong Families intervention promotes improvements in nutrition, activity and body weight in American Indian families with young children. *Public Health Nutrition*, *19*(15), 2850–2859. https://doi.org/10.1017/S1368980016001014

Tingey, L., Mullany, B., Chambers, R., Hastings, R., Lee, A., Parker, A., Barlow, A., & Rompalo, A. (2015). Respecting the circle of life: One year outcomes from a randomized controlled comparison of an HIV risk reduction intervention for American Indian adolescents. *AIDS Care*, *27* (9), 1087–1097. https://doi.org/10.1080/09540121.2015.1028879

Tong, E. K., Saw, A., Fung, L.-C., Li, C.-S., Liu, Y., & Tsoh, J. Y. (2018). Impact of a smoke-free-living educational intervention for smokers and household nonsmokers: A randomized trial of Chinese American pairs. *Cancer*, *124*(7), 1590–1598. https://doi.org/10.1002/cncr.31115

Tovar, A., Hennessy, E., Must, A., Hughes, S. O., Gute, D. M., Sliwa, S., Boulos, R. J., Vikre, E. K., Kamins, C. L., Tofuri, K., Pirie, A., & Economos, C. D. (2013). Feeding styles and evening family meals among recent immigrants. The International Journal of Behavioral Nutrition and Physical Activity, 10(84), 1–8. https://doi.org/10.1186/1479-5868-10-84

Tucker, C. M., Wippold, G. M., Williams, J. L., Arthur, T. M., Desmond, F. F., & Robinson, K. C. (2017). A CBPR study to test the impact of a church-based health empowerment program on health behaviors and health outcomes of black adult churchgoers. Journal of Racial and Ethnic Health Disparities, 4(1), 70–78. https://doi.org/10.1007/s40615-015-0203-y10

Ursua, R. A., Aguilar, D. E., Wyatt, L. C., Trinh-Shevrin, C., Gamboa, L., Valdellon, P., Perrella, E. G., Dimaporo, M. Z., Nur, P. Q., Tandon, S. D., & Islam, N. S. (2018). A community health worker intervention to improve blood pressure among Filipino Americans with hypertension: A randomized controlled trial. Preventive Medicine Reports, 11(6), 42–48. https://doi.org/10.1016/j.pmedr.2018.05.002

UyBico, S. J., Pavel, S., & Gross, C. P. (2007). Recruiting vulnerable populations into research: A systematic review of recruitment interventions. *Journal of General Internal Medicine*, *22*(6), 852–863. https://doi.org/10.1007/s11606-007-0126-3

Viswanathan, M., Ammerman, A., Eng, E., Garlehner, G., Lohr, K. N., Griffith, D., Rhodes, S., Samuel-Hodge, C., Maty, S., Lux, L., Webb, L., Sutton, S. F., Swinson, T., Jackman, A., & Whitener, L. (2004). Community-based participatory research: Assessing the evidence. *Evidence Report/Technology Assessment (Summary)*, *99*, 1–8.

Wallerstein, N., Oetzel, J., Duran, B., Belone, L., Tafoya, G., & Rae, R. (2008). CBPR: What predicts outcomes?. M. Minkler & N. Wallerstein, (Eds.), *Community-based participatory research for health: From process to outcomes*, (pp. 371–392). John Wiley & Sons.

Wallerstein, N., & Duran, B. (2008). The theoretical, historical, and practice roots of CBPR. In M. Minkler & N. Wallerstein (Eds.), *Community-based participatory research for health: From process to outcomes*, (pp. 25–40). John Wiley & Sons.

Wright, K., Giger, J. N., Norris, K., & Suro, Z. (2013). Impact of a nurse-directed, coordinated school health program to enhance physical activity behaviors and reduce body mass index among minority children: A parallel-group, randomized control trial. *International Journal of Nursing Studies*, *50*(6), 727–737. https://doi.org/10.1016/j.ijnurstu.2012.09.004

Wagner, F. A., Sheikhattari, P., Buccheri, J., Gunning, M., Bleich, L., & Schutzman, C. (2016). A Community-Based participatory research on smoking cessation intervention for urban communities. *Journal of Health Care for the Poor and Undeserved*, *27*(1), 35–50. https://doi.org/10.1353/hpu.2016.0017

Wieland, M. L., Weis, J. A., Hanza, M. M. K., Meiers, S. J., Patten, C. A., Clark, M. M., Sloan, J. A., Novotny, P. J., Njeru, J. W., Abbenyi, A., Levine, J. A., Goodson, M., Porraz Capetillo, M. G. D., Osman, A., Hared, A., Nigon, J. A., & Sia, I. G. (2016). Healthy immigrant families: Participatory development and baseline characteristics of a community-based physical activity and nutrition intervention. *Contemporary Clinical Trials*, *47*(March 2016), 22–31. https://doi.org/10.1016/j.cct.2015.12.004

Wilcox, S., Parrott, A., Baruth, M., Laken, M., Condrasky, M., Saunders, R., Dowda, M., Evans, R., Addy, C., Warren, T. Y., Kinnard, D., & Zimmerman, L. (2013). The faith, activity, and nutrition program: A randomized controlled trial in African-American churches. *American Journal of Preventive Medicine*, *44*(2), 122–131. https://doi.org/10.1016/j.amepre.2012.09.062

Williams, L. R., Ayers, S., Baldwin, A., & Marsiglia, F. F. (2016). Delaying youth substance-use initiation: A cluster randomized controlled trial of complementary youth and parenting interventions. Journal of the Society for Social Work and Research, 7(1), 177–200. https://doi.org/10.1086/685298

Wilson, T. E., Gousse, Y., Joseph, M. A., Browne, R. C., Camilien, B., McFarlane, D., Mitchell, S., Brown, H., Urraca, N., Romeo, D., Johnson, S., Salifu, M., Stewart, M., Vavagiakis, P., & Fraser, M. (2019). HIV prevention for Black heterosexual men: The barbershop talk with brothers cluster randomized trial. *American Journal of Public Health*, *10*(8), 1131–1137. https://doi.org/10.2105/AJPH.2019.305121

Wingood, G. M., & Diclemente, R. J. (1998). Gender-related correlates and predictors of consistent condom use among young adult African-American women: A prospective analysis. International Journal of STD & AIDS, 9(3),139–145. https://doi.org/10.1258/0956462981921891

Woods, G., Levinson, A. H., Jones, G., Kennedy, R. L., Johnson, L. C., Tran, Z. V., Gonzalez, T., & Marcus, A. C. (2013). The living well by faith health and wellness program for African Americans: An exemplar of community-based participatory research. *Ethnicity & Disease*, *23*(2), 223–229. Article ID 23530305

Yeh, M.-C., Heo, M., Suchday, S., Wong, A., Poon, E., Liu, G., & Wylie-Rosett, J. (2016). Translation of the diabetes prevention program for diabetes risk reduction in Chinese immigrants in New York City. *Diabetic Medicine: A Journal of the British Diabetic Association*, *33*(4), 547–551. https://doi.org/10.1111/dme.12848

Zoellner, J. M., Connell, C. C., Madson, M. B., Wang, B., Reed, V. B., Molaison, E. F., & Yadrick, K. (2011). HUB city steps: Methods and early findings from a community-based participatory research trial to reduce blood pressure among African Americans. *The International Journal of Behavioral Nutrition and Physical Activity*, *8*(1), 59. https://doi.org/10.1186/1479-5868-8-59

The Effect of an Entertainment-Education Intervention on Reproductive Health of Young Women of Color

Camille J. Saucier, Sapna Suresh, John J. Brooks, Nathan Walter, Aaron Plant, and Jorge A. Montoya

ABSTRACT

While teen pregnancy rates in the United States have been declining for decades, they remain the highest of all western countries. Within the U.S., Black and Latina teens experience disproportionate rates of unplanned pregnancy. *Plan A* is an entertainment-education video intervention that was developed to help address these disparities, in part by emphasizing the ability of young cisgender women to control when they become pregnant by using an effective contraception method. The intervention was developed in close collaboration with the target audience (Black and Latina women aged 18–19) to ensure that it was relevant, engaging, and motivational. We conducted an online study to: (a) investigate the effects of *Plan A* on attitudes toward the contraception methods covered in the video; (b) whether these effects varied by race/ethnicity or age, and; (c) if identification with characters in the video mediated these effects. The study used a posttest-only design where participants were randomly assigned to watch *Plan A* or to a neutral control condition. The sample included Black, Latina, and non-Latina White women aged 16 to 19 (N= 242), with younger and White women included for comparison purposes. Results indicated that exposure to *Plan A* significantly improved attitudes toward long-acting reversible contraceptives (LARCs) among all age groups and among young Black and Latina women, but not White women. These findings may be explained by participant's identification with the Black and Latina lead characters – both of whom model positive reproductive health behaviors.

Although overall pregnancy rates in the United States have declined since the 1990s, the adolescent pregnancy rate remains higher than in any other Western country as of the 2010 census (Sedgh et al., 2015). For adolescents, 75% of these pregnancies are unintended (Finer & Zolna, 2016). Notably, there are significant racial/ethnic disparities in birth rates, with Latina (26.7) and non-Latina Black (26.3) teens having birth rates twice as high per 1,000 females, as non-Latina White (henceforth referred to as White) teens (12.1) (Martin et al., 2019). These unintended pregnancies come at great personal cost to young mothers, as teen pregnancy can limit educational and professional achievement (Diaz & Fiel, 2016). Naturally, the risk of unplanned pregnancy increases as the rate of sexual intercourse rises and contraception usage falls. Comparing rates of sexual activity for U.S. teenagers, the data show little variance in the proportion of sexually active Latina, Black, and White female teens (Martinez & Abma, 2017). Thus, to understand why Black and Latina teens are disproportionately faced with unintended pregnancies, there is a need to look more carefully at gaps associated with contraception use.

Women's choice of contraception method is impacted by a range of factors. In addition to more conspicuous factors such as awareness, knowledge, and misperceptions regarding available methods (e.g., Barber et al., 2015; Jackson et al., 2016), the choice of contraception methods is associated with access to contraception (Cornet, 2013), attitudes toward healthcare providers (Kavanaugh et al., 2013), and racial/ethnic discrimination, which is negatively related to use of effective contraceptives (Kossler et al., 2011). A national study of women aged 18–19 found that Latina respondents reported less knowledge of available contraceptive options compared to White women (Craig et al., 2014). Targeted focus groups have also identified the existence of sexual health barriers such as inaccurate beliefs surrounding contraceptive side effects and correct usage among Black and Latinx teens (Galloway et al., 2017). These results indicate that a targeted intervention to improve the quality of information available to young women of color may go a long way in improving knowledge of effective contraceptives and, eventually, reducing disparities in unintended pregnancies.

A notable example of race-related disparities in contraception is related to Long-Acting Reversible Contraceptives (LARCs) including intrauterine devices (IUDs) and implants. LARCs, as an alternative to oral contraceptives and condoms, have the potential to dramatically reduce the incidence of unplanned pregnancies. Both etonogestrel implants and IUDs are safe and effective methods of contraception for adolescents that inherently offer significantly higher adherence rates compared to other contraceptive methods – and LARCs offer protection for 3–10 years, depending on the product (Usinger et al., 2016). Despite the potential benefits of these contraceptive methods, they continue to have low adoption rates among adolescents of all racial groups (Kumar & Brown, 2016). Adoption rates are especially low among Black (Dehlendorf et al., 2014) and Latina women (Rocca & Harper, 2012) compared to their White counterparts. These disparities were illustrated in a longitudinal study comparing sex and contraceptive use between White and Black women aged 18–19, suggesting that adolescent Black women were more likely to employ less effective contraceptive methods (e.g., condoms), compared to White women (Kusunoki et al., 2016). Given the misconceptions surrounding LARCs, our study focuses on mitigating the disparities in awareness of this contraceptive option.

Interventions that provide education and motivation to use effective contraception methods have shown promise in reducing unplanned teen pregnancies (Oringanje et al., 2016). To this end, an experimental design rooted in theories of entertainment-education and narrative persuasion (e.g., Bandura, 1986; Green & Brock, 2000) was employed to assess the impact of a culturally-tailored narrative intervention on attitudes toward LARCs among young Black and Latina women. The current research explores the attitudinal effects of *Plan A*, a narrative short video designed to provide information about contraceptive options such as LARCs, model positive behavior, and reduce unplanned pregnancies among 18–19-year-old Black and Latina cisgender women. The study also attempts to unpack factors that could facilitate learning and receptivity among the target audience.

Entertainment-education and health communication

An increasingly popular approach for addressing health disparities is *entertainment-education* (E-E), which utilizes entertainment media as a vehicle for prosocial messages (Singhal et al., 2003). Defined by Papa et al. (2000) as "media programs that intentionally incorporate one or more educational issues in an entertainment format in order to influence audience members' knowledge, attitudes, and overt behavior regarding an educational issue" (p. 32), E-E initiatives have proven effective in the domain of sexual and reproductive health around the globe (e.g., Sallar & Somda, 2011; Sypher et al., 2002). According to *social cognitive theory* (SCT), this is possible because humans can learn through both direct and vicarious experiences (Bandura, 2001a). In contrast to learning by doing, which requires significant time and effort to acquire and retain new knowledge, entertainment media can transmit a vast amount of information about social norms, behavior patterns, and contemporary lifestyles to geographically dispersed and/or isolated areas (Bandura, 2001b). By drawing on the symbolic modeling of people or characters seen on screen, individuals can acquire knowledge, adopt new behaviors, and enhance their own efficacy beliefs – all of which guide future decision-making (Bandura, 1986).

Though mass media is an ideal channel for wide-scale distribution of prosocial health behaviors, it is important to note that not all demonstrated behaviors are adopted by the audience. Rather, individuals must be sufficiently motivated to adopt a vicariously modeled action by weighing their outcome expectancies, or the positive and negative possibilities arising from their decision, in conjunction with their perceived ability to complete the same task (Bandura, 2001a). Naturally, one is motivated by the successes of others while adverse consequences usually deter imitation – and the ease with which the model accomplishes a task will increase one's self-efficacy beliefs (Bandura, 2001a).

In the context of contraceptive use, prior research has demonstrated that safer sex practices are more likely to be performed if a) the viewer perceives that the benefits associated with a preventive behavior outweigh the potential costs, and b) they judge that they can effectively do so, considering any social constraints (e.g., Futerfas & Nan, 2017; Walter et al., 2018). Thus, to acquire new behaviors, people often look to media exemplars who successfully navigate relevant tasks, such as talking with a partner about condom use or speaking to their health provider about long-term birth control options (Bandura, 1998). This type of vicarious learning is most effective when the viewer is emotionally and cognitively involved with the characters.

Character involvement is an umbrella term encompassing varied forms of relations with a character (e.g., identification, perceived similarity, and liking) that are distinguished by the depth of the perceived relationship between viewer and character as well as the extent to which the viewer becomes immersed in the character's experience (Moyer-Gusé, 2008). The most intimate form of character involvement, *identification*, describes a state wherein the viewer imagines becoming the character and shares the character's feelings, perspective, and motivations, allowing them to momentarily forget their role as an audience member (Cohen, 2001). As a result of this "psychological merging," the viewer is more likely to be emotionally and cognitively affected by a character's experience (Cohen, 2001).

To engage the audience and encourage identification with characters, an E-E intervention must present characters who demonstrate attractive qualities and possess key similarities with the viewers (Tal-Or & Cohen, 2016). In presenting characters that are both relatable and admirable, a narrative message can enhance its persuasive potential and encourage deeper involvement, which, in turn, is shown to enhance persuasion and encourage the adoption of story-consistent attitudes (Hoeken et al., 2016). Following this logic, identification with a character affords greater symbolic weight to the character's actions and their corresponding outcomes, which translates into adoption of story-consistent attitudes (Walter et al., 2017). As viewers connect with the characters, E-E capitalizes on the audience's involvement to positively influence viewers' knowledge, attitudes, beliefs, and behaviors (e.g., Murphy et al., 2011).

Notably, the theory of E-E has a considerable lineage of research that examines the impact of exposure to narratives on beliefs and behaviors associated with sexual and reproductive health. For instance, prior research has demonstrated how E-E interventions have encouraged dialogue about safe sex and one's sexual history (Moyer-Gusé et al., 2011), increased rates of cervical cancer screening (Baezconde-Garbanati et al., 2014), enhanced appraisals of condom efficacy (Collins et al., 2003), and promoted more favorable attitudes toward abortion (Mulligan & Habel, 2011).

This evidence suggests that even limited exposure to E-E content can influence a variety of cognitive and behavioral outcomes in a wide array of health contexts. The narrative intervention under study, *Plan A*, was designed in accordance with theories of E-E to improve the use of an effective contraception method, including dual contraception, as well as HIV/STI testing. Over the course of the narrative, four female friends help each other navigate sexual health challenges, including both the short- and long-term consequences of unplanned pregnancy. Two of the friends discuss contraception options with a physician, and explore the possibility of using a LARC method. One decides the IUD is the right method for her, because she is not ready to have another child. These narrative components should improve the audience's associated outcome expectancies, thereby encouraging more favorable attitudes toward LARCs. Accordingly, we propose the following hypothesis:

H1: Exposure to *Plan A* positively affects participants' attitudes toward LARCs (IUDs and implants).

Narrative persuasion interventions and racial disparities

While there is evidence to suggest that narratives can yield significant results in the context of health communication (Shen et al., 2015), not all health challenges or audiences are equally affected by narrative messages. In fact, there is a growing body of literature that points to narrative interventions as effective in serving minority populations (e.g., Unger et al., 2009). For example, a study by Murphy et al. (2013), comparing a narrative and a nonnarrative film intervention, found that a narrative featuring a Mexican-American family significantly improved both participants' posttest knowledge of cervical cancer and their attitudes toward getting a Pap test compared to the nonnarrative condition, especially among Mexican-American women compared to White women. These results have been corroborated by other studies, including an intervention in which an educational film narrative significantly increased Latinas' breast cancer knowledge and mammography self-efficacy (Borrayo et al., 2017). The film also improved behavioral norms regarding breast cancer screening from pretest to posttest, with the narrative intervention leading to greater feelings of self-efficacy among participants than among those in the non-narrative condition. Similar results have been demonstrated for Black women, utilizing a narrative video intervention developed to improve knowledge about breast cancer and increase preventive behaviors (Kreuter et al., 2010).

The success of these narrative interventions in mitigating race/ethnicity-based health disparities has, in part, been linked to cultural tailoring (Shen et al., 2015). Extant research suggests that culturally tailored, or culturally-appropriate, interventions that incorporate meaningful characteristics of the target audience into their health messages are more impactful than interventions which overlook these differences (e.g., Frank et al., 2015; Jensen et al., 2014). As indicated in a recent meta-analysis, meaningful cultural features include values, religious beliefs, and other social norms of a targeted ethnic/racial group as opposed to more superficial cultural features such as differences in language (Huang & Shen, 2016). In the context of *Plan A* and the intended 18- to 19-year-old minority female audience, cultural tailoring included developing relatable characters who encounter specific healthcare or relationship challenges exploring sexuality, values, and styles of interpersonal interaction that are unique to this audience. Given this specific tailoring efforts, we propose the following research questions:

RQ1: Are the effects of *Plan A* on attitudes toward LARCs (IUDs and implants) moderated by participants' race/ethnicity, such that Latina and Black women are more affected compared to White women?

RQ2: Are the effects of *Plan A* on attitudes toward LARCs (IUDs and implants) moderated by participants' age, such that older participants (18–19) are more affected compared to their younger (16–17) counterparts?

Lastly, based on the preceding empirical and theoretical rationales, as well as the nuanced tailoring of specific characters within the *Plan A* intervention, we propose a final research question:

RQ3: Are the effects of participants' race/ethnicity on attitudes toward LARCs (IUDs and implants) mediated by identification with the different characters, such that greater identification exerts more influence on attitudes?

The following section describes the formative research that was conducted to develop *Plan A*, as well as the efforts made to tailor the video to the audience of interest: Black and Latina women aged 18 to 19.

Study context: *Plan A* and formative research

In order to produce *Plan A* (see appendix for a synopsis), the project team conducted several types of formative research, including a literature review around sexual health disparities, focus groups with the population-of-interest, a clinical provider survey, and ongoing feedback collection from a review panel. First, the systematic literature review informed the video's messaging as well as the characters' modeled behaviors. The review focused on barriers and facilitators to preventing unplanned pregnancies and STIs among the target audience. Identified barriers included: incomplete knowledge or misperceptions about effective contraception methods; low use of dual contraception; difficulties with condom negotiation; low perceived risk for pregnancy; fatalistic attitudes about pregnancy; low perceived risk for STIs; and low rates of STI testing.

Second, our team worked closely with the target population to obtain input on *Plan A*, conducting three focus groups with reproductive health clients in October 2015. The first focus group met in Philadelphia with Black women aged 18–19 in English (n = 15). Two additional groups were recruited in Fresno with 18–19-year-old Latina participants. Of these two focus group studies, one was conducted in English (n = 15) and the other in Spanish (n = 11). During these focus groups, the moderator focused the discussion on video format and content along with knowledge, attitudes, and behaviors regarding pregnancy, contraception methods, emergency contraception, STIs, and patient-provider communication.

Next, an online survey of clinicians and health program managers ($n = 8$) at two clinics in Fresno and Philadelphia, respectively, identified recommendations which were incorporated into the *Plan A* narrative. Suggestions for the video included: empowering adolescent women to develop contraception plans, dispelling erroneous contraceptive beliefs, providing additional information on contraception methods, modeling healthy sexual relationships and condom negotiation, encouraging patients to be open with providers, and portraying the patient-provider relationship as a partnership. The video script was also reviewed by a reproductive health clinician for accuracy.

Lastly, a nine-person review panel consisting of target population members from Los Angeles and Philadelphia was assembled to provide regular feedback on the script and other program elements throughout video production. Feedback from the review panel with respect to the video content echoed that of the focus groups (e.g., inclusion of diverse characters, use of humor, high production value, and inclusion of realistic, relatable characters). The end-product resulted in a culturally tailored intervention designed to improve patient-provider communication around reproductive health as well as increase the use of effective contraception and STI testing among Black and Latina women aged 18 to 19 (for more information about the development of Plan A, see Plant et al., 2019).

Method

Design and participants

The experimental portion of the project was approved by the Institutional Review Board at the University of Southern California (Study number: UP-17-00807). The experiment used a posttest-only design where participants were randomly assigned to watch a 23-minute video (*Plan A*) or to a no-message control condition. Two hundred fifty-six self-identified female participants (16–19 years old) were recruited from Qualtrics and consented to participate in a "women's health study."[1] The data of 14 participants were excluded from further analyses because they turned in incomplete surveys or the time elapsed measurement indicated that they had not watched the video, reducing the effective sample size to 242 ($M_{age} = 17.93$, $SD = 0.96$).

As online panel members tend to be skewed toward particular demographic attributes, we used quotas for race/ethnicity to ensure sufficient representation for Black (76, 31.4%) and Latina women (94, 38.8%), as well as White women (72, 29.8%). The majority of participants reported having health coverage (146, 60.6%), and the median combined annual household income ranged from 40 USDk to 50 USDk. Sixty-three percent (151) of participants had at most a high school education, and the remainder had some college education. In terms of relationship status, 106 (44.0%) women indicated that they were in a long-term relationship, 72 (29.9%) were not in any relationship, 44 (18.3%) were in a casual relationship, and 19 (7.8%) were either married, engaged, or cohabiting.

Material

The narrative intervention, *Plan A*, consists of three vignettes that are separated by two brief, animated (< 60 second) health messages: the first message provides information about IUDs while the other informs viewers about contraceptive implants. The vignettes follow four friends named Eva, Michelle, Chela, and Nicole. Eva is a young Latina woman who has just moved into a new apartment with her boyfriend, Rick. Michelle, a young Black woman, is a single mother working to support her young daughter. Chela is exploring her sexuality with both men and women, while also dealing with her conservative Mexican family's expectations. Nicole, who is Black, is a pre-medical student with a part-time job at a pharmacy and a long-term boyfriend. To encourage stronger identification with the characters among the target audience, the characters were designed to reflect the lived experiences of the focus group and review panel participants. In the tradition of E-E (Singhal et al., 2003), the video uses these characters to model the positive and negative outcomes of intervention-relevant behaviors (e.g., having sex without a condom leads to an STI; using dual contraception helps people relax and enjoy sex; being open and honest with health providers helps identify an appropriate, effective contraception option). It also uses their dialogue to provide information about reproductive health and dispel misconceptions around contraception methods.

Measures

Attitudes toward LARCs

The attitudinal measures consisted of scales designed to measure participants' perceptions of LARCs. Adapted from Murphy et al. (2013), attitudes toward IUDs and attitudes toward implants were assessed with two separate scales. Each scale included seven items (e.g., the contraceptive method is "safe," "relatively inexpensive," and "very effective") ranged from (1) "completely disagree" to (7) "completely agree." The attitudes toward IUDs ($M = 3.99$, $SD = 1.28$, $\alpha = .87$) and implants ($M = 3.80$, $SD = 1.35$, $\alpha = .89$) scales had high reliability. In both cases, higher scores indicated a more favorable attitude toward the contraceptive.

Identification with characters

Based on previous measures of relative identification with multiple characters (e.g., Murphy et al., 2013), viewers of the *Plan A* video were asked the extent to which they identified with each of the four main characters. For each character, three core components of identification were assessed on a seven-point scale from (1) "not at all" to (7) "a great deal." The specific components included liking ("How much did you like X?"), familiarity ("How much do you feel like you know X?"), and similarity ("How similar are you to X?"). In these questions, each character was identified by name (e.g., "Nicole"), role (e.g., "the girl who works at a pharmacy"), and picture. The reliabilities of identification with Nicole ($M = 4.08$, $SD = 1.51$, $\alpha = .82$), Chela ($M = 3.97$, $SD = 1.53$, $\alpha = .85$), Michelle ($M = 3.95$, $SD = 1.48$, $\alpha = .80$), and Eva ($M = 3.89$, $SD = 1.59$, $\alpha = .82$) were satisfactory.[2]

Results

The first part of the results section reports on the main effect of exposure to *Plan A* followed by the role played by participants' race/ethnicity and age in moderating the observed effects. The results section concludes by examining whether the level of identification between *Plan A*'s characters and participants mediates the effects of the intervention on message-consistent attitudes.

To test H1 and RQ1, a two-way MANOVA was conducted, with the experimental condition (*Plan A*/control) and participant's race/ethnicity (Black/Latina/White) as independent variables, and attitudes toward IUDs and attitudes toward implants as dependent variables. In line with H1, the analysis revealed a significant multivariate effect of exposure to *Plan A* on research outcomes; Wilk's λ = .95, $F(2, 233) = 6.28$, $p = .002$, $\eta_p^2 = .05$. Further, the univariate analysis revealed that exposure to *Plan A* was positively associated with attitudes toward IUDs; $F(1, 239) = 12.61$, $p < .001$; and attitudes toward implants; $F(1, 239) = 4.95$, $p = .027$. In particular, after exposure to *Plan A*, on average, participants tended to report more favorable attitudes toward IUDs (M= 4.27, SD = 1.32) and attitudes toward implants (M= 3.99, SD = 1.42), compared to their counterparts in the no-video control condition (M_{IUD} = 3.71, SD_{IUD} = 1.17; $M_{Implant}$ = 3.61, $SD_{Implant}$ = 1.26). Thus, H1 was supported.

The same MANOVA model was used to test the potential moderation of participants' race/ethnicity (RQ1). The model retrieved a significant multivariate interaction between experimental condition and participants' race/ethnicity; Wilk's λ = .97, $F(4, 466) = 3.82$, $p = .023$, $\eta_p^2 = .03$. Likewise, the univariate analysis identified a significant moderation of race/ethnicity on attitudes toward IUDs; $F(2, 239) = 3.13$, $p = .043$; and attitudes toward implants; $F(2, 239) = 3.12$, $p = .046$. As illustrated in Figures 1, 2, White women (M= 4.30, SD = 1.31) tended to report more favorable attitudes toward IUDs and implants in the control condition compared to Latina (M= 3.58, SD = 0.98) and Black women (M= 3.24, SD = 0.97). However, the differences between White women (M= 4.30, SD = 1.11), Latina women (M= 4.28, SD = 1.43), and Black women (M= 4.22, SD = 1.37) were nonsignificant among participants who were exposed to *Plan A*. Consequently, with regard to RQ1, race/ethnicity was a significant moderator of attitudes toward LARCs.

To address the potential moderating role played by participants' age (RQ2), we used Model 1 in PROCESS (Hayes, 2018; 20,000 bootstrapped samples). Specifically, the PROCESS model treated the experimental condition (*Plan A*/control) as a predictor of research outcomes, with participants' age as a continuous moderator. Notably, the analysis failed to support age as a moderator of narrative effects for attitudes toward IUDs; b = .25, SE = .17, p = .13, 95% CI [−.08, .59], ΔR^2 = .009 and attitudes toward implants; b = −.00, SE = .18, p = .99, 95% CI [−.36, .36], ΔR^2 = .000. Thus, with respect to RQ2, the intervention was equally successful among its target population (ages 18–19) as well as younger individuals (ages 16–17).

Finally, to test the role played by identification in explaining the observed effects of *Plan A* (RQ3), we utilized a parallel mediation model (Hayes, 2018; PROCESS model 4; 20,000 bootstrapped samples). As depicted in Figure 3, Latina women were more likely to identify with Eva; b = 1.11, SE = .37, p = .003, 95% CI [.38, 1.83], whereas Black women were more likely to identify with Michelle; b = .82, SE = .37, p = .026, 95% CI [.10, 1.54]. In turn, identification with Eva and identification with Michelle were significant predictors of attitudes toward IUDs; b_{Eva} = .33, SE = .07, p = .0005, 95% CI [.19, .48]; b_{Michelle} = .21, SE = .08, p = .015, 95% CI [.04, .37]; and attitudes toward implants;; b_{Eva} = .26, SE = .08, p = .002, 95% CI [.10, .42]; b_{Michelle} = .24, SE = .09, p = .014, 95% CI [.05, .43]. In addition, the models also identified indirect effects of race/ethnicity on attitudes toward IUDs and attitudes toward implants through identification with Eva (b_{IUD} = .37, SE = .16, 95% CI [.11, .72]; b_{implant} = .28, SE = .14, 95% CI [.05, .58]) and Michelle (b_{IUD} = .17, SE = .10, 95% CI [.01, .44]; b_{implant} = .18, SE = .11, 95% CI [.01, .46]). Notably, as indicated in Figure 3, all other direct and indirect effects were

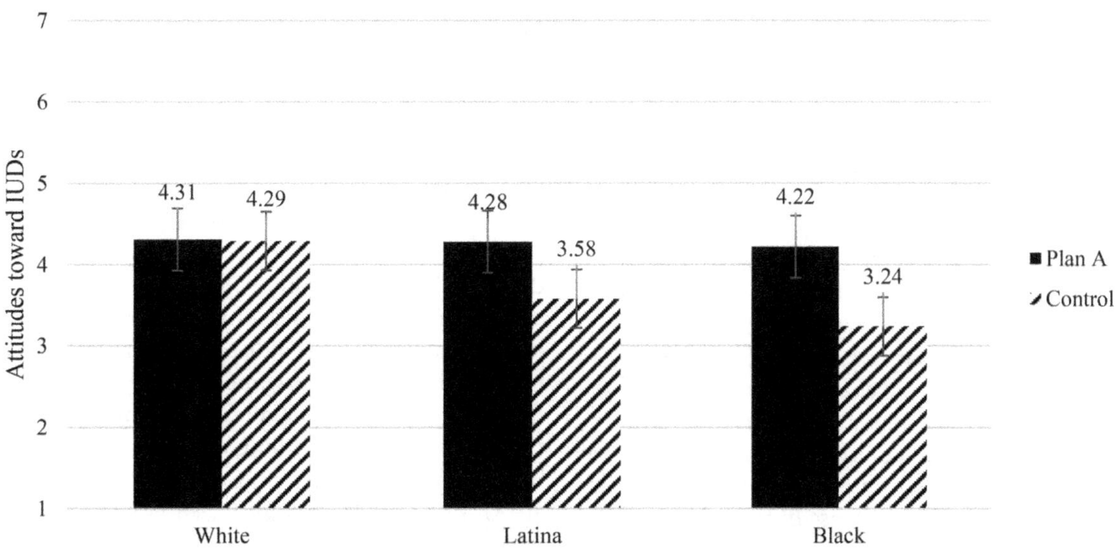

Figure 1. Means (and 95% CIs) for attitudes toward IUDs by experimental condition and participants' race/ethnicity.

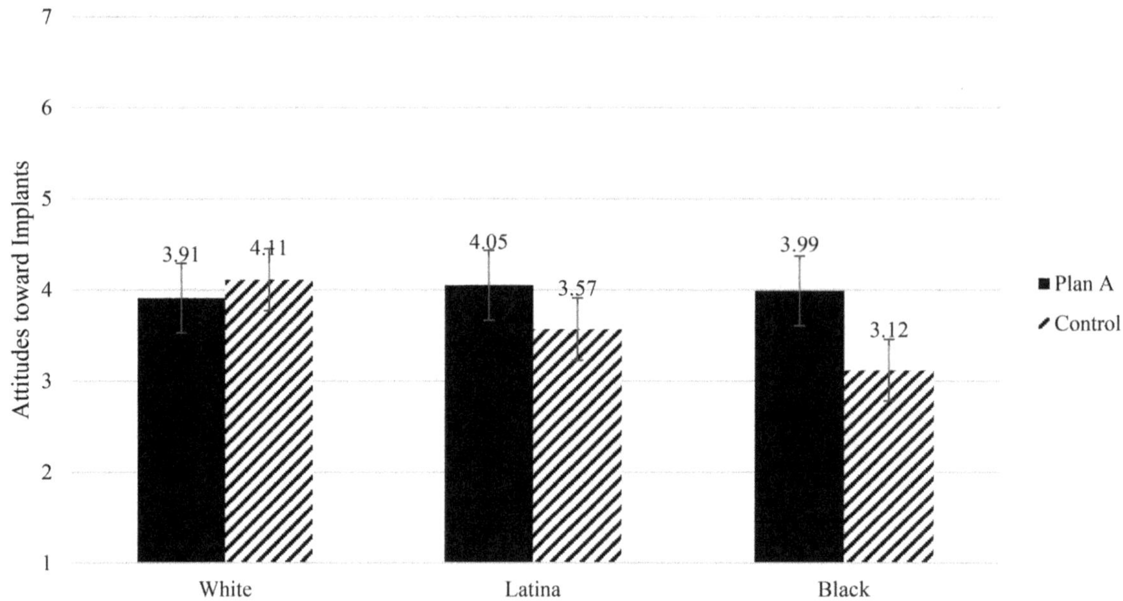

Figure 2. Means (and 95% CIs) for attitudes toward implants by experimental condition and participants' race/ethnicity.

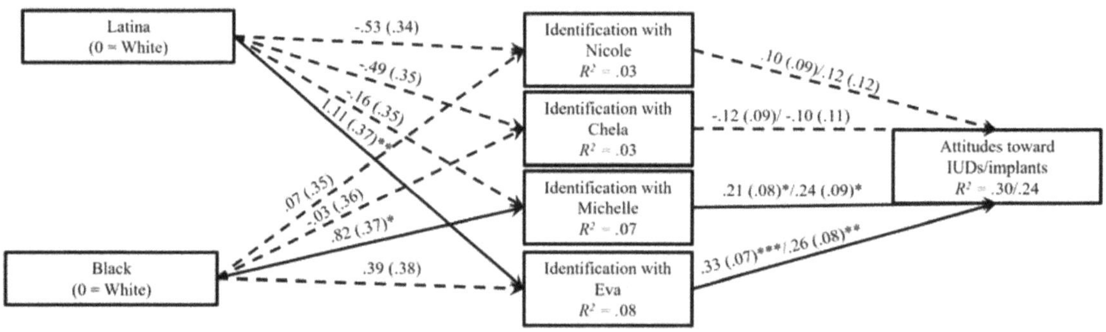

Figure 3. Unstandardized direct coefficient (and SEs) for the effects of race/ethnicity on identification with Plan A characters and attitudes toward IUDs/implants. * < .05, ** < .01, *** < .001. Dashed line indicated nonsignificant predictors and solid line represents significant predictors. Where two coefficients appear on the same line, the first represents an effect on attitudes toward IUDs and the second represents an effect on attitudes toward implants.

nonsignificant. Hence, there was only partial support for identification with characters as a mediator (RQ3).

Discussion

This study sought to identify the impact of a narrative short video tailored to young cisgender women of color on attitudes toward IUDs and implants, also known as LARCs. *Plan A*, a brief E-E intervention, endeavored to reduce unplanned pregnancies and encourage conversations about reproductive health, by emphasizing the benefits of effective contraception methods, including LARCs. Although traditional approaches to reproductive health campaigns often rely on didactic messages, *Plan A* instead communicates this information in an entertaining drama with relatable characters.

Our study investigated the impact of *Plan A* on attitudes toward LARCs. The results of our study showed support for H1, as exposure to *Plan A* significantly improved attitudes toward IUDs and implants. The increase in favorable attitudes after exposure to the E-E message presumably suggests that the audience paid attention to the information regarding the efficacy and suitability of LARCs – likely as a result of the positive outcomes modeled by relatable characters. Michelle, the young Black woman who chooses an IUD, highlights how liberated she feels because of the LARC – she already has a young daughter and is not ready for another child at this stage in her life. For Chela, the implant is explored with her doctor as a method that might be right for her, given that she reports challenges with remembering to take birth control pills.

With regard to RQ1, the results retrieved an encouraging pattern, as the effects of exposure to *Plan A* attenuated the disparity between White women, who showed a more favorable attitude toward LARCs in the control condition, and Black and Latina women, who displayed a nonsignificant difference in attitudes with White women after exposure to *Plan A*. These findings echo previous studies that demonstrated the efficacy of narratives in reducing differences in health-related attitudes between White women and women of color (Murphy et al., 2015). As with H1, this increased favorability is likely due to the characters in the narrative – because these young women of color were written to reflect the lived experience of members of the target population, it is natural that the audience might feel involved with the characters. This involvement would likely affect women of color more than their White counterparts.

Notably, the analysis did not support RQ2. Although *Plan A* was tailored to women aged 18 to 19, attitudes of participants in the 16 to 17 group were equally affected by exposure to the narrative. This is an encouraging finding as it suggests that the message resonates among younger audiences who may not yet consider using LARCs but can be informed about the benefits and availabilities of these contraceptive methods. That said, because the young women in the video are portrayed as only slightly older than the youngest participants in the study, participants' may have perceived them to be peers.

With regard to RQ3, the analyses only partially supported the role played by identification with story characters. Specifically, the effects of race/ethnicity on attitudes toward IUDs and implants were significantly mediated through identification with Eva and Michelle, but not Chela and Nicole. Although the role of identification with characters is well-established within the E-E literature (Bandura, 2004; Moyer-Gusé & Nabi, 2011; Murphy et al., 2013), this study suggests that the inclination to pay attention to and to form positive attitudes toward behaviors modeled by others was dependent on matching race/ethnicity between the viewer and the character. While both Black and Latina women benefited from exposure to the video, the underlying mechanism of narrative persuasion for these racial groups was different. Specifically, Black participants tended to identify with Michelle, a Black character, who models positive behavior by visiting a doctor and choosing a non-hormonal IUD. In turn, Michelle's decision to get an IUD benefits her romantic relationship by making her feel both safe and less inhibited. Latina participants, on the other hand, tended to identify with Eva, a Latina character, who initially models negative behavior by engaging in unprotected sex and contracting chlamydia from her boyfriend. However, she changes her behavior for the better after an informative discussion with her doctor about STI prevention.

Speculatively, the fact that participants identified more with Eva and Michelle than with Chela and Nicole, can be explained by differences in the representation of these characters. Eva and Michelle were the main protagonists in *Plan A* whereas Chela and Nicole played an important, albeit peripheral, role by providing positive and negative reinforcement for Eva and Michelle's decision-making throughout the film. According to this logic, people will be more likely to identify with the main characters and less likely to adopt the perspective of supportive characters. Alternatively, this gap can also be attributed to other features of the E-E intervention or the audience. Without a more careful analysis of identification and the audience's experience, however, it is difficult to know why some characters were more successful than others in modeling positive behavior and ultimately influencing message-consistent attitudes.

These results demonstrate the potential for E-E interventions to positively impact sexual health outcomes for Black and Latina adolescent women by helping to attenuate potential gaps in contraception perceptions. Although teens can be a notoriously difficult audience to persuade given their greater propensity for persuasive message reactance, narrative content appears to present a means to overcome this resistance (Moyer-Gusé & Nabi, 2010).

Limitations

Notwithstanding the aforementioned contributions, the current study has several limitations. A more controlled research design would have allowed us to make assertive claims about the impact of the intervention. In particular, the fact the experimental design did not include a pretest of participants' knowledge and beliefs regarding LARCs at baseline limits our ability to demonstrate a causal within-participants effect of exposure to *Plan A*. In choosing a posttest only design, we wanted to avoid alerting the participants to the topic of reproductive health prior to their exposure to *Plan A* (for a discussion of pretest effects, see Campbell & Stanley, 1963). After all, E-E programs are presumed to be effective because their persuasive intent is less pronounced than didactic, non-narrative messages (Moyer-Gusé, 2008). Given that exposure to *Plan A* was compared only to a neutral control condition, it is difficult to know whether *Plan A* is responsible for the retrieved effects or simply exposure to any type of intervention. With that in mind, however, it is important to note that the central purpose of the study was to assess whether *Plan A* could benefit young Black and Latina women. To this end, it is especially encouraging to see that the intervention had a more substantial effect on its target population – women of color – compared to White women, even within the same experimental condition. Relatedly, since the current study focused exclusively on short-term effects and self-report measures, it is unclear whether the observed effects would persist over a longer period and motivate a behavioral change. Optimistically, there is evidence to suggest that narrative interventions demonstrate their full potential when testing long-term effects and measuring actual behavior (Murphy et al., 2013; Oschatz & Marker, 2020). Yet, it remains to be seen whether this encouraging finding can also apply to the current intervention.

While much remains to be understood about the potential of narratives to mitigate disparities in reproductive health, the study showed significant support for the proposition that E-E can be effectively used in interventions designed for racial/ethnic minorities. The challenge for those working to address health disparities is how to best leverage narratives to make them both engaging and motivational. This study indicates that taking a highly collaborative approach with the intended audience can result in a promising E-E intervention.

Notes

1. The specific item was "Which of the following terms best describes your gender identity?" and the response options were "female," "male," and "other (with a textbox)." Respondents who chose "Male" were screened out. In addition, the questionnaire also assessed people's sexual orientation ("What best describes your sexual orientation?"). The majority or the sample self-identified as "heterosexual (60.7%)," followed by "bisexual (19.6%)," and "lesbian (5.4%)." Importantly, when responding to the sexual orientation item, 14.3% of the sample chose "Other" or "Prefer not to say."

2. Given the fact that identification has to be assessed separately for each of the four leading characters, we decided to use a shorter version of the identification scale (Murphy et al., 2013) rather than the complete 9-item version (Cohen, 2001).

Funding

The project described was supported by Grant Number TP2AH000036 from the HHS Office of Population Affairs. Contents are solely the responsibility of the authors and do not represent the official views of the Department of Health and Human Services or the Office of Population Affairs.

ORCID

Camille J. Saucier http://orcid.org/0000-0002-0408-2782
Nathan Walter http://orcid.org/0000-0002-8122-1221

References

Baezconde-Garbanati, L. A., Chatterjee, J. S., Frank, L. B., Murphy, S. T., Moran, M. B., Werth, L. N., Zhao, N., De Herrera, P. A., Mayer, D., Kagan, J., & O'Brien, D. (2014). Tamale Lesson: A case study of a narrative health communication intervention. *Journal of Communication in Healthcare*, *7*(2), 82–92. https://doi.org/10.1179/1753807614Y.0000000055

Bandura, A. (1986). The explanatory and predictive scope of self-efficacy theory. *Journal of Social and Clinical Psychology*, *4*(3), 359–373. https://doi.org/10.1521/jscp.1986.4.3.359

Bandura, A. (1998). Health promotion from the perspective of social cognitive theory. *Psychology and Health*, *13*(4), 623–649. https://doi.org/10.1080/08870449808407422

Bandura, A. (2001a). Social cognitive theory of mass communication. *Media Psychology*, *3*(3), 265–299. https://doi.org/10.1207/S1532785XMEP0303_03

Bandura, A. (2001b). Social cognitive theory: An agentic perspective. *Annual Review of Psychology*, *52*(1), 1–26. https://doi.org/10.1146/annurev.psych.52.1.1

Bandura, A. (2004). Health promotion by social cognitive means. *Health Education and Behavior*, *31*(2), 143–164. https://doi.org/10.1177/1090198104263660

Barber, J. S., Yarger, J. E., & Gatny, H. H. (2015). Black-White differences in attitudes related to pregnancy among young women. *Demography*, *52*(3), 751–786. https://doi.org/10.1007/s13524-015-0391-4

Borrayo, E. A., Rosales, M., & Gonzalez, P. (2017). Entertainment-Education narrative versus nonnarrative interventions to educate and motivate Latinas to engage in mammography screening. *Health Education and Behavior*, *44*(3), 394–402. https://doi.org/10.1177/1090198116665624

Campbell, D. T., & Stanley, J. C. (1963). *Experimental and quasi-experimental designs for research*. Rand McNally.

Cohen, J. (2001). Defining identification: A theoretical look at the identification of audiences with media characters. *Mass Communication and Society*, *4*(3), 245–264. https://doi.org/10.1207/S15327825MCS0403_01

Collins, R. L., Elliott, M. N., Berry, S. H., Kanouse, D. E., & Hunter, S. B. (2003). Entertainment television as a healthy sex educator: The impact of condom-efficacy information in an episode of friends. *Pediatrics*, *112*(5), 1115–1121. https://doi.org/10.1542/peds.112.5.1115

Cornet, A. (2013). Current challenges in contraception in adolescents and young women. *Current Opinion in Obstetrics and Gynecology*, *25*, 1–10. https://doi.org/10.1097/GCO.0b013e32835e06fd

Craig, A. D., Dehlendorf, C., Borrero, S., Harper, C. C., & Rocca, C. H. (2014). Exploring young adults' contraceptive knowledge and attitudes: Disparities by race/ethnicity and age. *Women's Health Issues*, *24*(3), 281–289. https://doi.org/10.1016/j.whi.2014.02.003

Dehlendorf, C., Park, S. Y., Emeremni, C. A., Comer, D., Vincett, K., & Borrero, S. (2014). Racial/ethnic disparities in contraceptive use: Variation by age and women's reproductive experiences. *American Journal of Obstetrics and Gynecology*, *210*(6), 526–531. https://doi.org/10.1016/j.ajog.2014.01.037

Diaz, C. J., & Fiel, J. E. (2016). The effect(s) of teen pregnancy: Reconciling theory, methods, and findings. *Demography*, *53*(1), 85–116. https://doi.org/10.1007/s13524-015-0446-6

Finer, L. B., & Zolna, M. R. (2016). Declines in unintended pregnancy in the United States, 2008-2011. *New England Journal of Medicine*, *374*(9), 843–852. https://doi.org/10.1056/NEJMsa1506575

Frank, L. B., Murphy, S. T., Chatterjee, J. S., Moran, M. B., & Baezconde-Garbanati, L. (2015). Telling stories, saving lives: Creating narrative health messages. *Health Communication*, *30*(2), 154–163. https://doi.org/10.1080/10410236.2014.974126

Futerfas, M. L., & Nan, X. (2017). Role of humor in the persuasiveness of entertainment narratives on unprotected sexual behavior. *Journal of Health Communication*, *22*(4), 312–318. https://doi.org/10.1080/10810730.2017.1284285

Galloway, C. T., Duffy, J. L., Dixon, R. P., & Fuller, T. R. (2017). Exploring African-American and Latino teens' perceptions of contraception and access to reproductive health care services. *Journal of Adolescent Health*, *60*(3), 57–62. https://doi.org/10.1016/j.jadohealth.2016.12.006

Green, M. C., & Brock, T. C. (2000). The role of transportation in the persuasiveness of public narratives. *Journal of Personality and Social Psychology*, *79*(5), 701–721. https://doi.org/10.1037/0022-3514.79.5.701

Hayes, A. F. (2018). *Introduction to mediation, moderation, and conditional process analysis: A regression-based approach* (2nd ed.). Guilford Publications.

Hoeken, H., Kolthoff, M., & Sanders, J. (2016). Story perspective and character similarity as drivers of identification and narrative persuasion. *Human Communication Research*, *42*(2), 292–311. https://doi.org/10.1111/hcre.12076

Huang, Y., & Shen, F. (2016). Effects of cultural tailoring on persuasion in cancer communication: A meta-analysis. *Journal of Communication*, *66*(4), 694–715. https://doi.org/10.1111/jcom.12243

Jackson, A. V., Karasek, D., Dehlendorf, C., & Foster, D. G. (2016). Racial and ethnic differences in women's preferences for features of contraceptive methods. *Contraception*, *93*(5), 406–411. https://doi.org/10.1016/j.contraception.2015.12.010

Jensen, J. D., King, A. J., Carcioppolo, N., Krakow, M., Samadder, N. J., & Morgan, S. (2014). Comparing tailored and narrative worksite interventions at increasing colonoscopy adherence in adults 50-75: A randomized controlled trial. *Social Science and Medicine*, *104*, 31–40. https://doi.org/10.1016/j.socscimed.2013.12.003

Kavanaugh, M. L., Frohwirth, L., Jerman, J., Popkin, R., & Ethier, K. (2013). Long-acting reversible contraception for adolescents and young adults: Patient and provider perspectives. *Journal of Pediatric and Adolescent Gynecology*, *26*(2), 86–95. https://doi.org/10.1016/j.jpag.2012.10.006

Kossler, K., Kuroki, L. M., Allsworth, J. E., Secura, G. M., Roehl, K. A., & Peipert, J. F. (2011). Perceived racial, socioeconomic and gender discrimination and its impact on contraceptive choice. *Contraception*, *84*(3), 273–279. https://doi.org/10.1016/j.contraception.2011.01.004

Kreuter, M. W., Holmes, K., Alcaraz, K., Kalesan, B., Rath, S., Richert, M., McQueen, A., Caito, N., Robinson, L., & Clark, E. M. (2010). Comparing narrative and informational videos to increase mammography in low-income African American women. *Patient Education and Counseling*, *81*, 6–14. https://doi.org/10.1016/j.pec.2010.09.008

Kumar, N., & Brown, J. D. (2016). Access barriers to long-acting reversible contraceptives for adolescents. *Journal of Adolescent Health*, *59*(3), 248–253. https://doi.org/10.1016/j.jadohealth.2016.03.039

Kusunoki, Y., Barber, J. S., Ela, E. J., & Bucek, A. (2016). Black-White differences in sex and contraceptive use among young women. *Demography*, *53*(5), 1399–1428. https://doi.org/10.1007/s13524-016-0507-5

Martin, J. A., Hamilton, B. E., & Osterman, M. J. K. (2019). Births in the United States, 2018. *NCHS Data Brief No. 346*, 1–8. https://www.cdc.gov/nchs/data/databriefs/db346-h.pdf

Martinez, G. M., & Abma, J. C. (2017). Sexual activity and contraceptive use among teenagers aged 15–19 in the United States, 2015–2017.

NCHS Data Brief No. 366, 1–8. https://www.cdc.gov/nchs/data/databriefs/db366-h.pdf
Moyer-Gusé, E. (2008). Toward a theory of entertainment persuasion: Explaining the persuasive effects of entertainment-education messages. *Communication Theory*, *18*(3), 407–425. https://doi.org/10.1111/j.1468-2885.2008.00328.x
Moyer-Gusé, E., Chung, A. H., & Jain, P. (2011). Identification with characters and discussion of taboo topics after exposure to an entertainment narrative about sexual health. *Journal of Communication*, *61* (3), 387–406. https://doi.org/10.1111/j.1460-2466.2011.01551.x
Moyer-Gusé, E., & Nabi, R. L. (2010). Explaining the effects of narrative in an entertainment television program: Overcoming resistance to persuasion. *Human Communication Research*, *36*(1), 26–52. https://doi.org/10.1111/j.1468-2958.2009.01367.x
Moyer-Gusé, E., & Nabi, R. L. (2011). Comparing the effects of entertainment and educational television programming on risky sexual behavior. *Health Communication*, *26*(5), 416–426. https://doi.org/10.1080/10410236.2011.552481
Mulligan, K., & Habel, P. (2011). An experimental test of the effects of fictional framing on attitudes. *Social Science Quarterly*, *92*(1), 79–99. https://doi.org/10.1111/j.1540-6237.2011.00758.x
Murphy, S. T., Frank, L. B., Chatterjee, J. S., & Baezconde-Garbanati, L. (2013). Narrative versus nonnarrative: The role of identification, transportation, and emotion in reducing health disparities. *Journal of Communication*, *63*(1), 116–137. https://doi.org/10.1111/jcom.12007
Murphy, S. T., Frank, L. B., Chatterjee, J. S., Moran, M. B., Zhao, N., De Herrera, A., & Baezconde-Garbanati, L. A. (2015). Comparing the relative efficacy of narrative vs nonnarrative health messages in reducing health disparities using a randomized trial. *American Journal of Public Health*, *105*(10), 2117–2123. https://doi.org/10.2105/AJPH.2014.302332
Murphy, S. T., Frank, L. B., Moran, M. B., & Patnoe-Woodley, P. (2011). Involved, transported, or emotional? Exploring the determinants of change in knowledge, attitudes, and behavior in entertainment-education. *Journal of Communication*, *61*(3), 407–431. https://doi.org/10.1111/j.1460-2466.2011.01554.x
Oringanje, C., Meremikwu, M. M., Eko, H., Esu, E., Meremikwu, A., & Ehiri, J. E. (2016). Interventions for preventing unintended pregnancies among adolescents. *Cochrane Database of Systematic Reviews*, *2*, 1–103. https://doi.org/10.1002/14651858.CD005215.pub3
Oschatz, C., & Marker, C. (2020). Long-term persuasive effects in narrative communication research: A meta-analysis. *Journal of Communication*, *70* (4), 473–496. https://doi.org/10.1093/joc/jqaa017
Papa, M. J., Singhal, A., Law, S., Pant, S., Sood, S., Rogers, E. M., & Shefner-Rogers, C. L. (2000). Entertainment-education and social change: An analysis of parasocial interaction, social learning, collective efficacy, and paradoxical communication. *Journal of Communication*, *50*(4), 31–55. https://doi.org/10.1111/j.1460-2466.2000.tb02862.x
Plant, A., Montoya, J. A., Snow, E. G., Coyle, K., & Rietmeijer, C. (2019). Developing a video intervention to prevent unplanned pregnancies and sexually transmitted infections among older adolescents. *Health Promotion Practice*, *20*(4), 593–599. https://doi.org/10.1177/1524839918778832
Rocca, C. H., & Harper, C. C. (2012). Do racial and ethnic differences in contraceptive attitudes and knowledge explain disparities in method use? *Perspectives on Sexual and Reproductive Health*, *44*(3), 150–158. https://doi.org/10.1363/4415012
Sallar, A. M., & Somda, D. A. K. (2011). Homosexuality and HIV in Africa: An essay on using entertainment education as a vehicle for stigma reduction. *Sexuality & Culture*, *15*(3), 279–309. https://doi.org/10.1007/s12119-011-9094-1
Sedgh, G., Finer, L. B., Bankole, A., Eilers, M. A., & Singh, S. (2015). Adolescent pregnancy, birth, and abortion rates across countries: Levels and recent trends. *Journal of Adolescent Health*, *56*(2), 223–230. https://doi.org/10.1016/j.jadohealth.2014.09.007
Shen, F., Sheer, V. C., & Li, R. (2015). Impact of narratives on persuasion in health communication: A meta-analysis. *Journal of Advertising*, *44*(2), 105–113. https://doi.org/10.1080/00913367.2015.1018467
Singhal, A., Cody, M. J., Rogers, E. M., & Sabido, M. (Eds.). (2003). *Entertainment-education and social change: History, research, and practice*. Routledge.
Sypher, B. D., McKinley, M., Ventsam, S., & Valdeavellano, E. E. (2002). Fostering reproductive health through entertainment-education in the Peruvian Amazon: The social construction of Bienvenida Salud! *Communication Theory*, *12*(2), 192–205. https://doi.org/10.1111/j.1468-2885.2002.tb00266.x
Tal-Or, N., & Cohen, J. (2016). Unpacking engagement: Convergence and divergence in transportation and identification. *Annals of the International Communication Association*, *40*(1), 33–66. https://doi.org/10.1080/23808985.2015.11735255
Unger, J. B., Molina, G. B., & Baron, M. (2009). Evaluation of Sweet Temptations, a fotonovela for diabetes education. *Hispanic Health Care International*, *7*(3), 145–152. https://doi.org/10.1891/1540-4153.7.3.145
Usinger, K. M., Gola, S. B., Weis, M., & Smaldone, A. (2016). Intrauterine contraception continuation in adolescents and young women: A systematic review. *Journal of Pediatric and Adolescent Gynecology*, *29*(6), 659–667. https://doi.org/10.1016/j.jpag.2016.06.007
Walter, N., Murphy, S. T., Frank, L. B., & Baezconde-Garbanati, L. (2017). Who cares what others think? The role of Latinas' acculturation in the processing of HPV vaccination narrative messages. *International Journal of Communication*, *11*, 4946–4964. https://ijoc.org/index.php/ijoc/article/view/6395/2206
Walter, N., Murphy, S. T., & Rosenthal, E. L. (2018). Narrative persuasion in a new media environment: The impact of binge-watching and second-screening. *Communication Research Reports*, *35*(5), 402–412. https://doi.org/10.1080/08824096.2018.1525348

Appendix Synopsis of *Plan A*

The first vignette opens with Eva, Chela, and Nicole helping Eva unpack her new apartment when Chela discovers condoms in one of the boxes – and Eva reveals that she has reunited with her ex-boyfriend Rick and that he will be moving in with her. As he walks in the front door, the girls depart, and Eva and Rick retire to the bedroom to celebrate their new place. However, despite Eva's repeated request that he wear a condom, Rick tries to negotiate his way out of it by imploring her to trust him, reminding her that she's using birth pills, and complaining about how condoms feel before she finally relents. Fast forward two weeks, and Eva is dealing with a burning sensation when she urinates. When she raises the issue with Rick, he states that he's feeling fine and accuses her of possibly giving him an STI. Eva then reaches out to Nicole, who advises her to get tested. During the appointment, the doctor informs Eva that she has chlamydia and provides information about the prevention and treatment of STIs before prescribing medication for both Eva and Rick. A week after the appointment, Rick and Eva have finished the medication, and Rick begins to pressure her to have sex without a condom again. This time, Eva holds her ground and Rick concedes to her wishes – but then Rick receives a call from a girl named "Tiffany" and the vignette ends with Eva looking at him in disgust.

The second vignette begins with Eva, Nicole, and Nicole's boyfriend John sitting together during a party at Eva's apartment and discussing her recent breakup with Rick. Michelle arrives at the party with pizzas, and Eva leaves to pay for them. She finds Chela in her bed with an unnamed man. While she's away, Michelle receives a text that her babysitter needs to leave early and heads home to relieve her. When Eva returns, they discuss how Michelle's life has changed since the baby – and how hard things have been without the support of the baby's father. They also reveal that Michelle has been flirting with a coworker but hasn't yet mentioned her daughter. At work the next day, Michelle is asked on a date by the coworker, Kevin, and explains that she has a 1-year-old named Mia. He reveals in turn that he is a single father to a 2-year-old named Cora. They bond over the struggles of single parenthood, and Michelle explains that she'd like to get back on birth control before they go any further. In the next scene, she visits a doctor who explains her contraceptive options and that women can control if and when they become pregnant. Michelle decides to try a non-hormonal IUD. We next see Michelle in Kevin's apartment, where they discuss her recent appointment and she explains how uninhibited she feels with her new contraceptive. However, when things begin to heat up, Michelle asks that they also use a condom, to which Kevin readily agrees. The vignette ends with Michelle regaling her friends with the details of her first time with Kevin before Chela reveals that she's met someone new: a girl named Trina.

The third and final vignette starts with Chela, Nicole, and Eva sitting on the grass in a park. Chela inquires whether Nicole and John are still having satisfying sex after two years together, and Nicole confirms that they do because they "tell each other what [they] want." Eva and Chela commiserate about how their parents are too conservative to openly discuss sex, and Chela confides that her parents do not even know she is sexually active – or that she is bisexual. She then explains how her relationship ended when Trina went back to college, and she has been lonely ever since. Shortly thereafter, John arrives with his friend, Lance, who immediately begins to flirt with Chela. She and Lance play 1-on-1 basketball as the sexual tension between them builds. The next scene opens with Nicole at work the next day when she receives a panicked call from Chela. Chela explains that she went home with Lance after their game and in the heat of the moment she forgot to use protection. Because she had been with Trina, she explains, she is no longer on birth control. Nicole urges her to come to the pharmacy to pick up an emergency contraceptive (Plan B), before cutting to the four young women sitting together in Eva's back yard. They discuss the effectiveness of Plan B, as well as Chela's desire to find a new contraceptive method. She discloses that she is hesitant to share her sexual behavior with a physician. Michelle explains how important it is to be honest with one's doctor, and then texts Chela the contact information for her provider. Chela meets with the doctor, who explains that STI transmission can occur with both male and female partners and suggests that the implant contraceptive might be a good option after Chela mentions that she often forgets to take her birth control pills. The final vignette ends with the four girls (and their boyfriends John, Kevin, and Lance) getting ready at Eva's apartment for a sporting event at their old high school. Suddenly, the doorbell rings and Eva opens the door to find a girl asking for Chela – to which Chela responds "Trina?" as the video cuts to black.

Still images from the Plan A video are included below:

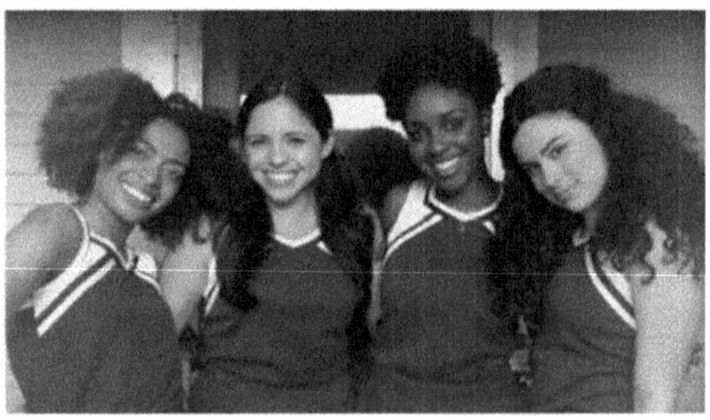

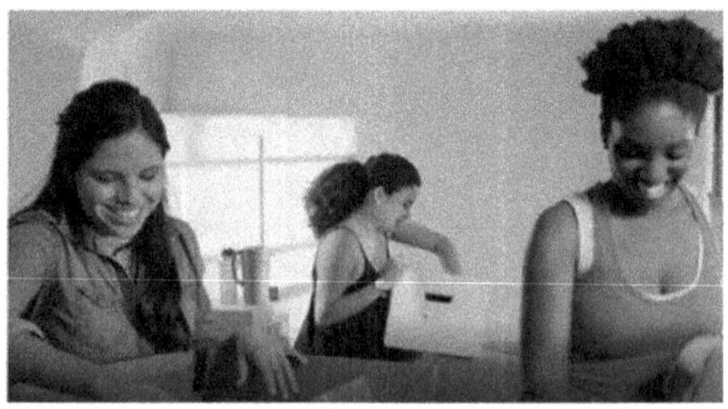

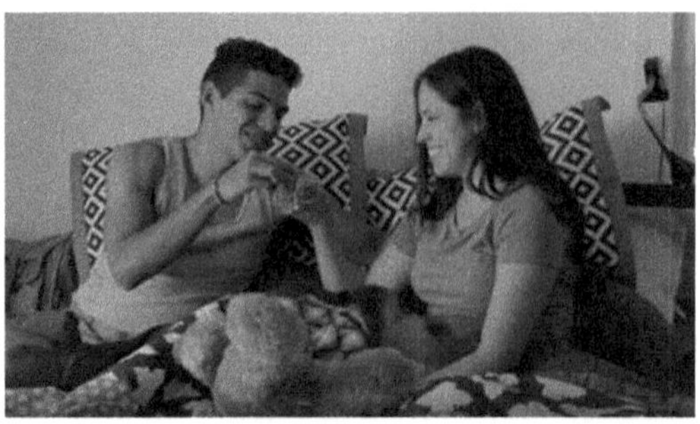

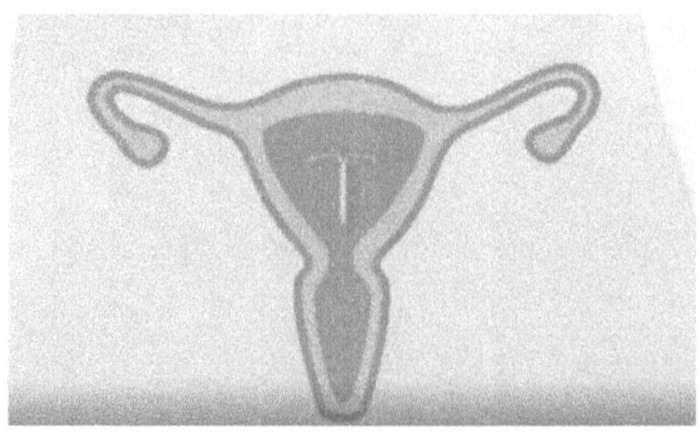

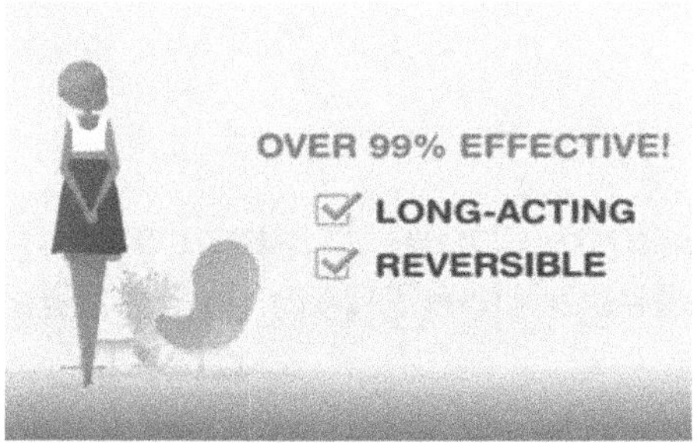
OVER 99% EFFECTIVE!
LONG-ACTING
REVERSIBLE

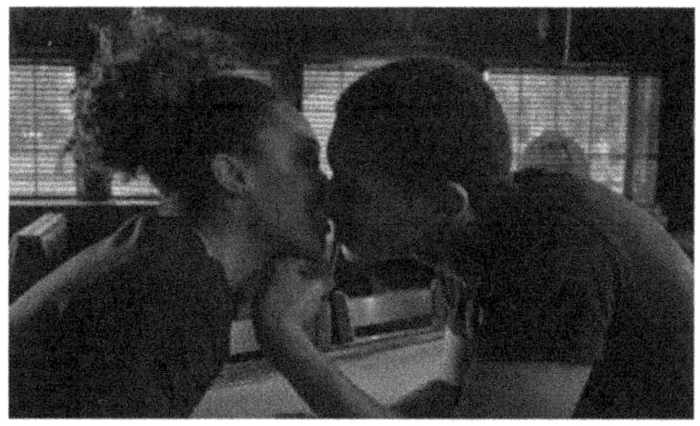

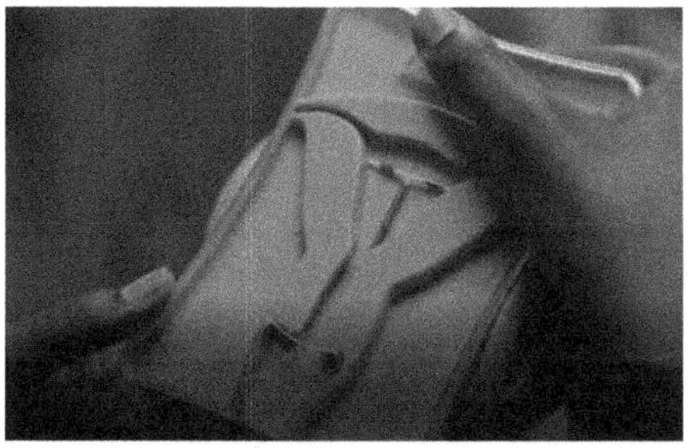

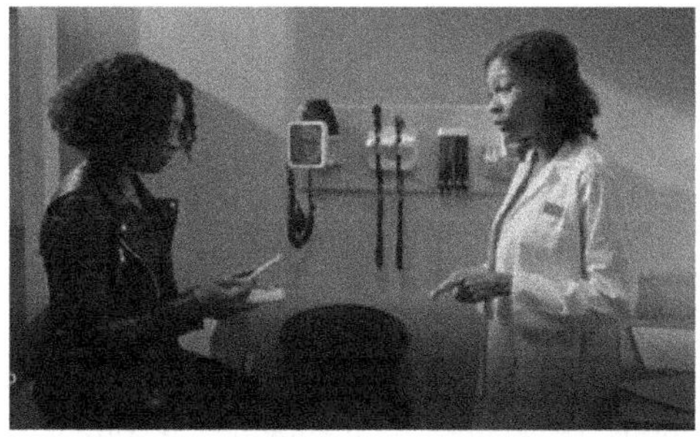

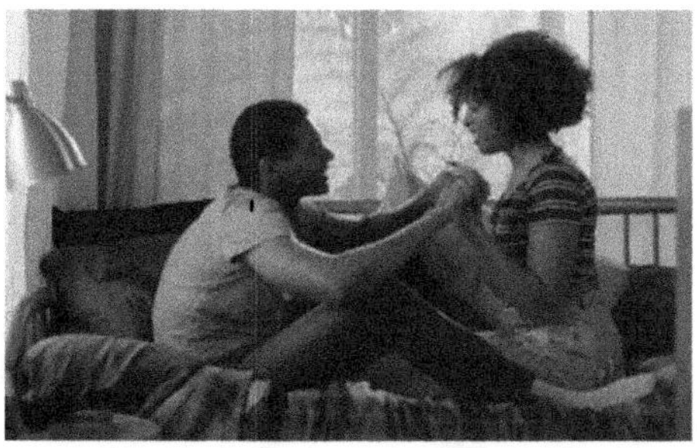

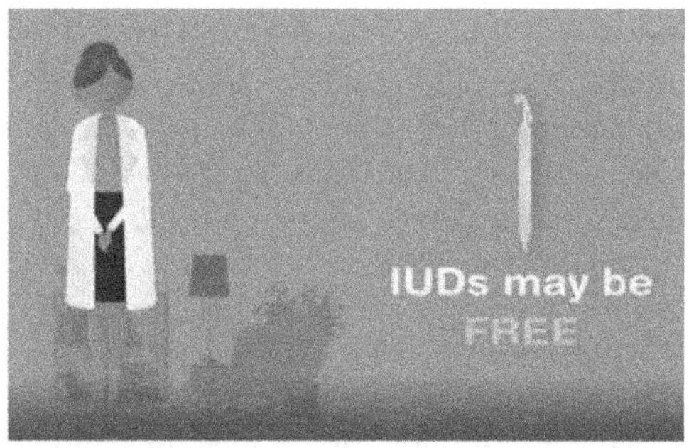
IUDs may be
FREE

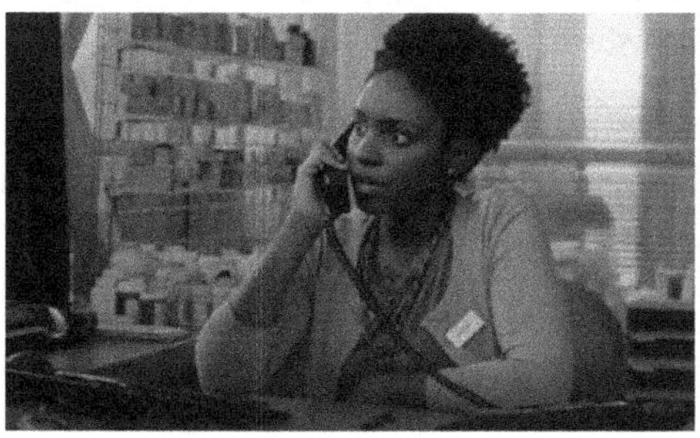

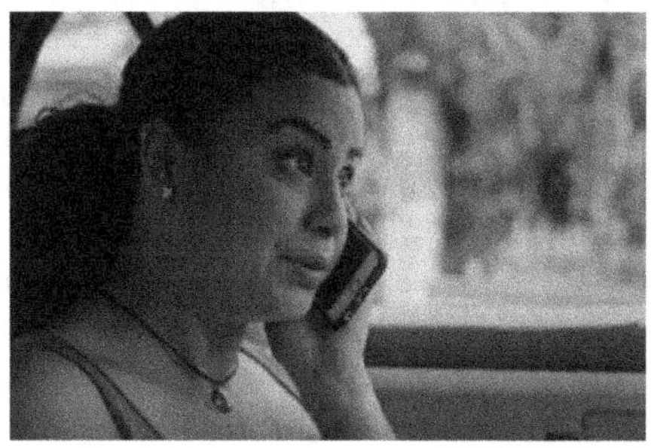

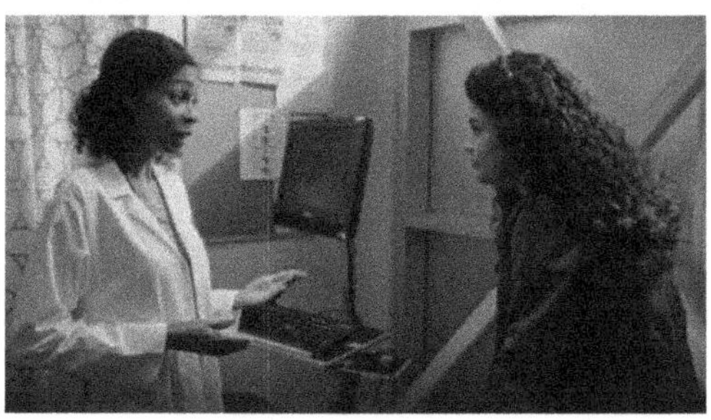

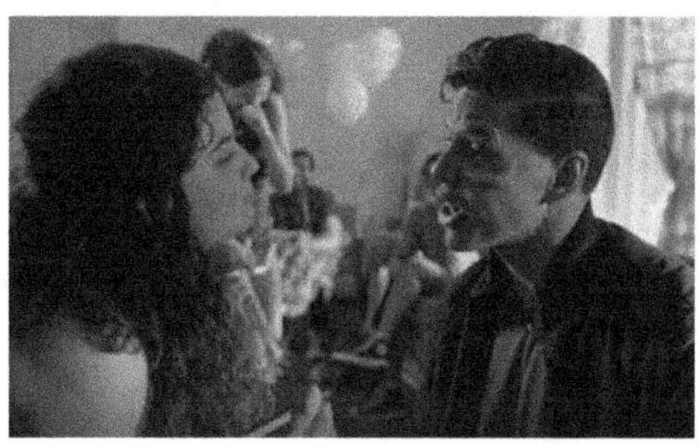

A Theoretically Based Analysis of Twitter Conversations about Trauma and Mental Health: Examining Responses to Storylines on the Television Show *Queen Sugar*

Diane B. Francis and LeChrista Finn

ABSTRACT

Entertainment programming in the United States has long addressed major public health issues. In the present study, we used a culture-centric approach to systematically investigate the role of television storylines in facilitating health-related conversations on social media. In particular, we examined Twitter conversations about sexual and police-involved trauma prompted by portrayals on the fictional television drama *Queen Sugar*. Guided by the culture-centric model of narratives in health promotion, we classified the tweets (N = 1,671) into four main thematic categories: identification, social proliferation, emotions, and intentions. The analysis also revealed several subthemes, including identification with characters and cultural elements, expressions of pain and joy, information seeking and sharing, and the need to address intergenerational trauma and promote intergenerational conversations. The data suggests that Twitter may provide a vehicle for engaging in difficult conversations. We discuss the theoretical and practical implications of the study for mental health communication with Black Americans.

Communication approaches, such as embedding messages in entertainment programming, could motivate people to engage in health-promoting behaviors, including discussing taboo topics or seeking help. Television storylines about social or health issues often generate offline and online conversations about the topic (Slater, 2002). In turn, these conversations are associated with changes in beliefs and behaviors (Southwell & Yzer, 2007). Nevertheless, we still have a lot to learn about the influence of entertainment narratives on audience's conversations, especially among minority populations and about difficult or taboo topics. In this study, we used the culture-centric model of narrative health promotion to investigate the role of storylines about sexual and police-involved violence portrayed on the television drama *Queen Sugar* in facilitating conversations on Twitter. The discussions – using the hashtag #QueenSugarTalks – aimed to address trauma and mental health in the Black community by encouraging people to talk about these issues. An examination of #QueenSugarTalks is essential because it has the potential to illuminate not only Black men and women's responses to the trauma narratives but also provide potential tools that could be utilized in mental health promotion among Black Americans. Additionally, the study contributes to extant research on the role of entertainment narratives in facilitating difficult conversations on social media.

Background and theoretical foundations

Exposure to trauma has become a global public health issue, given its pervasiveness worldwide (Magruder et al., 2017). However, Black people in the United States have long had to contend with adverse and traumatic experiences throughout their life course resulting from various types of historical and contemporary trauma (Mohatt et al., 2014). Black women are subjected to high rates of sexual trauma: More than 40% of adult Black women have experienced sexual coercion and other forms of unwanted sexual contact, and 20% have been raped at some point in their lifetime (West & Johnson, 2013). Concerns about law enforcement violence is also an inescapable issue for Black men and women. Black Americans are three times more likely to be killed by law enforcement officers than white Americans (Mapping Police Violence, 2020).

Traumatic experiences are associated with increased psychological distress and long-term mental and chronic health problems among individuals, directly and indirectly, exposed (Mouzon et al., 2016). Furthermore, family members who have not experienced traumatic experiences also feel the effects generations later through a process known as intergenerational transmission of trauma (Walters et al., 2011). Consequently, individual trauma becomes collective and compounded, affecting more members of a family and community (Mohatt et al., 2014). Traumatic experiences may also be contributing to increases in suicidal ideation and attempts and deaths by suicide among younger Black people (Lindsey et al., 2019). Joe (2006) observed that the risk of suicide for Black Americans extends into younger age groups with each passing generation. Despite all this, Black individuals are less likely to disclose traumatic experiences to family and friends, report to authorities, or seek professional help (Bakari, 2019).

Various interventions have been developed to address trauma and subsequent health issues among Black Americans, ranging from community and faith-based programs to cognitive-behavioral theory delivered over the Internet (Hays & Aranda, 2016; Jonassaint et al., 2017). Due to the broad audience reach and ability to target messages, fictional entertainment narratives represent an efficacious approach to move people to action on socially relevant issues such as trauma. Not only are entertainment narratives influential channels for communicating health messages, but they also spur viewers toward positive health-related behaviors and outcomes (Slater, 2002). Entertainment narratives may be particularly effective at stimulating conversations about taboo topics or health topics that people often avoid discussing. Empirical evidence from sexual health literature supports this idea. Experimental evaluations of storylines about sexually transmitted infections on the HBO series *Sex and the City* demonstrated a positive association between depictions of sexual discussions and actual discussion behavior two weeks after exposure (Moyer-Gusé et al., 2011). In another study, watching a teen pregnancy narrative led to more satisfying discussions about the topic among mother-daughter dyads (Moyer-Gusé et al., 2020). Extant research on celebrity health narratives also adds to evidence of an association between exposure to mediated health narratives and conversations (Francis, 2019; Francis et al., 2019).

The model of culture-centric narratives in health promotion offers another coherent framework of the mechanisms linking entertainment narratives to conversations (Larkey & Hecht, 2010). According to the model, identification and social proliferations are outcomes of exposure to narratives. Additionally, social proliferation follows from identification processes. Identification and social proliferations are then associated with attitudes and beliefs and behavior change. An essential contribution of the model is its treatment of the mediators at the personal and sociocultural levels. Although the model was developed to guide and test the design of intentional narrative-based health promotion interventions, the model can be used to understand and explain narrative effects in other contexts, such as those from fictional television programs.

Researchers have acknowledged the central role identification plays in the processing of narratives. An extensive body of research supports the idea that people tend to look too similar to others when examining their own beliefs and behaviors (Brown, 2015; Moyer-Gusé, 2008). Identification with characters is associated positively with increased attention, less counterarguing, and behavioral modeling (Moyer-Gusé, 2008). However, identification is not only an individual-level phenomenon as primarily studied in the media effects literature (Larkey & Hecht, 2010). Cultural identification, or identification with cultural elements in the story, is posited to influence downstream outcomes as well, suggesting that cultural cues in the characters' behavior or language attune viewers to the culture depicted in the story (Larkey & Hecht, 2010). In a study by Murphy et al. (2013), Mexican American women exposed to a narrative video featuring a Mexican American family discussing the Pap test, HPV, and cervical cancer, reported greater identification with the characters. In that same study, however, African American women also reported identification, though to a lesser extent than Mexican American women. African American women perceived the characters as relatable and the story to be culturally resonant. Thus, both Mexican American and African American women identified with the cultural cues in the story and the characters' behavior. In this study, we examine identification at the personal and sociocultural levels. In line with prior research, identification with characters refers to instances of perceived similarity, liking, and parasocial interaction or feelings of empathy for the characters. At the sociocultural level, we examine identification with the cultural elements in the story by looking at factors beyond demographic similarities that may not be readily observable but that audience members can still identify with, including similar experiences with trauma or depictions of conversations with family and friends.

Larkey and Hecht (2010) model also describes the process of social proliferation, which refers to the uptake and diffusion of ideas or behaviors through discussion, rehearsal, and reciprocal support. Reciprocal support processes include a sense of caring and obligation amongst those who discuss the topic as well as emotional support in the form of sympathy or empathy that is expressed or exchanged (Larkey, 2015). More and more, individuals are seeking and sharing information and support through online means. In particular, Twitter has emerged as one of the leading social media platforms for discussions about engagement with and support for mental health issues (McClellan et al., 2016). One study found that one of the main reasons cited for using Twitter was to receive support for mental health conditions (Berry et al., 2017). Another study documented how Twitter users communicated support to Black men following rapper Kid Cudi's depression announcement (Francis, 2019). In this study, we refer to and assess social proliferation at the personal and sociocultural levels as the concept taps into not only the discussion and diffusion of ideas but also reciprocal support. At the personal level, we examine instances of liking and gratitude, and encouragement and empathy. At the sociocultural level, we examine information sharing and seeking.

Beyond identification and social proliferation, emotions also play a role in how audiences respond to narratives and their persuasive impact. Although emotions are not illustrated in the culture-centric model, Larkey and Hecht (2010) argued for investigations of how emotions influence the persuasive process as part of the work on narratives in culture-centric health promotion. Individuals develop emotional connections with characters and vicariously experience the feelings, perspectives, and goals of the character (Moyer-Gusé et al., 2011) and respond through emotional support (e.g., empathy for the character) or expressions. In the Murphy et al. (2013) study described previously, they found that Mexican American and African American women reported more negative and more positive emotions than European American women. In online contexts, emotions can take the form of emotional support (such as communicating empathy for others) or emotional expressions (communicating about how the user feels) (Myrick et al., 2016). Studies show that emotions are strongly associated with communication behaviors, including online information seeking and conversations (Francis et al., 2019). Recent research has also found empirical evidence for the social sharing of emotions and group-based emotions (Kessler & Hollbach, 2005; Myrick et al., 2016), which are relevant to our understanding of emotions on social media. Brock (2020) argues that much of Black people's conversations in digital spaces revolve around joy and pain. Brock (2020) notes that "Black digital identity draws in equal measure on expressions of joy and pain in everyday life in American racial ideology, which are articulated as cultural critiques enacted online" (p. 12). In this study, we explore emotions in the form of joy and pain.

Current study

The purpose of the current study was to systematically investigate Twitter conversations related to storylines about sexual and police-involved trauma on the television drama *Queen Sugar*. We focus on audience responses to the storylines by using the hashtag #QueenSugarTalks to engage in conversations about trauma and mental health in the Black community. Consequently, we were interested in the influence of entertainment narratives on conversations about trauma and mental health and how audiences made sense of the storylines about significant health and social issues. Our research questions were: 1) In what ways did audience members and Twitter chat participants identify with the characters, story, or cultural elements within the show? 2) In what ways did they engage in social proliferation? 3) In what ways did they respond emotionally to the images and information portrayed on the show? 4) What insights were raised in terms of behavioral intentions?

Methods

Queen Sugar, which airs on the network OWN, follows a Black family, the Bordelon siblings, in rural Louisiana. Since its premiere in September 2016, the show has addressed a range of social and health issues relevant to the Black community. To date, the show's primary audience is Black women (Williams, 2019). During its fourth season (June to September 2019), *Queen Sugar* introduced two subplots whereby two characters disclosed their traumatic experiences to family and friends. The August 21, 2019, episode examined in this study follows Darla as she reveals to Violet that she was raped while in college. After Darla's revelation, Violet then discloses her own experience of being raped by her husband when she was younger. The second subplot follows Micah and Blue's traumatic interactions with a police officer. The young men then share details of their interactions with other male family and friends.

Data for the study were collected from August 21 to 25, 2019. Hours before the airing of the August 21 episode, *Queen Sugar* producers launched the #QueenSugarTalks hashtag campaign. The hashtag was used to engage audience members in a direct Twitter chat "to discuss important topics like trauma touched on in the show with leading voices in their respective field" and talk more broadly about trauma and healing in the Black community. The official Twitter chat occurred from 6–9 p.m. Eastern Standard Time. The producers invited several prominent Black people to answer questions from audience members. They included #MeToo founder Tarana Burke, author and talk show host Iyanla Vanzant, music superstar and activist Common, and Central Park Five member Yusef Salaam.

We collected all publicly available tweets from the start of the conversation's announcement on August 21 through midnight on August 25. We chose this timeframe because it enabled us to capture the direct involvement in the question-and-answer segments of #QueenSugarTalks chat and live tweets of viewer responses to the episode. The timeframe also meant we could capture any lagging tweets from people who were not part of the live chat session. Prior research has shown that Twitter activity increases precipitously in the first 24 hours in response to planned events, then wanes or returns to low levels of activity in the days after (Francis, 2019; McClellan et al., 2016). The tweets were collected using NVIVO's NCapture software. The software allowed for reliable access to Twitter's public stream to retrieve a live feed of the hashtag conversations. We only collected tweets with the #QueenSugarTalks hashtag because of the specific research questions guiding the study. Audience members on Twitter usually use a range of hashtags to respond to *Queen Sugar* programming (e.g., #QueenSugar and #GimmeSugar). The extraction of tweets using the #QueenSugarTalks hashtag allowed us to ascertain engagement with the specific storylines and hashtag conversation. The #QueenSugarTalks hashtag generated 15,148 tweets over the five days. The majority of the tweets (89%, n = 13, 477) were retweets. The remaining 11% (n = 1,671) were unique tweets. We analyzed these unique tweets for this study. The project was exempted from review by the Institutional Review Board for the participating university.

We used a thematic analysis approach to analyze the data collected through #QueenSugarTalks. Thematic analysis involves a six-step process, from coding to theme development to refinement (Braun & Clarke, 2006). First, we read and re-read the tweets multiple times to become familiar with the conversations' content. Second, we developed a thematic codebook based on the culture-centric model described above. The purpose of the codebook was to identify instances of the thematic categories appearing in the tweets. We used the coding scheme to operationalize the key study's concepts: identification, social proliferation, emotions, intention (defined below). Third, we coded the tweets for themes across overt and latent aspects of the data. We used in vivo coding. During the coding process, we also identified subthemes within each of the thematic categories. The specification of subthemes allowed for more in-depth analysis that delved into the latent content from the broader conversations. As themes were determined a priori according to concepts from the culture-centric model, we did not need to adhere to Braun and Clarke (2006) fifth step of defining and naming the themes. The report produced here is the final step in the thematic analysis process.

Within the thematic category of identification, we coded for identification with characters and identification with cultural elements in the story. Identification with characters was defined as tweets conveying liking, empathy, similarity, and feeling like you know or wanting to be like the character. Identification with cultural elements was defined as tweets expressing recognition of events and characters in the story that resonated with the person's culture, events that could happen in their community, or how watching the story made them want to do something in their community. For social proliferation, we focused on reciprocal support. Reciprocal support was defined as tweets expressing liking or gratitude for the conversation, conveying encouragement or empathy, and information sharing and seeking. Information sharing was defined as tweets providing information to others; information seeking was defined as tweets directly asking questions of the moderators and participants or asking others more broadly for guidance. Emotions were defined as tweets expressing positive (e.g., joy, hope) or negative (e.g., pain, sadness, anger, fear) reactions to either the specific storyline or the overall conversation. Intentions were defined as tweets conveying information about what can or should be done to address individual and collective trauma.

After testing and finalizing the codebook on a sample of tweets, the lead author coded the full dataset. The unit of analysis was the entire tweet, and each tweet could contain more than one thematic category. To verify coding and reduce bias, a research assistant read and reviewed the tweets and checked the coding against the data set. Any discrepancies were discussed and resolved between them. Below, we indicated the percentage of tweets coded for each thematic category or subtheme. The percentages were calculated from the full sample (N = 1,671). The percentages do not total 100% because tweets could be coded into more than one category.

Results

Using a culture-centric approach, we examined four thematic categories emerging from Twitter conversations about trauma and mental health and informed by storylines in the television show *Queen Sugar*. The four thematic categories were: 1) identification, 2) social proliferation, 3) emotion, and 4) intentions. Identification was further broken down into two subthemes: identification with characters and identification with cultural elements in the story. Emotions also included two subthemes of expressions of positive and negative reactions. Reciprocal support included four subthemes: 1) liking and gratitude, 2) encouragement and empathy, 3) information sharing, 4) information seeking. Finally, intentions included: 1) addressing intergenerational trauma, and 2) fostering intergenerational conversations. Table 1 shows the definition and exemplar tweets. We report the quantitative and qualitative data alongside one another. Each of these thematic categories and subthemes is detailed below.

Identification

More than a third (39%) of the tweets expressed some form of identification. More of the tweets addressed cultural identification (25%) than character identification (16%). However, some cultural identification tweets referenced how the characters' portrayal of the traumatic events closely resembled what they saw in their everyday lives. To that end, we first report on identification with characters and then on identification with cultural elements in the story.

Identification with characters

The Twitter chat participants expressed identification with the main characters in the storylines – Darla and Violet, Micah and Blue. Participants voiced concern and empathy for Darla and compassion and respect for Violet. Participants talked about loving Darla's character and showed how they connected emotionally to her. An example of this is one tweet saying, "My heart breaks for Darla. She represents so many young women … the inability to consent is more common than spoken." Twitter participants sometimes addressed the characters as if they were friends in real life, blurring the lines between fiction and reality. For example, in their tweets, participants sometimes appeared to be speaking directly to the characters. An example of this is a tweet telling Darla: "Darla, you were raped." The tweets revealed that participants were emotionally invested in Darla and Violet's conversation and overall relationship. The tweets about the interactions between the two women were revealing: "I think Darla and Violet need this moment. I know Darla is clearly going through it, but Violet needs to realize that talking about things is important;" "Maybe Darla and Aunt Violet can seek help together." And "Everybody needs an Aunt Violet in their life." Although the tweets mostly mentioned Darla and Violet, some talked about Micah and Blue. Some expressed anxiety for Micah and Blue. Tweets also connected the characters' decisions to disclose their traumatic experiences. Sample tweets included: "That baby [Blue] has seen so much. And still, the light within him shines brightly;" and "It took time, but Micah was finally able to share his personal experience. And he did it to help the community address the issues they've been facing." Overall, they identified more so with Darla and Violet as individual characters than with Micah and Blue.

Identification with cultural elements

Conversation participants most identified with Micah and Blue's interactions with the police officer at the cultural level. Some participants compared what they saw portrayed in these storylines with their personal, family, or community experiences. They particularly connected the portrayals to what has been happening in the wider Black community. Sample tweets included: "Micah's first brush with law enforcement was a realization for him as a Black man – how quickly an interaction with the police can escalate." Another said, "When we saw Micah pulled over & abused by a white police officer, it hits home because we understand the real dangers that we and our loved one's face." Some tweets, though, saw the stories not only as mere portrayal but as a step toward identifying ways to heal as a community. For example, one tweet said, "Similar to Darla and Micah on #QueenSugar, the Black community often experiences traumatic events that can alter the trajectory of their lives. But if we can courageously face our trauma, we might be able to heal the pain we've been holding onto for years." While viewers mostly identified with Darla and Violet on a personal level, Micah and Blue's interactions with the police officer resonated with some participants at the sociocultural level. Thus, how the Twitter conversation participants connected with the characters or the storyline was essential to understanding how they made sense of what was depicted.

Social proliferation and reciprocal support

The majority of tweets concerned social proliferation and, more specifically, reciprocal support. Three quarters (74%) of all tweets expressed some form of reciprocal support. Reciprocal support tweets were less a direct response to the Queen Sugar episode, characters, and the story. Instead, these tweets focused much more on the overall #QueenSugarTalks conversation, including engagement with the celebrities and public figures invited to talk about trauma and mental health in the Black community. Twitter chat participants also responded and connected to each other's experiences during the conversation. About a third (34%) of the tweets indicated liking or gratitude for the discussion. Tweets conveying encouragement, empathy, sympathy, or caring for chat participants accounted for 16% of the sample. Information sharing (13%) and seeking (8%) represented other forms of reciprocal support.

Liking and gratitude

Reciprocal support emerged in the form of participants expressing liking the conversations and being thankful that it was happening. Although this was the most prevalent way of expressing support during the Twitter conversation, many tweets were single words or phrases such as amen or yes or thank you. Examples of liking and gratitude included: "This thread is life-giving" and "So much insight and wisdom being shared." Some participants expressed appreciation for the conversation's ability to raise awareness of trauma: "Thank you all for bringing awareness to the social issues."

Encouragement and empathy

Participants also offered encouragement and empathy for those experiencing traumatic experiences. Many tweets of such expressions had general statements such as "we must be courageous and face it." However, other tweets focused on encouragement and empathy specifically directed toward people who were sharing their experiences. For example, one tweet expressing empathy said: "Sis, I am sorry you are holding both of those things. Counseling could be a big help, but I would also suggest that you give full attention to each of them individually. Those are separate hurts that both need your attention." Encouragement also came from health care professionals who joined the conversation. One such professional said: "As a psychologist, watching these #QueenSugarTalks tweets is warming my soul! Keep the conversation going and normalize these experiences."

Information sharing

The #QueenSugarTalks conversation was a way to talk about trauma and healing in the Black community broadly. Inevitably, it was expected that the discussion would include information about ways to address these issues and about healing.

Thus, both the chat moderators and Twitter participants gave information and advice about a range of topics. Some of the topics covered included: having a plan if someone is going to talk about their trauma, the importance of having a support system, and asking for help. They also suggested utilizing experts at each stage of the disclosure process. Some tweets provided suggestions on what questions to ask when someone with trauma is in need. Participants also wanted others to know of the realities of the healing process, including potential difficulties along the way. For example, one tweet said: "If you want to heal, you can't phone it in. You've got to get down in the mud, get dirty, and deal with the facts." Finally, they cautioned participants that healing takes time: "Healing isn't a straight line. Neither is growth. #QueenSugar has normalized that for me, for all of us.

Information seeking

As with information sharing, a significant part of the #QueenSugarTalks conversation was participants asking questions. A broad range of questions emerged during the discussion. Some participants wanted to know what trauma is, how it is defined. Others quested about how to deal with similar situations to what the characters were experiencing. They also wanted information on how to seek help both for themselves and how to help others. One tweet asked: "How can we take that leap to seek help? How can we best utilize our empathy to help someone else seek help?" Other topics of interest included what comes next after disclosure and the potential recurrence of trauma. Several participants asked about supporting others through trauma, including youth and young people. For example, a tweet asked: "I have often thought that there is a lot of anxiety and depression among our youth, especially the young men. Your thoughts, and how do we effectively address them? For those who were interested in help-seeking but concerned about it being taboo, participants wanted information on countering such taboos. Finally, supporting those who are not interested in therapy was something that participants wanted to know about as well. An example of this included: "How do you properly support and encourage someone to deal with trauma when they aren't interested in therapy but still want help." In the end, the conversation seemed to bring up more questions than either moderators and participants could answer.

Emotions

Throughout the #QueenSugarTalks conversation, Twitter chat participants expressed both positive and negative emotions. However, these emotional expressions were often not distinct from their other reactions and responses (e.g., identification with the characters or information sharing). Forty percent of tweets were identified as expressing positive or negative emotions. Nevertheless, there were more expressions of pain (27%) than of joy (11%).

Expressions of pain

The conversations and show brought up a range of negative feelings from the conversation participants. Expressions of pain were reflected through a shared sense of personal, intergenerational, historical, and contemporary experiences. Emotions emerging in the conversation included shame, guilt, fear, and anxiety. Examples of these emotions included: "I was also ashamed to admit for a long time that throughout the #Ferguson uprising, I was in therapy every week. Ain't no shame now. It saved my life" and "For a long time I felt guilty for letting the abuse happen" and "I was checking in on my partner and brother so often and almost freaking out every time they took a little too long to answer. I feared for their lives constantly. That trauma has had long-lasting effects." One of the more prominent examples of emotional expressions was through disclosures and sharing of similar experiences to what happened to the characters. Some tweets included people disclosing and detailing their own experiences with trauma and the pain they felt. Examples of such tweets were: "I didn't need to be shamed or told to be abstinent. I just needed to be seen. And heard. And cared for" and "Literally just talked about trauma at my therapy session this morning. I am definitely working on accepting it as trauma and not something I was supposed to experience due to culture" and "I'm a Black man who probably still has PTSD from police stops in my youth. I see a police officer in my community, and I don't feel safe. I feel triggered, on alert, fearful for my life. Micah's story breaks me." Throughout, participants were expressing pain toward both individual and collective trauma.

Expressions of joy

While there were expressions of pain, participants expressed positive emotions about the conversations and moving past trauma. More specifically, the discussions and the episode brought up a range of positive feelings. Some tweets conveyed hope and optimism for what the conversation might produce. For example, one tweet said: "Hope this conversation is helping others as is helping me." Beyond hope, expressions of joy have become a central aspect of Black people's expressions on social media. Many of the positive tweets conveyed the importance of joy in the healing process. Further, joy was most often connected to expressions and the importance of healing. Examples of such tweets included: "Joy and healing go so well together" and "Give yourself room for joy" and "Joy is transformational" and "Our joy is as much an act of resistance as anything else." In essence, participants were expressing joy toward individual and collective healing.

Intentions

About a third (31%) of the tweets addressed the question of what's next in some form. The prevailing concerns were to address intergenerational trauma and how to foster intergenerational conversations.

Address intergenerational trauma

A significant touchpoint of the conversation for participants was the importance of recognizing and addressing how trauma has affected generations of Black people and families. For example, one tweet said: "Studies show trauma is passed down from one generation to the next. It makes sense since we absorb whatever our mother's wombs eat/experience/feel. So, we're living with compounded trauma in our communities." Another said, "My grandmothers went to their graves with their trauma. My mom probably will too. They believed you don't 'air your dirty laundry.' And I don't judge them. I get why. But that has created a cycle of pain that's hard to break when you can't pinpoint the source." Participants were also interested in what can be done to protect future generations. One such example tweet said: "All of this resonates so much, especially about not passing on that trauma to my daughter. I truly want to show her a better way of dealing with trauma by being open and transparent about my struggles and wins." Participants connected the conversation about the intergenerational transmission of trauma back to the show: "The Darla/Violet talk, I hope it inspires us (parents) to be very careful what and who we encourage our children toward." The participant also said they hope the talk encouraged parents to discuss these issues with their children.

Promote intergenerational conversations

While #QueenSugarTalks participants valued the conversations, they saw this as a start. Some called for taking the conversations offline and into the community. They argued that such discussions could be a way to foster collective healing and action. For example, one tweet said: "We need more conversations like this! The more we talk, the more we heal." While one tweet acknowledged that "Intergenerational conversations are taking place and leading to change," others noted that "Such a necessary conversation and to focus on healing as a community. So many of our youth are experiencing more than one traumatic experience during their childhood years."

Intergenerational conversations, online or offline, emerged as a mechanism aiding in healing from trauma.

Discussion

Research on social media conversations about health represents a burgeoning area of health communication inquiry. Studies about health-related discourses on Twitter have examined tweets covering broad topics (e.g., depression) as well as conversations that emerge following the specific mediated event. For this study, we examined Twitter conversations about sexual and police-involved trauma prompted by storylines in the television show *Queen Sugar*. We used the culture-centric model of narrative health promotion to classify the tweets into four main thematic categories: identification, social proliferation, emotions, and intentions. Our analysis of more than 1,500 unique tweets using the hashtag #QueenSugarTalks revealed that participants identified with the characters portrayed in the storylines and with the cultural elements. They engaged with the conversation by seeking information and advice and asking a range of questions. While the discussions brought forth positive and negative emotions, participants also expressed interest in addressing intergenerational trauma and moving the conversation away from social media and into individuals' homes and communities.

A primary aim of the study was to utilize a narrative-based theory to investigate the potential persuasive impact of the *Queen Sugar* storylines. The culture-centric model of narratives in health promotion was developed to guide the design and testing of intentional behavior change messages (Larkey & Hecht, 2010). However, people often have multiple opportunities for exposure to narratives, including those that appear in the media. And while the model considers that people can be exposed to narratives in various ways, to our knowledge, this is one of the first studies to utilize the model to assess narratives in a television program that was not designed to promote specific health behaviors. Ours is also the first study to use the model to examine a qualitative dataset; research testing various components of the model often utilize quantitative measures. Our study adds to the utility of the model and shows that the model could be used to examine a broad range of culture-centric narratives and their impact. Future studies on the effects of exposure to narratives in the media should consider the model, aiming to specify the utility of other components of the model not examined here.

A secondary aim was to assess Twitter as a tool to discuss difficult topics. Despite efforts to increase public concern about trauma and mental health among diverse peoples and communities, barriers to open discussions remain. Talking about mental health and trauma is still taboo in many Black communities (Williams, 2014). Nevertheless, evidence suggests some narrative-based strategies may activate discussions about trauma and mental health among Black people. It is possible that the nature of the medium (i.e., social media) is what is prompting viewers to engage in these conversations. People may be open to discussing difficult or taboo topics on social media than in face-to-face conversations. People are also willing to express positive and negative emotional reactions to the storylines and the characters in their Twitter conversations. Through our analysis, we found that participants first expressed concern and worry upon seeing Darla and Violet together. Still, their reactions were more positive after learning that both women were raped. That is, their Twitter reactions changed from negative to positive as both women shared about their histories of sexual assault. Regular viewers of the show commented that Violet's character has not always been kind to Darla. Thus, they were concerned when the two women were placed in a scene together. However, the characters' shared traumatic experiences, and Violet's empathy for Darla, prompted the shift in responses. Our findings of a transition from negative to positive reactions can be explained through identification processes. As viewers identified with Violet, they empathized with what she went through and understood better her perspective on the situation.

Also emergent in the conversations were discussions about collective healing. The findings illustrate support for a strengths-based healing centered approach to addressing trauma and mental health with Black Americans. Ginwright (2018) proposed the healing centered approach to move from the deficit-based, individually-focused trauma-informed care toward an asset-based approach. A healing centered approach "views trauma not simply as an individual isolated experience, but rather highlights how trauma and healing are experienced collectively" (Ginwright, 2018). Additionally, the approach is holistic, involves culture, spirituality, civic action, and collective healing, and is facilitated through healing centered engagement. Unlike the trauma-informed approach, healing centered engagement re-centers culture as a central feature in well-being and advances a collective view of healing (Ginwright, 2018). Furthermore, the healing-centered approach starts with the assumption that groups of people – whether at the family, neighborhood or community-levels – share similar traumatic experiences. As our study indicates, communication plays a vital role in understanding how "trauma and healing are experienced collectively" (Ginwright, 2018). The healing centered approach, and healing centered engagement, is an emerging framework but builds on prior work in positive psychology. To our knowledge, this is the first health communication study to utilize the healing centered approach. However, the approach holds promise for continued health communication research to identify effective ways of engaging Black people in conversations about trauma and mental health. Research is also needed to develop hypotheses and research questions linking healing centered approach to communication and health outcomes.

Our study contributes to growing research on social media conversations about health. Moreover, our study indicates the continued need for theory-driven analysis to identify the processes by which conversations may lead to change. Trauma and mental health are difficult topics to talk about. Yet, some studies indicate that Black Americans may be willing to talk about these issues on social media (Brock, 2020; Francis, 2019). Twitter, in particular, has emerged as one of the leading social media platforms for conversations about and engagement with mental health topics among Black Americans (Francis, 2019). The discourse on Twitter may constitute part of the process of normalizing these conversations and experiences. As one tweet reiterated, "Keep the conversation going and normalize these experiences." Mental health advocates and practitioners need to be aware that media narratives often prompt these social media conversations. Their involvement may be critical to understanding how online discourse about health topics translate to real-world impact among Black Americans.

Recent theoretical work on the relationship between media exposure and conversations is also important to consider when considering this study's findings. Our study provided evidence that Twitter users attended to the storylines presented on *Queen Sugar* and were motivated by the storylines to actively participate in the conversations. Engaging in social media conversations about mental health and trauma could be a means of either discussion-generated elaboration or anticipatory elaboration. Discussion-generated elaboration "suggests that the act of engaging in discussion forces meaningful information processing" (Eveland, Jr., 2004). This information processing, or elaboration, is likely to increase learning and recall of the health topic. Anticipatory elaboration, on the other hand, refers to the process whereby people who are expecting to engage in discussions about health later on "will invest more heavily in processing the information upon first being exposed to it because they want to be prepared to engage in later discussion of this information" (Eveland, Jr., 2004). These two processes were observed in discussions about political content (Eveland, Jr., 2004). While we cannot say for sure that these processes were indeed happening in the conversations examined in the study, it's possible that people were taking part in the discussions to learn more or to gain ideas for what to say in a future conversation. Anticipatory elaboration of content about healing from trauma may be a beneficial construct to consider in future research on the relationship between social media conversations and everyday offline interpersonal interactions.

The television show and the subsequent Twitter conversations offered a unique opportunity to theoretically examine, at individual and sociocultural levels, audience engagement with entertainment narratives that address health issues of concern to Black Americans. In contrast to other nonmedical fictional programming dealing with trauma and mental health, *Queen Sugar* particularly emphasized the everyday problems and realities experienced by Black men and women in the United States. The show has been explicit in its pro-social use of television to inform the public about these issues affecting the Black community. The issue of coping with and disclosing traumatic experiences is nuanced and complex, and the show has been an outlier in the amount of time and depth of detail devoted to this sobering topic, including its depictions of family and friends disclosing and discussing traumatic experiences. Data from May 2020 showed that anxiety and depression among Black Americans increased after the video emerged of George Floyd's death (Fowers & Wan, 2020). In 2020, the deaths of Breonna Taylor, Ahmaud Arbery, and George Floyd, among others, sparked global outrage and protests. For Black people, viewing images of these deaths has also produced its own form of trauma. At the same time, people are continually engaging with conversations about these events on social media. Future investigations on discussion-generated elaboration or anticipatory elaboration in health contexts would add much to our understanding of motivations for engaging in social media conversations about health and the implications of such discussions.

Several limitations must be acknowledged for our study. First, the #QueenSugarTalks hashtag provided a rich dataset; however, we only analyzed one hashtag. Analysis of multiple hashtags could give a more nuanced, perhaps longitudinal, understanding of how people respond to culture-centric narratives. However, as the current study explicitly focused on responses to media portrayals of Black American's traumatic experiences, the hashtag provided a solid case for examination. Second, we were not able to examine demographic data of those who participated in the Twitter conversation. Past research on social media users gives us confidence that many of those who used the hashtag had some familiarity with the television show; many would probably identify as Black or African American. Third, another limitation with social media data is that not everyone who participates in conversations is visible and counted. The study relied only on what was classified as unique tweets emerging from Twitter accounts. The audience for the Twitter chat may have been even bigger, given that the majority of tweets captured by the software were retweets of the conversation. While the full stream of tweets would enable us to have a larger sample size, other studies (Francis, 2019) have found that successful analysis of a convenient sample of tweets is sufficient to conduct methodologically sound research. Despite these limitations, our study suggests that Twitter may provide a vehicle for engaging in difficult conversations.

Acknowledgments

We thank the Black community on Twitter. This work would not be possible without them.

ORCID

Diane B. Francis http://orcid.org/0000-0001-8603-3046
LeChrista Finn http://orcid.org/0000-0003-1654-8866

References

Bakari, R. (2019). Black quiet noise: Breaking the silence on sexual assault within the Black community. *Journal of Black Sexuality and Relationships*, *5*(3), 25–41. https://doi.org/10.1353/bsr.2019.0001

Berry, N., Lobban, F., Belousov, M., Emsley, R., Nenadic, G., & Bucci, S. (2017). #WhyWeTweetMH: Understanding why people use Twitter to discuss mental health problems. *Journal of Medical Internet Research*, *19*(4), e107. https://doi.org/10.2196/jmir.6173

Braun, V., & Clarke, V. (2006). Using thematic analysis in psychology. *Qualitative Research in Psychology*, *3*(2), 77–101. https://doi.org/10.1191/1478088706qp063oa

Brock, A., Jr. (2020). *Distributed blackness: African American cybercultures* (Vol. 9). NYU Press.

Brown, W. J. (2015). Examining four processes of audience involvement with media personae: Transportation, parasocial interaction, identification, and worship. *Communication Theory*, *25*(3), 259–283. https://doi.org/10.1111/comt.12053

Eveland, Jr., W. P. (2004). The effect of political discussion in producing informed citizens: The roles of information, motivation, and elaboration. *Political Communication*, *21*(2), 177–193. https://doi.org/10.1080/10584600490443877

Fowers, A., & Wan, W. (2020). Depression and anxiety spiked among Black Americans after George Floyd's death. *Washington Post*. https://www.washingtonpost.com/health/2020/06/12/mental-health-george-floyd-census/?arc404=true

Francis, D. B. (2019). "Twitter is really therapeutic at times": Examination of Black men's Twitter conversations following hip-hop artist Kid Cudi's depression disclosure. *Health Communication*, 1–9. https://doi.org/10.1080/10410236.2019.1700436

Francis, D. B., Stevens, E. M., Noar, S. M., & Widman, L. (2019). Public reactions to and impact of celebrity health announcements: Understanding the Charlie Sheen effect. *Howard Journal of Communications*, *30*(5), 479–494. https://doi.org/10.1080/10646175.2018.1532852

Ginwright, S. (2018). The future of healing: Shifting from trauma informed care to healing centered engagement. *Occasional Paper*, *25*. https://medium.com/@ginwright/the-future-of-healing-shifting-from-trauma-informed-care-to-healing-centered-engagement-634f557ce69c

Hays, K., & Aranda, M. P. (2016). Faith-based mental health interventions with African Americans: A review. *Research on Social Work Practice*, *26*(7), 777–789. https://doi.org/10.1177/1049731515569356

Joe, S. (2006). Explaining changes in the patterns of Black suicide in the United States from 1981 to 2002: An age, cohort, and period analysis. *Journal of Black Psychology*, *32*(3), 262–284. https://doi.org/10.1177/0095798406290465

Jonassaint, C. R., Gibbs, P., Belnap, B. H., Karp, J. F., Abebe, K. Z., & Rollman, B. L. (2017). Engagement and outcomes for a computerised cognitive-behavioural therapy intervention for anxiety and depression in African Americans. *BJPsych Open*, *3*(1), 1–5. https://doi.org/10.1192/bjpo.bp.116.003657

Kessler, T., & Hollbach, S. (2005). Group-based emotions as determinants of ingroup identification. *Journal of Experimental Social Psychology*, *41*(6), 677–685. https://doi.org/10.1016/j.jesp.2005.01.001

Larkey, L. (2015). Toward a measure of reciprocal support in health promotion. *Annals of Behavioral Science and Medical Education*, *12*(2), 58–64.

Larkey, L. K., & Hecht, M. L. (2010). A model of effects of narrative as culture-centric health promotion. *Journal of Health Communication*, *15*(2), 114–135. https://doi.org/10.1080/10810730903528017

Lindsey, M. A., Sheftall, A. H., Xiao, Y., & Joe, S. (2019). Trends of suicidal behaviors among high school students in the United States: 1991–2017. *Pediatrics*, *144*(5), 5. https://doi.org/10.1542/peds.2019-1187

Magruder, K. M., McLaughlin, K. A., & Elmore Borbon, D. L. (2017). Trauma is a public health issue. *European Journal of*

Psychotraumatology, *8*(1), 1375338. https://doi.org/10.1080/20008198.2017.1375338

Mapping Police Violence. (2020). *Mapping police violence*. https://mappingpoliceviolence.org/

McClellan, C., Ali, M. M., Mutter, R., Kroutil, L., & Landwehr, J. (2016). Using social media to monitor mental health discussions - evidence from Twitter. *Journal of the American Medical Informatics Association*, *24*(3), 496–502. https://doi.org/10.1093/jamia/ocw133

Mohatt, N. V., Thompson, A. B., Thai, N. D., & Tebes, J. K. (2014). Historical trauma as public narrative: A conceptual review of how history impacts present-day health. *Social Science & Medicine*, *106*, 128–136. https://doi.org/10.1016/j.socscimed.2014.01.043

Mouzon, D. M., Taylor, R. J., Nguyen, A. W., & Chatters, L. M. (2016). Serious psychological distress among African Americans: Findings from the national survey of American life. *Journal of Community Psychology*, *44*(6), 765–780. https://doi.org/10.1002/jcop.21800

Moyer-Gusé, E. (2008). Toward a theory of entertainment persuasion: Explaining the persuasive effects of entertainment-education messages. *Communication Theory*, *18*(3), 407–425. https://doi.org/10.1111/j.1468-2885.2008.00328.x

Moyer-Gusé, E., Chung, A. H., & Jain, P. (2011). Identification with characters and discussion of taboo topics after exposure to an entertainment narrative about sexual health. *Journal of Communication*, *61*(3), 387–406. https://doi.org/10.1111/j.1460-2466.2011.01551.x

Moyer-Gusé, E., Woods, K., Rader, K., & Luong, K. T. (2020). Talking about TV: Mother-daughter viewing and discussion of an entertainment narrative about teen pregnancy. *Health Communication*, *35*(10), 1200–1209. https://doi.org/10.1080/10410236.2019.1623642

Murphy, S. T., Frank, L. B., Chatterjee, J. S., & Baezconde-Garbanati, L. (2013). Narrative versus nonnarrative: The role of identification, transportation, and emotion in reducing health disparities. *Journal of Communication*, *63*(1), 116–137. https://doi.org/10.1111/jcom.12007

Myrick, J. G., Holton, A. E., Himelboim, I., & Love, B. (2016). #stupidcancer: Exploring a typology of social support and the role of emotional expression in a social media community. *Health Communication*, *31*(5), 596–605. https://doi.org/10.1080/10410236.2014.981664

Slater, M. D. (2002). Entertainment education and the persuasive impact of narratives. In M. C. Green, J. J. Strange, & T. C. Brock (Eds.), *Narrative impact: Social and cognitive foundations* (pp. 157–181). Lawrence Erlbaum Associates Publishers.

Southwell, B. G., & Yzer, M. C. (2007). The roles of interpersonal communication in mass media campaigns. *Communication Yearbook*, *31*(1), 420–462. https://doi.org/10.1080/23808985.2007.11679072

Walters, K. L., Mohammed, S. A., Evans-Campbell, T., Beltrán, R. E., Chae, D. H., & Duran, B. (2011). Bodies don't just tell stories, they tell histories: Embodiment of historical trauma among American Indians and Alaska natives. *Du Bois Review: Social Science Research on Race*, *8*(1), 179–189. https://doi.org/10.1017/S1742058X1100018X

West, C., & Johnson, K. (2013). Sexual violence in the lives of African American women. *VAWnet, a project of the National Resource Center on Domestic Violence*, 1–14. https://vawnet.org/material/sexual-violence-lives-african-american-women-risk-response-and-resilience

Williams, S. (2019). Queen sugar's women directors: Nourishing complex images. *Feminist Media Studies*, *19*(7), 1043–1046. https://doi.org/10.1080/14680777.2019.1667073

Williams, S. L. (2014). Mental health service use among African-American emerging adults, by provider type and recency of use. *Psychiatric Services*, *65*(10), 1249–1255. https://doi.org/10.1176/appi.ps.201300329

"After Philando, I Had to Take a Sick Day to Recover": Psychological Distress, Trauma and Police Brutality in the Black Community

Deion S. Hawkins

ABSTRACT

Unfortunately, encounters between Black Americans and law enforcement frequently feature violence, resulting in a myriad of negative health influences including increased rates of race-based mortality, chronic stress and trauma. Despite police brutality's increased media coverage, there is a dearth of empirical research surrounding violence at the hands of law enforcement and how it impacts the health of the Black community. Police departments across the country fail to release official data or information related to police brutality; however, technological advancements, such as social media and smart phones, have revolutionized information seeking and dissemination related to brutality. Drawing on Critical Race Theory (CRT), this qualitative study used phenomenological interviews to better understand how Black Americans interpret stories of police brutality and the impact such stories have on one's mental health. Analysis confirmed previous quantitative research, revealing the Black community can be traumatized by viewing graphic images or videos of police brutality. Interviewees reported a constant fear of dying, hyper alertness and lack of coping mechanisms. Findings from this study not only should be used to build health communication models that can address mental health issues, but also should be used as a blueprint to improve police-community relations. Implications are drawn from this study for addressing the issue of police violence in the Black community. Policy recommendations are suggested.

Police misconduct is not new, but technological advancements such as social media, smartphones and body cameras now allow an unprecedented amount of access to information related to police violence. Police killings of Black Americans are often video recorded and displayed for all to see via social media and traditional news outlets; these recordings often serve as a catalyst for protests, call for systemic change and the prosecution of the officers responsible (Dawson, 2018). In the past five years, the American Psychological Association (APA) has propelled themselves to the forefront of police brutality. In addition to releasing reports and statements in 2016 that condemned police violence, in 2020, the APA declared racism as a public health emergency (Mills, 2020). In a press release, Sandra L. Shullman, president of the APA, vocalized her concerns stating "we are living in a racism pandemic, which is taking a heavy toll on our African American citizens. The health consequences are dire" (p. 1).

Previous research adequately documents the notion that Black Americans experience police brutality more than other demographics (Bor et al., 2018; J. E. Devylder et al., 2018; Hattery & Smith, 2018), but one area remains elusive- understanding the effects of police killings on Black Americans' mental health (Bor et al., 2018; J. E. Devylder et al., 2018). When it comes to reckoning the toll of police brutality on Black Americans' mental health, accountability requires adequate record-keeping and access to valid data, but since reporting of police brutality is not federally mandated, only 3% of precincts provide information (Davis & Lowery, 2015). While the number of U.S. law enforcement agents killed while on duty is documented; official, reliable and verifiable data related to individuals killed *by* law enforcement are virtually nonexistent (Krieger, Chen, et al., 2015).

Interactions between police officers and civilians are increasingly commonplace in America, but far too often these encounters turn deadly, especially for African-Americans, who are nine times more likely to be killed by police than other Americans (Feldman et al., 2017; Swaine et al., 2016). Previous research suggests police brutality is not an issue of class but of race. Using forty years of data, a study found high-income Black Americans are just as likely to be killed by police officers as low-income Black Americans (Krieger, Kiang, et al., 2015). Still, even these troubling statistics are likely to under-estimate the scale of the problem (Krieger, Chen, et al., 2015). Simply put, little to no information surrounding police violence is being disseminated from law enforcement, and they are frequently the only individuals with all the necessary information (Davis & Lowery, 2015; Krieger, Chen, et al., 2015; Swaine et al., 2016). Furthermore, few studies have centered the voices of Black Americans and explored the health-related consequences of living with the constant threat of racialized police violence. Hence, more research into police brutality – particularly from a health communication perspective – is needed.

Police brutality: A brief explication

There is no single, universally agreed-upon definition of police brutality. At best, the current literature uses two concepts loosely related to police brutality: excessive force and death by legal intervention. The use of force by law enforcement is legal under certain circumstances, such as in self-defense or to protect other individuals. However, there is no federal definition of "excessive force." Instead, officers are guided by "the Use-Of Force Continuum." (National Institute of Justice, 2020). Alpert and Dunham (2004) write, "excessive force refers to situations where government officials legally entitled to use force exceed the minimum amount necessary to diffuse an incident." (p. 21). Outside of excessive force, the government classifies a death at the hands of law enforcement as "death by legal intervention." Death by legal intervention is defined as the killing of a person by a law enforcement officer or other peace officer with specific legal authority to use deadly force acting in the line of duty, excluding legal executions (Gilbert & Ray, 2015). According to the Center For Disease Control (CDC, 2018), death by legal intervention is the third leading cause of violence-related deaths, clearly indicating a threat to public health and worthy of exploration via a health communication lens.

Police brutality can be defined as a police act that harms, dehumanizes or degrades its target. Excessive use of physical violence constitutes brutality, but not all brutality stems from excessive force. Police brutality also includes: false arrests, verbal abuse, intimidation and corruption (Alpert & Dunham, 2004). Some scholars agree that brutality extends past physical violence and includes emotional violence, verbal assault and psychological intimidation (Alang et al., 2017). It is also important to note that brutality *does not require intent;* dehumanization and degradation can occur in the absence of intent.

Police brutality and public health

Police violence has been increasingly recognized as public health issue in the United States (Alang et al., 2017; Bor et al., 2018; J. E. Devylder et al., 2018). Even if an officer has the most noble and innocuous intentions, accidents can still harm one's health. In fact, the CDC has the National Center For Injury Prevention and Control, an entire branch dedicated to examining and responding to the public health influences of accidents, unintentional injuries, and violence (CDC, 2018). In 2014, the World Health Organization also added "violence" as a category associated with the prevention of health risks stating that "violence is the use of physical force or power, threatened or actual, against oneself, another person or against a group or community, which either results in or has a high likelihood of resulting in injury, death, psychological harm, or deprivation," (World Health Organization, 2014, p. 217). Police brutality harms health both directly and indirectly.

Direct health impacts of brutality

The most direct connection between excessive police force and health is as a cause of injury and death (Alang et al., 2017). Krieger et al. write, "police violence events involve mortality and affect the well-being of the families and communities of the deceased," (Krieger, Kiang, et al., 2015, p. 1). Victims of brutality, ranging from George Floyd, Breonna Taylor, and Tamir Rice, succumbed to their injuries related to police brutality. On the other hand, Krieger, Chen, et al. (2015) explain that while fatal acts are the most salient and heinous, less severe forms of police violence are even more common, and these acts also directly influence health outcomes. For example, emergency room reports found that broken bones are often a direct consequence of interactions with law enforcement (Krieger, Chen, et al., 2015).

Indirect impacts of police brutality

Beyond the clear consequence of direct injury and increased race based mortality, police killings also indirectly affect the Black community by harming mental health. Krieger and colleagues (Krieger, Kiang, et al., 2015) write,

> Combine excessive police violence with inadequate prosecution of such violence, and the ties that bind citizens and their democratically elected governments become deeply frayed, with vicious cycles of distrust and violence fueling dysfunctional policing and dysfunctional governance more generally The direct effects and spill-over effects matter for public health and medicine alike, as reflected in the impact on emergency medical services, trauma units, mental health, and the trust required to deliver and implement any government- sponsored program, public health or otherwise. (p. 43)

There is little research surrounding the influence of witnessing brutality specifically, but exposure to violence in the Black community has been well researched (Gillikin et al., 2016; Jenkins, 2002; Sheats et al., 2018). Inner city youth frequently report elevated stress and symptoms of PTSD (Gillikin et al., 2016), and between 26% and 70% of African-Americans have been exposed to violent incidents, such as gang violence or witnessing a shooting or abuse at the hands of law enforcement (Jenkins, 2002). Three previous studies (E. Devylder et al., 2015; Koyanagi et al., 2016; Smith-Lee & Robinson, 2019) analyzed the psychiatric impact of police encounters and found that perceived unfair treatment and aggressive policing significantly affected the prevalence of mood and anxiety disorders. Another study revealed that police presence and associated perceived threat of police harassment or violence was considered a top neighborhood stressor (Sewell & Jefferson, 2016).

Next, trauma is an additional outcome closely related to witnessing violence. Judith Herman (2015) notes that psychological trauma is an affliction of the powerless; when trauma occurs, the victim is rendered helpless. Notably, Herman (2015) states that trauma and violence are not synonymous; violence can lead to trauma, but not all violence is inherently traumatizing. Traumatic events must involve a threat to one's life, bodily integrity, or a personal encounter with violence and death. She writes, "traumatized people do not have a normal baseline level of alert. Instead, they have an elevated baseline of arousal, their bodies are always on alert for danger," (p. 36).

As a response to alleviate trauma, multiple fields, including public health and communication, have advocated for the use of trauma-informed approaches. In their study documenting Black men's exposures to police violence, Smith-Lee and Robinson (2019) note the importance of utilizing a trauma-informed approach when analyzing the Black community's perception of law enforcement. A joint report by the CDC and National Center for Trauma-Informed Care (NCTIC), outlined six principles that ought to guide a trauma-informed approach: safety, trustworthiness/transparency, peer support, collaboration/mutuality, empowerment/choice and cultural, historical & gender issues (CDC, 2020). When applied correctly, trauma informed approaches can increase awareness of the impact of trauma and help individuals understand the community where they work (CDC, 2020). Furthermore, the APA has recently outlined the importance of "citizen psychologists," clinicians who give voices to marginalized voices and who "aspire to understand the power and privilege lying at the core of multicultural tensions and the impact of this oppression," (2017, p. 46).

Previous research strongly suggests that violence, regardless of who enacts it, breeds trauma and distress within a community, but a research void exists. First, most of these studies are quantitative, asking respondents to indicate trauma and reactions to events using a scale. However, Herman (2015) notes trauma exists within specific social settings and is steeped in one's understanding of feelings, actions and motives; this perspective is a linchpin of qualitative research (Lindlof & Taylor, 2019). Second, previous research does not allow respondents to give their own definition of trauma and how it manifests, and this study is one of the first to explicitly document the Black community's perceptions and reactions to police brutality. Finally, at best, previous research stops at the surface level, neglecting the opportunity to engage in a rich discussion about the relationships between race, police brutality, mental health and trauma. In short, research suggests violence and trauma can lead to negative mental health outcomes, but no research provides Black respondents the opportunity to explain how or why this is the case.

Critical race theory (CRT) and public health

Often used in education and legal studies, Critical race theory (CRT) is a race-equity methodology rooted in social justice (C. Ford & Airhihenbuwa, 2018). At its core, CRT argues that we must reconceptualize our understanding of race and racism; racism is not always overt acts of racial discrimination at the individual level. Instead, CRT promotes a framework that identifies and targets the subtle and systemic ways in which racism, especially Anti-Blackness, operates in our country (Crenshaw et al., 2010). L. Ford and Airhihenbuwa (2010) contend that race is often ignored in public health/health communication. They argue CRT can and should be applied to better understand race-based health disparities and outline four distinct characteristics associated with critical race theory and public health: (1) race consciousness, (2) contemporary mechanisms, (3) centered to margins and (4) praxis (L. Ford & Airhihenbuwa, 2010).

One of the leading scholars of CRT, Kimberlé Crenshaw, has adequately documented CRT's direct connection to police brutality. For example, in 1993, Crenshaw argued the acquittal of Rodney King's assailants was not merely a one-time act of injustice, but instead, it highlighted a criminal justice system ripe with systemic inequities. Crenshaw (1993) explains that our court system is not neutral nor colorblind, and in the case of Rodney King, lawyers purposely sought to isolate the video from its actual context. By doing so, jurors viewed the video of his beating through the lens of racist stereotypes of Black male aggression and anger. Jurors no longer saw a Black man fighting for his life – they saw a Black man fighting police who were vulnerable victims (Crenshaw, 1993). This application of CRT can still be applied nearly 30 years later. As Crenshaw (2020) argued to the Congressional House Oversight Committee regarding police brutality against Black women, intersectionality is crucial in any work driven by CRT.

Even though race is a well-known sociodeterminant of health, public health and health communication scholars frequently present studies that do not respond to structural racism (L. Ford & Airhihenbuwa, 2010). Ford and Airhihenbuwa write, "although race is salient to public health in a variety of ways, the field's theoretical and methodological conventions inadequately address the complexity with which structural racism influences both health and the production of knowledge about populations, health, and health disparities" (p. 531). An application of CRT to police brutality allows one to better understand structural racism's influence on police violence, a well–documented health disparity.

Research question

Previous quantitative literature (Bor et al., 2018; J. E. Devylder et al., 2018) indicatesexposure to brutality and witnessing violence can lead to adverse mental health symptoms for Black Americans. However, to my knowledge, no prior study has used CRT and interviews to capture the lived realities, experiences and perceptions of Black Americans of all genders as it relates to police brutality. Thus, the following research question guided the study:

RQ: How do Black Americans feel after viewing/hearing instances of police brutality?

Methods

Recruitment & participants

Black Americans above the age of 18 were eligible to participate in the study. This study (1,195,331-1) was approved by the Institutional Review Board at George Mason University. Respondents were recruited using convenience and snowball sampling. I posted the solicitation message on various social media websites including Facebook and Twitter and emailed the message to multiple national academic organization listservs, such as the National Communication Association, Pi Kappa Delta, the National Forensic Association. Next, the solicitation message was sent to multiple advisors and presidents of Black student organizations at universities in the area. Lastly, I located a key informant in an underserved area of the Washington D. C. and through network sampling, he provided me with the contact information for multiple individuals who live in the community. Originally, there was a dearth of Black women respondents, but because of the importance of intersectionality (Crenshaw, 1993) and #SayHerName campaign, I encouraged Black women to reach out to their networks and prompt participation.

Twenty-seven semi-structured interviews were conducted in Spring 2018. The average interviewee was 26 years old with ages ranging from 19 to 43. Educational attainment ranged from high school to a terminal degree (MD, PhD). Fourteen respondents identified as men, eleven as women and two identified themselves as non-binary/third gender.

Data collection

When possible, participants had a choice as to how they were interviewed. Of the 27 interviews, 22 were conducted in person while the remaining 5 were completed via telephone. Telephone interviews were recorded using a call-recording application on the principal investigator's smart phone. As sole author, I conducted all interviews, which had an average time of 43 minutes, but ranged from 31 to 97 minutes. All names were changed to pseudonyms. All participants provided verbal and electronic informed consent.

A semi-structured interview guide was used to collect data. The construction of the interview guide and the interview themselves were guided by trauma-informed approaches, and the researcher completed a trauma training to better assist respondents during their interview. The first set of questions centered on capturing demographic data (e.g., age, gender, education). The second set of questions focused on respondents' exposure to stories related to police brutality (e.g., "Tell me about some stories of police brutality," "What do you remember most about these stories? Why? "Where do you go to learn more about stories of police brutality? Why?"). The third set of questions focused on the mental health impact of consuming information and watching videos related to police brutality (e.g., "After you heard about this case, how did you feel? Please explain why."). I probed for clarification when necessary. Interviews were conducted until data saturation, or the point where little to no new information related to respondent experiences was achieved (Glaser & Strauss, 2017).

Data analysis

All interviews were recorded and transcribed within two weeks of completion. Data were analyzed to isolate themes and reveal a patterned response and meaning in the data Braun and Clarke (2006). Thematic analysis allows a researcher to better understand the experiences, meanings and reality of their respondents (Braun & Clarke, 2006). This study utilized Smith's (1995) five-part thematic analysis process. First, although I conducted and transcribed all of the interviews, I re-read the transcripts to famialrize myself with the data and get a preliminary understanding of respondents' experiences. Second, while reading transcripts, I made detailed notes and identified potential themes. Owen (1984) notes themes should meet the criteria of recurrence, repetition and forcefulness. Third, building on Owen (1984) and using my notes, I filtered and inductively coded to isolate the most prevalent themes in the data. Lastly, after identifying themes, I selected rich, thick quotations to illustrate and support the themes.

Once the coding process was complete, I shared my findings with three senior faculty in my department, and in turn, they affirmed my themes, revealing a form of researcher triangulation (Creswell & Poth, 2018). Finally, since I was the sole coder, in order to maximize validity, I engaged in member checks (Creswell, 2014) and shared my themes with two respondents; they confirmed the themes accurately reflected their experience and reality.

Findings

Analysis yielded four themes: (1) debilitating sadness, (2) hyperarousal/chronic fear of dying, (3) constant sense of helplessness and (4) lack of healthy coping mechanisms.

Debilitating sadness

When asked about their feelings after viewing videos or images, nearly every participant indicated intense sadness as the primary emotion. For example, one respondent, Charlie, said, "Bro, I am not even a crier, but shit, seeing people who look like you, your friends, your family (pause) . . . .constantly get killed without punishment. Of course, it gets to you. I'm human bro (pause) . . . . So, yea . . . . I cried." Another respondent, Chanelle, stated, " I feel a wave of emotions. Anger. (pause) Hmmmm . . . .it's stronger than anger. Rage, I'd say. But that rage always ends up turning into sadness. So, you get pissed off and next, you cry." Although virtually every interviewee revealed sadness as the primary emotion, their responses to handling such sadness varied. Some respondents maintained a strong façade, articulating that while they were sad, they did not have the luxury of grieving:

> Of course, I felt sad. I think any Black person in America felt sad after Trayvon. But I couldn't let my sadness get in the way. That meant they won. I couldn't let White people know they had broke me down. Grandma always said you can never let them see you sweat. -Lena, Black female.

> It's a part of being Black in America man. There have been hella times where I wanted to just lay around and do nothing, but I can't. If I had a penny for every time some fucked up shit happened to me cause I was Black, I would be rich. Bill Gates type rich. -Mark, Black male

While Lena and Mark portrayed tenets of strength and perseverance, several respondents expressed the polar opposite. Exposure to police brutality ushers in sadness, often resulting in emotional strain and breakdowns:

> Sometimes I feel disgust toward cops and at random times, I find myself literally sobbing. I think what if that were me? What if that were someone in my family? It's so personal even if I don't know that person specifically, I know someone similar to that person. -Imani, Black female

Imani's experience is just the tip of the iceberg. Further analysis shows a pattern of sadness after consuming media related to police brutality:

> Philando Castile. I was rrreeallly sad. Philando was the boiling point. I cracked. I literally had to leave my desk at work and take a break. When I came back, my White coworkers told me I was overreacting because I didn't know him. Which pissed me off. What they don't get is that Philando could be anyone in my family. It's not just Philando, it's that I fear my brothers could be shot in cold blood at any moment. That's why I was so damn sad. -Chanelle, Black female

Chanelle shared how police brutality impedes her ability to function at work. Others shared her frustrations. After consuming information related to police brutality, a dark cloud of sadness hangs over the heads of Black Americans. This emotional plague often hinders Black Americans' ability to complete daily tasks:

> Oh yea bro, I was sad, I don't even know if sad is the right word. Bro, after Tamir Rice, I straight up looked at my 10 year old brother and cried. He didn't get it and he had never seen me cry before. I couldn't do shit for legit like two to three days. I missed hella assignments, and tried to explain to professors why I was struggling. Bro, at least I was honest. I told them the video had me feeling some type of way. Guess what they did? Nothing. They told me I was making excuses and the only deaths that are excused are my immediate family. -Charlie, Black male

> I remember I walked into work, face cut up and people were like what's wrong? What happened? I told them I had been in a fight. But really, I had been beat up by a police officer who assumed I was someone else. I appreciated them asking me if I was ok, but I wasn't really comfortable telling them, you know? We had previous conversations that let me know, they didn't really think Black Lives Mattered. Corporate world is a whole other beast. I couldn't explain to them that I was innocent and was profiled. It was frustrating as hell. I had to deal with the cop himself, then, had to deal with ignorant White people. And after Philando, I had to take a sick day to recover. That's how sad I was man. I've never felt anything like that before in my life. -Darius, Black male

> There are days when you just don't feel like getting out the house and don't go anywhere. Because everybody is going to have an opinion and wants to share that opinion regardless of if you wanna hear it or not. I wasn't for it. I did not have the energy to talk about race. So I just stayed in the house for days. -Nicole, Black female

This finding is incredibly important for a myriad of reasons. First, as mentioned above, police brutality is interfering with the Black community's ability to conduct daily tasks. Nicole's statement revealed that her sadness forced her to stay in the house. Long term, intense sadness is linked to a multitude of negative health outcomes including depression, suicide and substance abuse (Tebeka et al., 2017). Second, in addition to this, many respondents feared losing their jobs for being too vocal about police brutality, further exacerbating stress. As Chanelle explained:

> Being Black at work means you have to constantly chose. You can say what's really on your heart and risk the job, or keep quiet and make these coins. It's a lose-lose either way. I know one of my friends quit their job because their boss said something about Eric Garner, but then he was broke. So, he was stressed more. Like I said, It's a lose-lose.

Chanelle's statement alludes to systemic racism in the workplace, a well-documented phenomenon for many Black Americans, especially in corporate and business settings (Holder et al., 2015). Third, this finding suggests Black Americans encounter sadness on two fronts-the first wave occurs once the actual image, story or video is consumed. However, analysis indicates the second wave of sadness occurs *after* one has had dismissive conversations with White peers. Paired together, these constant acts of racism, brutality and emotional dismissal, create the perfect storm for chronic stress. Fourth, this research demonstrates that Black Americans do not need to know the victim directly to feel sadness. Witnessing police violence on TV or a computer screen is enough to spark debilitating sadness in the participants.

Hyperarousal/chronic fear of dying

Similar to intense sadness, interviewees discussed their chronic fear of dying at the hands of law enforcement. In turn, this fear prompts a permanent state of hyperarousal. Herman (2015) contends after traumatic events, our bodies never return to a normal level of alertness/arousal; the Black community is always on alert for danger at the hands of police and constantly feel like they are going to die when they encounter a police officer:

> Whenever I see cops, I tense up. One time cops pulled up to me when I was in a car and my friend looked at me with the straightest face and said "one of us is about to die. I was so shocked and I said "that's not funny." But he was serious. He really thought one of us was going to die. -Mary, Black female

> There is not a single time where I can sit in a car and hear a siren or see a cop light flash, that I'm not fearful. I get so tense. I imagine it's like what soldiers feel when they hear anything that sounds like a bomb. When I hear sirens, I start to look around and hope that someone else is around. Because If I were to get shot, I would want someone to be able to tell the truth. People are straight up dropping at the hands of police. I never want to be in that situation. -Luke, Black male

Mary and Luke both expressed increased tension in their bodies as a response to interacting with police officers. Luke's statement also reveals he feels emotionally "triggered" when he sees a cop's lights and/or sirens; as Luke articulated, such a reaction is well documented in veterans who are diagnosed with PTSD (Mcdonald et al., 2019). Mary mentioned an intense encounter while a friend was with her, but others expressed the constant fear of being alone and shot in cold blood:

> I get very anxious and scared when I'm by myself. There is no one else to see what's going on. No one else that could step in if necessary. One of my greatest fears is being stopped by police when I'm alone. I literally have nightmares about it. (DH: Can you tell me more about these nightmares?) After Alton Sterling, I had a fucked up dream. (Interviewee: Oh man. Sorry. Can I cuss? DH: Say exactly what you want. Be yourself.) I'm a barber. So one time I had a dream that I was standing outside the shop and a cop came up and I don't remember how or why, but I got choked out. Woke up sweaty and scared as hell. -Derek, Black male

Although Derek did not mention it, night sweats and nightmares are two common manifestations of PTSD (Mcdonald et al., 2019). When a probing question related to PTSD was asked, Derek explained, "I never thought of it like that. I know my homies who went to Iraq have nightmares, but damn, it never occurred to me that that may be what's happening to me. " Similar to Derek, others expressed hyperarousal when alone:

> I'm always scared and alert honestly. I walk around on campus and I use my iPad to listen to music. I always have my iPad with me. It's weird because I think about how I need to hold my iPad to make sure cops know it's an iPad. Especially at night. I'm afraid the police are going to see me holding my iPad and assume it's something else and before I have time to explain what it is, I'm afraid I would be shot. I always have my headphones in too. I replay this terrible scenario in my head over and over again. A cop is yelling at me to stop, but since my headphones are in, I can't hear him and keep walking. He thinks I am running away and shoots me in my back (long pause). So sometimes, I won't listen to music at all. I have to be aware of my surroundings at all times. -Corey, Black male

When asked why he felt this way, like Derek and Luke, Corey reiterated the multiple cases of police brutality where unarmed Black men were shot and killed by law enforcement. The examples above tell hypothetical situations, but many revealed nearly fatal encounters with police officers:

> One time I was going home with one of my friends and we were 5mph over the speed limit. We got pulled over by the police. While she was talking to one officer, I had no idea there was another officer so when she was told to get out the car, I was going to get out the car too. But the officer that was on my side . . . . . .he had his gun out. I didn't know what to do. I thought to myself, it's just 5 mph over the limit and next thing I know, I had a gun at my face. I thought I was going to die. I tried to turn on my camera but he yelled at me and told me I couldn't move. So I sat back in my seat and didn't move a muscle. Now, I count the number of cops I see every day. -Nicole, Black female

Some participants particularly Black women, voiced fears that small things such as a "nasty" look, shift of tone, increased volume or communicative use of hands, could lead to a fatal interaction, increasing their awareness of body movements and facial expressions.

> Police need to do a better job and understand that we are scared and why we are scared. We are alert for a damn reason. They need to do a better job at understanding communities. The argument that they fear for their life is a piss poor excuse. I fear for my life every day. I live in a predominantly White neighborhood. I fear for my life on a daily basis, but that doesn't give me the go ahead to just punch somebody in the face. If I look at a cop wrong, I feel like I become his target practice. -Tiffany, Black female

> Black people . . . I don't know . . . .we are just more expressive. Or at least I think so. And I'm Jamaican so I have an accent and speak loudly (laughter) and use my hands. One time I left a bar and was accused of taking some White girl's purse. I was pissed because first of all, I have no reason to steal. Second of all, I had no idea what the hell they were even talking about. They showed me a picture and I said don't nobody want that ugly ass purse. (laughter). A cop came up to ask me a question and I told her, mam I'm wearing a dress, where can I hide the purse? She said she felt threatened because I was using my hands to talk. (eye roll) So I put my hands behind my back. Then, she told me my tone was aggressive. It's like we damned if we do, damned if we don't. Always gotta be on yo toes with cops. A damn shame, but it's true. Tell the truth and shame the Devil (laughter). It aint fair but I wanna stay alive. - Charlotte, Black female

Tiffany and Charlotte's experiences support the notion that hyperarousal is heavily experienced by both Black men and women, highlighting the importance of #SayHerName.

Constant sense of helplessness

Charlotte's latter remarks of "damned if we do, damned if we don't" encapsulates the feeling of helplessness and powerlessness. Herman (2015) argues trauma is most often inflicted on those without power, leaving the victim helpless. Heightened locus of control and increased self-efficacy are foundational concepts of many health models (Brincks et al., 2010). However, when it comes to curbing police brutality and the negative health impacts, the Black community feels powerless. Analysis reveals Black Americans feel like they have no control over interactions with police; regardless of their tone, behavior or actions, law enforcement will continue to plague the community with violence. Many interviewees revealed first-hand accounts of police brutality where their health was placed at risk at the hands of law-enforcement:

> I'm convinced there is nothing you can do to change a cop's mind. I've seen it happen too many times. I was out on U Street with some friends when cops came up to ask us questions. Felt like an interrogation. No answer was enough. No matter what we said or did, the cops were going to assume we were up to no good. We followed every rule. Yes sir, No sir, made no sudden movements. Kept our hands visible at all times. Did everything we were taught and still, somehow, some way, a cop ended up slamming my friend on the ground. Fractured one of his ribs. We all sat there shocked. We wanted to help him, but we knew that jumping in meant the cop was going to shoot us. So we just sat there man, helpless. Waiting for my friend to be uncuffed. – Chad, Black male

For many respondents, including Chad, the sense of helplessness was not just a hypothetical situation sparked by viewing videos of police brutality, instead, the feeling of powerlessness was rooted in a negative previous experience with officers. During the interviews, others mentioned that they were willing to place themselves in harms way to *avoid* calling law enforcement:

> It's a sad reality to accept that no matter how you dress, how you talk, a police officer will always judge you and think you're a threat. I don't think we have control over if we are going to get beat or not. Black folks could literally read a how to survive book and do every step, but cops would still find some reason to make the situation worse. We are always in a catch 22. If we talk too much, we are talking back. If we talk too little, we are suspicious. I do everything in my power to avoid cops. Listen, someone broke in my house and I refused to call the police. I be damned. (DH: Why did you refuse to call the police?) Because I think they would have assumed I was the robber and shot me.

-Lena, Black female

Lena's experience illuminates a dreary reality for many Black Americans- she feels safer in her home with a burglar than a cop. Others elaborated on their violent encounters with law enforcement, and how that has morphed into helplessness at best, and at worst, a constant fear of being in danger:

> (DH: Talk me through what happened next. What do you remember?) My dad told him he was reaching in the glove box and the officer was just standing there and shouted "is there a weapon the glove box" and pointed his gun at us. The other officer hit the glass and told me to roll down my window. My dad rolled the window down and I was terrified. My dad is the strongest man and I know, but I watched my father, a man I looked up to and admire, I'm looking at this person who turned into not weak, but turned into a very docile being. I felt like in that moment if something were to happen, the person who I looked to to protect me, wouldn't be able to do so. We were weak. Vulnerable. The cops harassed both of us, pointed a gun at us, and we couldn't do anything about it. Coming to that realization shook me to my core. I have felt unsafe since then. I have never felt so helpless in my life. -Tiffany, Black female

More troubling, analysis also revealed interviewees viewed this form of helplessness as a cycle they had no control over, completely eradicating any locus of control or self-efficacy:

> It's definitely a cycle. Things are a hot issue for three months. Black boy gets murdered. Cops don't get arrested. If they do get arrested, they are acquitted. Black boy gets buried. It's all gonna be wrapped

> up and done, but never really wrapped up because it happens again. It's never done for us. -Charlotte, Black female

> Every time I see a video, I feel an intense sadness. It feels like you are in the world's worst (pause) cycle I guess. Some kind of sick joke. It's like damn, it happened again. Like nothing is ever going to change. Things may look like they are getting better, but then even when they are arrested, the sadness continues because you know they aren't going to get charged. We are left there left to dry again and there aint shit we can do about it. -Virginia, Black female

This theme supports the notion that police brutality serves as a catalyst for many negative psychological health outcomes. In social work and psychology, two fields directly linked to health communication, the sentiments echoed above are known as "learned helplessness," a condition often seen in individuals who experience severe intimate partner violence, state sanctioned torture or constant war (O'Rourke et al., 1980). The impact of learned helplessness on one's health and well-being is well documented. Individuals who are confronting learned helplessness often face elevated rates of depression, increased suicide attempts, heightened stress levels, and less desire to take steps to improve their physical health (Bargai et al., 2007; Maier & Seligman, 2016; Trindade et al., 2020). Next, similar to the finding related to sadness, this analysis reveals psychological distress occurs at two stages– (1) the initial incident and (2) the frequent acquittal of law enforcement. Black Americans are not dealing with a one-time instance of a negative health outcome, but, instead, are constantly having to deal with the pain of brutality. In an attempt to reckon with the pain of brutality, the Black community desperately needs effective coping strategies, but the next theme illustrates coping is virtually non-existent.

Lack of healthy coping

As participants continued to express their experiences and how they process stories of brutality, another finding emerged. The participants rarely cope with their psychological distress and trauma related to police brutality. The majority of respondents explicitly stated they never cope with these issues:

> (pause) I don't think I do cope. What does coping even look like? I don't really ever want to accept things like this as normal. Like I said, I've become numb to some it. Sometimes that makes me feel terrible, the fact that I can hear a story and my only thought is it happened again. Being that flat about it (pause) that scares me. Damn, you got me thinking now (laughter). Yea, I don't cope. Maybe me going numb is coping? I don't know. -Meka, Black female

Meka's story illustrates a flat affect, expressing a numbness related to hearing stories of brutality. Some interviewees felt like even if they knew *how* to cope, there is not *time* to cope:

> I don't think we ever unpack the pain that we are going through. We are expected to be the activists, but no one ever asks if we are okay? People come to us and ask "what do we do next?" But I need to decompress. People expect us to have all the answers and sometimes, I don't want to give the answers. Sometimes, I don't want to talk about brutality. When brutality happens, every Black person becomes an ambassador, people expect you to raise awareness. But that means we never get to truly cry or express our emotions. We have to suck it up and advocate. -Taylor, gender non-binary

Meka and Taylor shared their realities as it relates to lack of coping, but other responses highlighted some coping mechanisms. For those that did report methods of coping, social support in the form of friends was the most common response:

> I'm the type of person who needs to talk things out. Umm and not on social media though, but actually going to my core group. Friends that I can be vulnerable with who can help me find the language and guidance. They let me know that I still have people who care about me and don't view my Blackness as a target. -Mary, Black female

> Thank God I have a solid group of friends. Watching someone die on camera is rough. But my friends helped me get through it. (DH: how so? Did you guys talk about what happened?) Yea I guess we talk about the case, but it really turns out to be a conversation about how much we hate the police (laughter). It may not be healthy, but it's all we got. -Dejuan, Black male

Finally, some participants in the study explicitly called for the Black community to seek the help of licensed mental health professionals:

> We need to see professionals. Trained professionals. A check up from the neck up (laughter) I actually tried to go to one before, but it did not go well. My therapist was White. Lilly White (laughter). And she literally told me my feelings weren't valid. She told me that I should avoid social media if I was getting overwhelmed. Chile, I looked at that women like she was crazy. Like she had three heads. I'm pissed she got my money (laughter). -Chanelle, Black female

Although Chanelle takes a lighthearted approach, her quotation exposes a lack of culturally competent mental health providers. If there is any hope to mitigate the impact of brutality, clinicians must validate the experiences of Black Americans. Michelle shared her perspective on coping strategies and how the Black community has a morbid history of carrying trauma.

> Talking to a professional would be great. Everyone copes in their own ways. I think talking to a professional would help guide steps in the direction of healthy coping, the direction at which to go. I just had a conversation with one of my best friends about this. Trauma is inflicted upon us by other people, and we have the unfortunately responsibility of living with it. It's now a part of who we are, a part of our journey. Letting feelings fester is not going to help anyone at all. It's not our fault but it is our problem. -Michelle, Black female

Discussion

This study is one of the first qualitative studies to document how police brutality translates to psychological impacts I investigated how Black Americans interpret stories of police brutality and the resulting psychological distress and trauma related to police violence. This was accomplished by interviewing Black Americans and documenting their perception of their mental health. Framing police violence as a health communication, and therefore, a public health issue, has critical implications. The findings warrant further discussion.

Insight/Implications

First, police brutality undoubtedly harmed the mental health of the participants, and the findings expose multiple theoretical and knowledge gaps in the field of health communication. Analysis from this study suggests the field of health communication ought to embrace CRT and because trauma has a direct impact on how one's past shapes their present, we ought to integrate more literature surrounding the Black experience, in both historical and contemporary contexts. Regarding knowledge, much of the current health communication research surrounding aspects of mental health studies disclosure, social support, and stigma. Findings from this study suggests we need more research about trauma in the Black community, and how the community copes with police brutality specifically. Most importantly, health communication desperately needs trauma-based communication models that can frame brutality as a health communication issue.

Next, in addition to advocating for a more racially equitable approach to *studying* health communication, this study advocates for a shift in how scholars teach health communication. I implore scholars to infuse CRT in their courses, asking students to analyze racism as a system that depends on racial stratification opposed to individual acts of discrimination. Health communication courses should (1) explore mental health in the Black community, (2) deconstruct the historical roots of racial inequity in healthcare and (3) create trauma-informed syllabi that can equip students, especially Black students, with the skills to engage in robust discussions surrounding police brutality. Currently, many individual based health models/theories relay on self-efficacy and locus of control, but these concepts were diminished for the participants. Therefore, I argue police brutality is best addressed through adopting CRT and communal or ecological frameworks; frameworks such as People and Places (Maibach et al., 2007) are more equipped to address brutality. Similar to the APA's (American Psychological Association, 2017) call to focus on ecological factors and sociocultural contexts, this study suggests this health outcome is predicated on systemic factors, thus, a critical approach that analyses how systems and environment operates is ideal. Simply put, following CRT, this study reinforces the notion that racism is a mechanism of oppression that depends on inequity in society's systems and structures; therefore, adopting an ecological model that utilizes CRT is uniquely equipped to tackle this systemic issue.

On the other hand, if brutality was to be addressed as an individual behavior, findings suggest the onus of this behavior change is on law enforcement, not the Black community. Yet, as the recent cases of George Floyd and Breonna Taylor reveal, police departments often double down on their protocol. They refuse to admit fault, and frequently blame the Black community for acts of violence. Unfortunately, if both assailant (law enforcement) and victim (Black community) feel as if they have no control over the health behavior of brutality, it is destined to continue.

Second, participants reported clear markers of trauma throughout the duration of the study, and this finding aligns with previous research (Bor et al., 2018; Smith-Lee & Robinson, 2019). However, this study is one of the first to document the cyclical of nature of psychological distress for many Black Americans. For the participants, trauma and distress were not a one-time event, instead, a constant struggle that impacts one's mental health. Initially, the distress is related brutality itself, as the act of witnessing violence was enough to spark trauma. However, participants also reported elevated distress once (1) cops were acquitted and (2) they had to have conversations *about* incidents related to brutality with white Americans, especially in the workplace. The lived experiences of the participants revealed a vicious cycle for many Black Americans- murder, acquittal and dismissal. Therefore, any efforts to mitigate the mental health impacts of brutality must adapt a multi-pronged approach and be implemented at various times in the cycle. For example, one may not feel distress after seeing a story of brutality because law enforcement was arrested and charged, but they could start to experience distress if the cop is found not guilty.

Third, the study highlights the dire impact of police brutality on the community even when there is no direct connection to the victim. Previous research (Bor et al., 2018; J. E. Devylder et al., 2018) was predicated on not knowing the victim, *but* whether the victim lived in the same neighborhood or state. This analysis shows viewing a video of a case hundreds of miles away can negatively influence mental health. For example, multiple respondents reported the murder of Philando Castile prompted a level of sadness that they had never experienced. Simply, the state sanctioned murder of Black bodies hinders the mental health of Black Americans *even* when the person is a complete stranger. In addition to this, findings from the study suggest that consuming media, including videos, social media posts and news coverage about police brutality can serve as a trigger for the Black community. Therefore, I argue social media sites and news station across the country have a moral obligation to better monitor stories of police brutality. If the act of viewing or hearing about another case of brutality is enough to wreak emotional distress for the participants, the media choosing to show such traumatic stories is not just morally irresponsible, it is dehumanizing for Black Americans and a threat to our nation's public health.

Practical suggestions

Overall, it is important to articulate the various ways this research can help curb the negative health impacts of police brutality. Three recommendations emerged from my analysis: (1) push for more culturally competent mental health clinicians, (2) de-escalation training and (3) media content warnings. Analysis showed the tangible influences of brutality on the Black community, but most disheartening, were the blatant dismissals of those feelings. One respondent even indicated being ridiculed by a mental health clinician. The American Psychological Association and the National Association of Social Work should mandate formal culturally competence trainings for mental health care providers that include instruction about race-based trauma. It is important to note that we must not only increase the number of clinicians available, but also equip them with the trauma training and knowledge to mitigate the impact of brutality and its resulting race based trauma, specifically. Trauma, including vicarious trauma, has psychological and physiological impacts, and thus, clinicians must be better equipped to help heal the effects on the nervous system (Van der Kolk, 1989). Again, I argue race based trauma ought to have its own specific training since previous research clearly indicates it is different than PTSD (Alang et al., 2017; Gillikin et al., 2016; Smith-Lee & Robinson, 2019). Second, de-escalation tactics for law enforcement officers who interact with the public should be mandated by the federal government. Currently, de-escalation is not mandated, local law enforcement agencies are "encouraged" to undergo such trainings. Lastly, if images and stories are fueling intense adverse reactions, media companies should install more stringent content warnings about the potential influences of viewing graphic imagery concerning police violence.

Limitations and future research

The findings of the study must be interpreted with limitations in mind. First, despite conducting member checks and ensuring triangulation, the analysis of the data relied on one coder, but different researchers may code interviews in vastly different ways (Clark et al., 2018). Next, as with any qualitative study utilizing interviews, the findings are not designed to be generalized, instead, they only represent the lived experiences and realities of the 27 participants. The final limitation is a bit unorthodox, but valid qualitative research requires reflexivity. In order to ensure a smooth IRB approval and protect the well-being of the participants, I prepared various resources that would help respondents cope with their traumatic experiences. However, I did not account for the toll the stories would take on myself. For weeks, I listened, transcribed and analyzed stories of individuals who looked like me being systematically oppressed, brutalized and killed. Eventually, hearing people's lived experiences of how they fear death every day was an emotionally taxing endeavor.

Even with limitations, the study gave voice to a marginalized population and provided information that is ripe for further research. For example, it is important to understand how police officers perceive their self-efficacy and locus of control related to police brutality; a study analyzing how law enforcement views the health impacts of their actions would be an important addition to health communication. Second, findings suggest a high level of communal grief and community spill over of negative mental health impacts; more research is needed to understand *why* Black Americans have such a visceral reaction to the stories of strangers. Lastly, in terms of mental health, we need to better understand the concept of learned helplessness in the Black community. When looking at the analysis, there were some stark parallels to issues found in intimate partner violence research (Palker-Corell & Marcus, 2004). How can one ever feel safe in a world where their skin color makes them a target? Is it possible to mitigate this constant fear of death?

Conclusion

Police brutality is an issue rooted in communication and health, yet research is sparse. Applying Critical Race Theory, this study captured how 26 Black Americans felt after consuming information related to police brutality. Analysis revealed that the circulated information of police brutality fuels psychological distress and trauma in the Black community.

ORCID

Deion S. Hawkins http://orcid.org/0000-0003-3032-0462

References

Alang, S., McAlpine, D., Mccreedy, E., & Hardeman, R. (2017). Police brutality and Black health: Setting the agenda for public health scholars. *American Journal of Public Health, 107*(5), 662–665. https://doi.org/10.2105/ajph.2017.303691

Alpert, G., & Dunham, R. (2004). Police use of force: The history of research. *Understanding Police Use of Force*, 17–53. https://doi.org/10.1017/cbo9780511499449.002

American Psychological Association. (2017). *Multicultural guidelines: An ecological approach to context, identity, and intersectionality*. APA.org. https://www.apa.org/about/policy/multicultural-guidelines.pdf

Bargai, N., Ben-Shakhar, G., & Shalev, A. Y. (2007). Posttraumatic stress disorder and depression in battered women: The mediating role of learned helplessness. *Journal of Family Violence, 22*(5), 267–275. https://doi.org/10.1007/s10896-007-9078-y

Bor, J., Venkataramani, A. S., Williams, D. R., & Tsai, A. C. (2018). Police killings and their spill over effects on the mental health of black Americans: A population-based, quasi-experimental study. *The Lancet, 392*(10144), 302–310. https://doi.org/10.1016/s0140-6736(18)31130-9

Braun, V., & Clarke, V. (2006). Using thematic analysis in psychology. *Qualitative Research in Psychology, 3*(2), 77–101. https://doi.org/10.1191/1478088706qp063oa

Brincks, M., Feaster, D. J., Burns, M. J., & Mitrani, V. B. (2010). The influence of health locus of control on the patient-provider relationship. *Psychology, Health & Medicine, 15*(6), 720–728. https://doi.org/10.1080/13548506.2010.498921

Center For Disease Control (Ed.). (2018, June 21). *Mortality mapping help - Section 2.1*. Retrieved August 3, 2020, from https://www.cdc.gov/injury/wisqars/mapping_help/injury_type.html#:~:text=Legal%20intervention%20refers%20to%20deaths,and%20performing%20other%20legal%20actions.

Center For Disease Control. (2018, August 8). *Violence prevention home page*. Retrieved August 3 2020, from https://www.cdc.gov/violenceprevention/index.html

Center For Disease Control. (2020, September 17). *Infographic: 6 guiding principles to a trauma-informed approach*. Centers for Disease Control and Prevention. https://www.cdc.gov/cpr/infographics/6_principles_trauma_info.htm.

Clark, J. A., Cavatorta, F., & Yaghi, M. (2018). Coding in qualitative research. In *Political science research in the Middle East and North Africa: Methodological and ethical challenges* (pp. 17–31). Essay. Oxford University Press, Inc.

Crenshaw, K. (1993). Reel Time/Reel Justice. In R. Gooding-Williams (Ed.), *Reading Rodney King: Reading urban uprising* (pp. 56–72). Routledge.

Crenshaw, K. (2020). An overdue reckoning with structural racism in policing, house oversight committee on oversight and reform. *116th Congress*.

Crenshaw, K., Gotanda, N., Peller, G., & Thomas, K. (2010). *Critical race theory: The key writings that formed the movement*. The New press.

Creswell, J. W. (2014). *Research design: Qualitative, quantitative, and mixed method approaches*. Sage.

Creswell, J. W., & Poth, C. N. (2018). *Qualitative inquiry and research DESIGN: Choosing among five approaches*, Sage.

Davis, A., & Lowery, W. (2015, October 7). *FBI director calls lack of data on police shootings 'ridiculous,' 'embarrassing'*. Retrieved August 31 2020, from https://www.washingtonpost.com/national/fbi-director-calls-lack-of-data-on-police-shootings-ridiculous-embarrassing/2015/10/07/c0ebaf7a-6d16-11e5-b31c-d80d62b53e28_story.html

Dawson, A. (2018). A space for countering colorblind discourse: Constructions of police-perpetrated homicides of African-American males. *Critical Studies in Media Communication, 35*(3), 300–313. https://doi.org/10.1080/15295036.2018.1436763

Devylder, E., Lukens, E. P., Link, B. G., & Lieberman, J. A. (2015). Suicidal ideation and suicide attempts among adults with psychotic experiences. *JAMA Psychiatry, 72*(3), 219. https://doi.org/10.1001/jamapsychiatry.2014.2663

Devylder, J. E., Jun, H., Fedina, L., Coleman, D., Anglin, D., Cogburn, C., Link, B., & Barth, R. P. (2018). Association of exposure to police violence with prevalence of mental health symptoms among urban residents in the United States. *JAMA Network Open, 1*(7), e184945. https://doi.org/10.1001/jamanetworkopen.2018.4945

Feldman, M., Gruskin, S., Coull, B. A., & Krieger, N. (2017). Killed by police: Validity of media-based data and misclassification of death certificates in Massachusetts, 2004–2016. *American Journal of Public Health, 107*(10), 1624–1626. https://doi.org/10.2105/ajph.2017.303940

Ford, C., & Airhihenbuwa, C. (2018). Commentary: Just what is critical race theory and what's it doing in a progressive field like public health? *Ethnicity & Disease, 28*(1), 223–230. https://doi.org/10.18865/ed.28.S1.223

Ford, L., & Airhihenbuwa, C. O. (2010). Critical race theory, race equity, and public health: Toward antiracism praxis. *American Journal of Public Health, 100*(S1), S30–S35. https://doi.org/10.2105/ajph.2009.171058

Gilbert, K. L., & Ray, R. (2015). Why police kill black males with impunity: Applying public health critical race praxis (PHCRP) to address the determinants of policing behaviors and "justifiable" homicides in the USA. *Journal of Urban Health, 93*(S1), 122–140. https://doi.org/10.1007/s11524-015-0005-x

Gillikin, C., Habib, L., Evces, M., Bradley, B., Ressler, K. J., & Sanders, J. (2016). Trauma exposure and PTSD symptoms associate with violence in inner city civilians. *Journal of Psychiatric Research, 83*, 1–7. https://doi.org/10.1016/j.jpsychires.2016.07.027

Glaser, B. G., & Strauss, A. L. (2017). The constant comparative method of qualitative analysis*. In *The discovery of grounded theory: strategies for qualitative research* (1st ed., pp. 101–116). Essay. Routledge. https://doi.org/10.4324/9780203793206-6

Hattery, A., & Smith, E. (2018). *Policing black bodies: How black lives are surveilled and how to work for change.* Rowman & Littlefield.

Herman, J. L. (2015). *Trauma and recovery.* BasicBooks.

Holder, M., Jackson, M. A., & Ponterotto, J. G. (2015). Racial microaggression experiences and coping strategies of Black women in corporate leadership. *Qualitative Psychology, 2*(2), 164–180. https://doi.org/10.1037/qup0000024

Jenkins, J. (2002). Black women and community violence. *Women & Therapy, 25*(3–4), 29–44. https://doi.org/10.1300/j015v25n03_03

Koyanagi, A., Oh, H., Stickley, A., Haro, J. M., & Devylder, J. (2016). Risk and functional significance of psychotic experiences among individuals with depression in 44 low- and middle-income countries. *Psychological Medicine, 46*(12), 2655–2665. https://doi.org/10.1017/s0033291716001422

Krieger, N., Chen, J. T., Waterman, P. D., Kiang, M. V., & Feldman, J. (2015). Police killings and police deaths are public health data and can be counted. *PLOS Medicine, 12*(12), e1001915. https://doi.org/10.1371/journal.pmed.1001915

Krieger, N., Kiang, M., Chen, J. T., & Waterman, P. 2015. Trends in US deaths due to legal intervention among black and white men, age 15–34 years, by county income level. *Harvard Public Health Review, 3* (RACISM (Winter 2015)), 1–5. Retrieved 2020, from https://www.jstor.org/stable/48503126

Lindlof, R., & Taylor, B. C. (2019). *Qualitative communication research methods.* SAGE Publications.

Maibach, E. W., Abroms, L. C., & Marosits, M. (2007). Communication and marketing as tools to cultivate the public's health. *A Proposed "People and Places" Framework. BMC Public Health, 7*(1). https://doi.org/10.1186/1471-2458-7-88

Maier, S., & Seligman, M. E. (2016). Learned helplessness at fifty: Insights from neuroscience. *Psychological Review, 123*(4), 349–367. https://doi.org/10.1037/rev0000033

Mcdonald, D., Sasangohar, F., Jatav, A., & Rao, A. H. (2019). Continuous monitoring and detection of post-traumatic stress disorder (PTSD) triggers among veterans: A supervised machine learning approach. *IISE Transactions on Healthcare Systems Engineering, 9*(3), 201–211. https://doi.org/10.1080/24725579.2019.1583703

Mills, K. (2020, May 28). *'We are living in a racism pandemic,' says APA President.* American Psychological Association. https://www.apa.org/news/press/releases/2020/05/racism-pandemic

National Institute of Justice. (2020). *Overview of police use of force.* Retrieved August 3, 2020, from https://nij.ojp.gov/topics/articles/overview-police-use-force

O'Rourke, T. M., Tryon, W. W., & Raps, C. S. (1980). Learned helplessness, depression, and positive reinforcement. *Cognitive Therapy and Research, 4*(2), 201–209. https://doi.org/10.1007/bf01173651

Owen, W. F. (1984). Interpretive themes in relational communication. *Quarterly Journal of Speech, 70*(3), 274–287. https://doi.org/10.1080/00335638409383697

Palker-Corell, A., & Marcus, D. K. (2004). Partner abuse, learned helplessness, and trauma symptoms. *Journal of Social and Clinical Psychology, 23*(4), 445–462. https://doi.org/10.1521/jscp.23.4.445.40311

Sewell, A. A., & Jefferson, K. A. (2016). Collateral damage: The health effects of invasive police encounters in New York city. *Journal of Urban Health, 93*(S1), 42–67. https://doi.org/10.1007/s11524-015-0016-7

Sheats, J., Irving, S. M., Mercy, J. A., Simon, T. R., Crosby, A. E., Ford, D. C., Merrick, M. T., Annor, F. B., & Morgan, R. E. (2018). Violence-related disparities experienced by black youth and young adults: Opportunities for prevention. *American Journal of Preventive Medicine, 55*(4), 462–469. https://doi.org/10.1016/j.amepre.2018.05.017

Smith, J. A. (1995). Semi-structured interviewing and qualitative analysis. In J. A. Smith. R. Harré, & L. V. Langenhove (Eds.), *Rethinking methods in psychology* (pp. 10–26). SAGE Publications Ltd. https://doi.org/10.4135/9781446221792.n2

Smith-Lee, J. R., & Robinson, M. A. (2019). "That's my number one fear in life. It's the police": Examining young Black men's exposures to trauma and loss resulting from police violence and police killings. *Journal of Black Psychology, 45*(3), 143–184. https://doi.org/10.1177/0095798419865152

Swaine, J., Laughland, O., Lartey, J., & McCarthy, C. (2016, February). *About the counted: Why and how the Guardian is counting US police killings.* Retrieved August 3, 2020, from https://www.theguardian.com/us-news/ng-interactive/2015/jun/01/about-the-counted

Tebeka, S., Pignon, B., Amad, A., Strat, Y., Brichant-Petitjean, C., Thomas, P., Vaiva, G., Roeland, J.-L., Benradia, I., Etain, B., Rolland, B., Dubertret, C., & Geoffroy, P. (2017, September 21). *A study in the general population about sadness to disentangle the continuum from well-being to depressive disorders.* Retrieved August 23, 2020, from https://www.sciencedirect.com/science/article/pii/S0165032717313162

Trindade, A., Mendes, A. L., & Ferreira, N. B. (2020). The moderating effect of psychological flexibility on the link between learned helplessness and depression symptomatology: A preliminary study. *Journal of Contextual Behavioral Science, 15*, 68–72. https://doi.org/10.1016/j.jcbs.2019.12.001

Van der Kolk, B. (1989). Psychobiology of the trauma response. In B. Lerer & S. Gershon (Eds.), *New directions in affective disorders* (pp. 443–446). Springer-Verlag.

World Health Organization. (2014). Retrieved 2020, from https://www.who.int/violence_injury_prevention/violence/status_report/2014/en

OPEN ACCESS

A Subjective Culture Approach to Cancer Prevention: Rural Black and White Adults' Perceptions of Using Virtual Health Assistants to Promote Colorectal Cancer Screening

Melissa J. Vilaro, Danyell S. Wilson-Howard, Jordan M. Neil, Fatemeh Tavassoli, Mohan S. Zalake, Benjamin C. Lok, François P. Modave, Thomas J. George, Folakemi T. Odedina, Peter J. Carek, Aubrey M. Mys, and Janice L. Krieger

ABSTRACT

In the US, Black adults are less likely than White adults to be screened for colorectal cancer (CRC). This study uses a subjective culture approach to describe and compare perceptions of a CRC screening intervention delivered via virtual health assistants (VHAs) among rural Black and White study participants. We analyzed 28 focus groups with Black (n = 85) and White (n = 69) adults aged 50–73. Participants, largely recruited through community engagement efforts, tested the VHA intervention on mobile phones provided by the research team. Moderated discussions were recorded, transcribed, and analyzed using thematic analysis. All groups preferred the VHA to be friendly. Other important cues included trustworthiness, authority, and expertise. Black participants expressed a preference for receiving information about their CRC risk from the VHA compared with White adults. Black participants also expressed the importance of sharing the intervention and the CRC screening messages with younger members of their networks, including family members who could benefit from screening messages before reaching the recommended age for screening. The key similarities and differences between Black and White adults' perceptions of the intervention that were identified in this study can help inform future efforts to develop effective communication strategies and reduce cancer screening inequities.

On August 28, 2020, actor Chadwick Boseman died from colorectal cancer (CRC). Boseman was beloved for his moving portrayals of historical figures, such as Jackie Robinson and Thurgood Marshall, as well as his embodiment of the larger-than-life Marvel superhero Black Panther. The loss of this accomplished celebrity sparked mourning across society; it also sparked a collective dialogue about CRC.

Screening is important for prevention and early detection of CRC, which can reduce CRC incidence and mortality by 30%–60% (Lin et al., 2016). Among the pervasive health inequities associated with CRC outcomes, it is clear that Black adults are less likely to be screened than White adults (May et al., 2020). The goal of the current study was to describe and compare perceptions of CRC screening among adults at average risk of CRC and to identify appropriate strategies and messages to facilitate guideline-concordant screening.

Racial inequities in colorectal cancer screening

Chadwick Boseman's death made the news because he was a celebrity. However, he is only one of the 70,000 Black adults in the US expected to die from CRC in 2020 (DeSantis et al., 2019). Improving guideline-concordant screening is particularly important for this community. In Florida, 69% of all adults follow screening guidelines, but screening rates among Non-Hispanic Black adults (67%) and Non-Hispanic White adults (74%) differ. CRC incidence rates and mortality rates also differ: Non-Hispanic Black men have a higher incidence of CRC than Non-Hispanic White men (48.9 vs. 41.3 per 100,000), and Non-Hispanic Black women have a higher incidence than Non-Hispanic White women (36.7 vs. 31.3 per 100,000). Mortality rates follow a similar pattern, with higher rates among Non-Hispanic Black men (20.6 vs. 15.5 per 100,000) and women (14.0 vs. 10.9 per 100,000).

Due to a constellation of factors, therefore, Black adults experience a greater burden of CRC. Yet when detected early CRC has a 5-year survival rate of 90%. The best way to reduce inequities is thus to promote regular screening. That means there is urgent need for a nuanced understanding of screening perceptions among diverse populations in order to develop and provide effective and culturally tailored health promotion messages regarding guideline-concordant CRC screening.

Theoretical underpinnings: Critical race theory and subjective culture

Critical race theory (CRT; Ladson-Billings, 2013) centers race as a primary driver of understanding inequity. Interventions aiming to improve health equity, such as by developing culturally tailored approaches to reduce cancer inequities, must reposition race as central rather than peripheral (Resnicow et al., 1999). Five key CRT tenets map onto assumptions that can help guide development of culturally tailored health interventions: First, racism is a normal experience in US society, and racism should be assumed to shape Black patients' healthcare experiences. Second, many attempts to address racism are symbolic, and what is actually needed are practical solutions that add tangible value to Black communities. Third, race is a social construction, and health scholars should consider both the limits and the benefits of using race as a variable. Fourth, race is a product of other social forces, meaning that race operates in the context of multiple other identities, such as gender and social status. Fifth, interventions must include voice and counternarrative. This means that interventions should incorporate diverse perspectives through qualitative inquiry or storytelling to ensure that cultural narratives (which may differ both across and within cultures) are at the forefront.

This study uses a subjective culture approach to facilitate description and comparison of the complexities of racial identity and culture across and within groups. Subjective culture is defined as unique shared values, beliefs, and practices that can shape behavior and influence acceptance of health messages (Pasick et al., 1996). Subjective culture acknowledges that contextual factors shape access to and uptake of healthcare. It also enables scholars and practitioners to design health messages based on group members' cultural preferences.

Applying a subjective culture approach to cancer screening interventions

Many interventions address racial disparities in cancer screening in part by determining intervention effectiveness across different racial categories or identifying within-group predictors of screening. Subjective culture, of course, encompasses more than ethnic and racial identity. Oetzel et al. (2007) describe how examination of culture is generally lacking within cancer screening interventions, as well as how subjective culture can profoundly shape preferences for specific sources of screening information among minoritized groups. To achieve equity in cancer outcomes, it is vital to understand exactly how race and culture inform preferences for intervention content and delivery, as well the mechanisms that make interventions successful (or not) across and within racial groups.

Culture, source cues, and CRC screening

Studies show that racial discordance in healthcare interactions – in which patient and provider perceive each other as belonging to a different race – reduces patient compliance with medical recommendations, lowers patients' perceptions of the quality of medical care, and reduces both communication satisfaction and perceptions of trust in providers among patients (LaVeist et al., 2003; Shen et al., 2018). Although we know that racial discordance is negatively associated with patient health outcomes, the ways that race is socially constructed as a source cue in healthcare interactions are poorly understood. Culture plays a role in teaching people how to identify and respond to certain cues related to the source of a message. Because some source cues may improve cognitive processing of cancer prevention information while other cues may hinder information processing (Claypool et al., 2012) the role of race as a source cue is a particularly important to explore.

Culture provides a foundation for connecting knowledge about the source of information, such as race, to perceptions of factors critical to a healthcare provider's credibility, such as authority, expertise, trustworthiness, and friendliness. The literature views authority cues as being transmitted by observable formal positions indicating particular education (Metzger et al., 2003). Expertise cues are commonly connected to demonstrations of experience, credentials, or skill (O'Keefe, 2002). Friendliness cues are thought to influence message acceptability, as if people are subconsciously thinking, "People I like usually have correct opinions on issues" (Chaiken, 1987, p. 4). Friendliness cues, therefore, are cues that demonstrate likability – an important component of social exchanges that induces a positive, emotional experience and can put receivers at ease, increasing their willingness to change attitudes and behaviors regarding cancer prevention (Whelehan et al., 2017). Meanwhile, trustworthiness cues are associated with perceptions of the message source being truthful, honest, or unbiased (Tseng & Fogg, 1999).

Source cues associated with virtual health assistants

A key healthcare challenge is that while racial concordance between patient and provider promotes positive health outcomes, the US healthcare system doesn't have enough healthcare providers from minoritized populations to meet demand. Under these circumstances, there may be an opportunity for technology to support the delivery and reception of cancer screening interventions. Virtual human technology, and the use of virtual health assistants (VHAs) in particular, makes it possible for interdisciplinary teams to customize race-concordant virtual characters to deliver screening recommendations. Previous research has demonstrated that VHAs can be tailored to engender positive source cues that invoke feelings of trust among users and increase truthfulness of disclosures (Zhou et al., 2014). Today's VHAs have the ability to embody high-quality patient-provider communication practices, including elicitation of individual preferences and empowerment in the decision-making process, while promoting CRC screening options. The subjective culture and CRT frameworks make it clear that such VHAs must be co-developed with community members – in this case, Black men and women – to embody culturally sensitive CRC screening messages. Thus, we pose the following research questions:

(1) How does race shape perceptions of the source of CRC screening messages.
(2) How does race shape intentions to engage in CRC screening?

Methods

This study was part of a larger clinical trial aiming to promote CRC screening among rural adults in the United States. The current analysis reports on data collected during the preclinical trial deployment phase, which engaged community members in an iterative process of informing message development and adaptations of a digital intervention using principles of user-centered design. User-centered design emphasizes iterative development that seeks continual feedback from the target audience throughout the development process (McCurdie et al., 2012).

Focus group discussions were used to elicit study participants' perceptions of a CRC intervention (Meet ALEX) and of the VHA that delivered the content. Focus groups were stratified by gender. Most focus groups were also stratified by race; however, due to the community-engaged nature of the research, some groups included both Black and White participants. In total, 28 audio and video recorded focus groups, each moderated by a trained research coordinator matched to participants based on race and gender, were conducted between January 2017 and November 2018.

Participants

To be eligible for the study, participants had to be between 50 and 73 years of age, self-identify their primary race as Black or White, and be proficient in English. We analyzed focus group data from 154 Black ($n = 85$) and White ($n = 69$) adults living in rural North Florida at the time of the study, including Black women ($n = 53$), Black men ($n = 32$), White men ($n = 26$), and White women ($n = 43$). Participants' average age was 63 ($SD = 6.7$) years. Most were unmarried with some level of college education (Table 1).

Table 1. Participant characteristics.

Variable		*N*	%
Gender	Women	96	62.3%
	Men	58	37.6%
Race	Black	85	55.2%
	White	69	44.8%
Income	<$10,000–$19,999	42	27.3%
	$20,000–$34,999	21	13.6%
	$35,000–$74,999	21	13.6%
	≥$75,000	17	11.0%
	Preferred not to answer or missing	53	34.4%
Marital status	Married	54	35%
	Single, divorced, widowed, or separated	100	65%
Education	Grade 1–8	1	0.7%
	Some high school or technical, vocational school	15	9.7%
	High school graduate or GED certificate	20	13.0%
	Some college or college graduate	76	49.4%
	Post-graduate training	33	21.4%
	Preferred not to answer or missing	9	5.8%
Total		154	100%

Procedures

Following IRB approval from University of Florida (IRB201601642), we used a purposive participant recruitment strategy. While the most successful recruitment efforts were done in person, we utilized a number of strategies, including recruitment via farm share programs, senior centers, a university-affiliated research registry, flyers placed in clinics and churches, and word of mouth.

Each focus group contained 2 to 8 participants, and each participant provided written informed consent before providing feedback. Each group responded to a single iteration of the evolving intervention prototype. Over the course of the study period, the prototypes progressed from printed representations of VHA characters with professionally recorded voice scripts to a fully interactive prototype intervention delivered by a race- and gender-matched VHA via an app housed on its own secure server and preloaded on Samsung JX7 smartphones. Sterilized headphones were provided to each participant so they could interact privately with the app. Focus group discussions were recorded and transcribed verbatim using a paid transcription service; transcripts were managed with NVivo 12 Pro (QSR International, 2018). Paper questionnaires were used to collect participant characteristics and health behaviors, with the data entered manually into Qualtrics by researchers immediately following each focus group.

Data analysis and prototype development

We used a team science approach (described elsewhere) to develop and test evolving versions of the intervention (Griffin et al., 2019). The team consisted of computer scientists, health communication scholars, medical researchers, and a community advisory board. To facilitate comparative analysis of Black and White participant feedback, we adapted an existing codebook developed during a previous examination of VHA credibility cues. The codebook was updated to capture CRC prevention behaviors and intentions discussed during the focus groups. Training of the coding team consisted of two coders coding 20% of the transcripts and calculating inter-rater reliability (IRR) using the NVivo comparison query function. The team's IRR was found to have a Kappa statistic above 0.8, indicating acceptable agreement. The primary coder then coded all remaining transcripts for source cues (i.e., perceptions of the VHA as source) and for behavioral intentions related to CRC prevention.

This paper assesses four of the multiple source cues that have been identified as contributing to VHA credibility (Vilaro et al., 2020). These cues were selected by researchers in advance based on prior research and because they represent source characteristics that seem likely to be perceived differently among groups with different experiences of healthcare interactions. We also coded for three distinct behavioral intentions among participants.

We used the case classification and crosstabs functions of NVivo 12 Pro to facilitate comparisons of coded data by race and gender. A constant comparison approach was used to iteratively review participant comments coded to each theme for similarities and differences across groups. Comparisons were made by identifying predominant themes within a group and comparing them against the predominant themes in another. When gender differences were identified in addition to racial differences, these were noted and are also described in the results. Otherwise, differences and similarities are described based on nuances between the comments of Black and White participants.

Results

Source perceptions

Our first research question describes and compares Black and White adults' perceptions of the race-concordant VHA that was communicating the CRC screening messages. Four source cues were explored: (a) authority, (b) expertise, (c) friendliness, and (d) trustworthiness. All the focus groups perceived all four cues as important characteristics of a VHA delivering cancer prevention messages. In addition, the data also revealed nuanced and distinct preferences associated with racial and gender identity (Table 2).

Authority

All participants wanted the VHA to represent a medical authority. Participants suggested that the VHA should have a formal position or appearance that indicates authority: "You should go with the most authority you can realistically bring" (White man [WM], Participant ID 96 [P96]). However, there were subtle differences between conversations in Black and White focus groups.

First, Black participants openly endorsed the authority of the VHA as a medical expert, with comments suggesting this perception was desirable and acceptable: "She looked like a doctor" (Black woman [BW], P34, P43, P45). Also: "His voice was knowledgeable and patient, um, kind of, has some authority ... but he wasn't judgmental. I had a positive response to it, yeah" (Black man [BM], P17). Benefits of the VHA being a medical authority included expanded access to information. For example:

> They have all that information just readily [available], as opposed to a doctor that may not think of something ... I would definitely go for that 'cuz I like all that information coming in ... basically be an expert authority on different things. (BW, P10)

The VHA's position as a medical authority was signaled by clothing: "She dressed – because her appearance, you knew that she was, like, a doctor or a nurse" (BW, P30). Even when they acknowledged that additional consultation with a traditional medical authority might be warranted, overall, Black participants recognized the VHA as an authority.

In contrast, White participants described the VHA as a supplemental or alternative authority that should not be relied on more than one's own doctor. They said, for example, "I'd like to have it linked to the doctor. I'd like to have the doctor be copied on what I'm finding out through this thing" (WM, P96). White participants' comments suggested that the VHA might not meet their needs as patients and that they did not see the VHA as a doctor; they often referenced a different category of health professional, such as a nurse, or explicitly stated the VHA was not a doctor. White participants also described the VHA's authority in terms of how connected it was to the traditional healthcare system (e.g., their real medical doctor) and specifically how it could facilitate communication with their own real-life doctor. For example, one participant commented,

> That would give you some credibility, that the doctor believes it ... 'cause so many times when you're in with the doctor, you're rushed. But if you had time to go through some stuff [with the VHA] and then get with your doctor, you could maybe ask some more educated questions. (WM, P97)

White men in particular were less likely to describe the VHA as an authority, saying, "He's not an authority. He's an authority on the subject, but he's not an authority as a doctor or a nurse or a policeman or something. He is helping us to make a decision" (WM, P95).

Expertise

Expertise is a construct closely related to authority. While both source cues are influenced by perceptions of credentials and training, expertise includes perceptions of skill. Our study participants used various cues to evaluate skill and technical expertise, including perceptions of the VHA's age, clothing, and years of training and the quality of the external sources informing the intervention. Participants also described the type of technical skills a VHA should possess, including diverse communication skills and an ability to serve as a second opinion. All participants indicated that the VHA should be a knowledgeable expert and appear professional.

Among Black participants, looking professional was described as an important component of expertise: "I want them to look like they think they know something" (BW, P5). Black women, in particular, frequently described the VHA as a professional. Professionalism, by its formal definition, denotes positive perceptions of "technical skill or competence related to a specific trade or profession" (Merriam-Webster, n.d.). Appearing skillful and fulfilling visual expectations of professionalism were important cues that signaled expertise. Perceptions of the VHA's clothes were a cue for expertise and professionalism among Black men and all woman. Clothes provided cues to the type of expertise, such as nurse, doctor, patient advocate, or medical assistant, and participants discussed how different types of medical professionals have different years of training and thus different skills and levels of expertise. Age seemed to evoke similar conceptualizations of expertise across all groups. Overall, Black men engaged in very little discussion of the VHA's expertise, in terms of frequency of comments, with only two Black men touching on the topic.

Participants also discussed having a broad knowledge base about individualized patient needs and a connection to a diverse medical community as components of expertise. Black women, White women, and White men all mentioned listening and communication as a type of expertise that the VHA was able to provide: "At least [the virtual person] heard you, and she's gonna answer you ... you're putting out that information. Then you're getting feedback" (BW, P9). The communicative role of expertise was also described as the ability to understand a diversity of patient needs and make patients feel heard. This included desires for the VHA to have an "alternative medicine" background indicative of a broader education, to be able to engage in empathetic listening, and to be able to provide the "right answer" to patients. Nobody wanted the "canned" answer, which was linked to perceptions of low expertise and inability to meet patient needs.

Participants across groups perceived the VHA as a valuable point of access to a second medical opinion. We interpreted this as a point of expertise for the VHA, given participant comments

Table 2. Insights and strategies for improving perceptions of VHA credibility derived from focus groups with adults 50–73 years old.

VHA Cue	Definition	Insights/Communication Strategies	Participant Quotes
Trust	The degree to which a message recipient believes the VHA is conveying the truth as they know it. Indicates a positive belief about the perceived reliability or dependability of the VHA (includes perceived fairness or lack of bias)	Similarities: Participants desired a VHA connected to a trusted source. Trust of this study's VHA was contextualized by perceptions of the local university hospital. Perceptions of the VHA costing money, or of any money-making intentions, lowered trust. Differences: White participants would trust the VHA if it came directly from their doctor. White adults' privacy concerns were balanced by the potential benefits of personalized information. Black adults reported that a VHA who could provide help with health questions, normalize fears, and reduce uncertainty enhanced trust. Black men responded positively to interacting with the Black male VHA. Potential communication strategies: Race and gender concordance may be particularly important for Black men. For Black participants, trust included interpersonal considerations such as friendliness and ability to alleviate uncertainty. White participants commented on the structural ways their privacy and security might be violated.	**BW**: I think we all agree we would be more likely to use it because it came from UF. (P7) **BW**: Yes, because of the rep. They have a good reputation. (P8) **BM**: Like I say, bein' as that he was a brother-doctor look, it was more acceptable to listen to it opposed to another type. (P150) **BM**: Yeah. I was just looking at her picture that we've been talking about. It seems like more – not the doctor part, but this person can explain it to me more. (P107) **WW**: You know, maybe you do voices for different regions, you know, because people relate and sort of trust, you know. Hopefully nobody's from New York, but if you have a New Yorker (indicates accent) or somebody from Massachusetts speaking, people are going to go, what? Where are they? (P9) **WW**: If my doctor told me at an appointment, "I recommend that you do this," then I would find a way to do it. (P10). **WM**: Well, the question is how do I trust it. And when it presents itself as "I'm a person" when I know, but, and I'm looking at it, and it's very, very clear, this is not a person, that uh, that leads me to not trust it. (P42) **WM**: I would want to not only put in my information once I trusted the system. I would want to put in what happened to my dad, and my great-aunt, and my uncles and my sisters, brother, cousins. (P96)
VHA Cue	Definition	Insights/Communication Strategies	Participant Quotes
Expertise	The degree to which a message recipient believes the VHA to be knowledgeable about a topic, with a specific level of skill derived from training or experience	Similarities: Visual attributes of the VHA (e.g., age, clothing) were important cues to expertise. The VHA's ability to integrate relevant patient information and communicate on a variety of topics during the interaction was viewed as a type of expertise. Listening skills were considered an area of VHA expertise. Differences: Black adults primarily commented on the VHA's professional appearance. Only a few Black males discussed expertise. Only White adults wanted to evaluate the external sources of information that informed the messages (e.g., seeing a diploma on the wall, or hearing the message was backed by research) as a way to assess the VHA's expertise. Potential communication strategies: Visual expectations of expertise can be cued by different features (appearance vs. evidence). Gender may play a strong role in perceptions of expertise and can be explored further.	**BW**: She sounded young. Like she was too young to be a doctor giving us this important advice. (P18) **BW**: I think with the virtual human, I think they have all that information just readily, as opposed to a doctor that may not think of something, you know, so. I would definitely go for that 'cuz I like all that information type thing coming in. (P10) **BM**: If you wanted the [virtual] doctor to seem an expert, I probably would have done a better job on the animation . . . I hadn't seen many doctors dressed that way. He had his shirttail out . . . but his voice was very clear, and his diction was really good. (P19) **BM**: Like it was informative, . . . seem like he had some kinda medical background to speak on it, and that's what I looked at. (P150) **WW**: I would enjoy it – because the virtual human is backed by the research and profession, it's not just a website or some testimony. (P88) **WM**: But a virtual doctor with a resource of background information that can bring this together, I think would actually be better than an actual doctor. (P95) **WM**: A patient advocate. They would know things, but would they articulate my needs of why I'm there? I'd like the doctor's opinion then. Eight years of schools of schooling as opposed to three years of junior college. (P81)
VHA Cue	Definition	Insights/Communication Strategies	Participant Quotes

(Continued)

Table 2. (Continued).

VHA Cue	Definition	Insights/Communication Strategies	Participant Quotes
Authority	The degree to which the VHA is observed to have credentials or training as a medical authority. Perception of the VHA having a formal position/job indicating specific education or requiring relevant experience (e.g., doctor)	Similarities: Black and White participants both wanted the VHA to represent a medical authority. When the VHA was perceived as a community health worker, it was a less acceptable source of screening messages. Differences: Black adults accepted and endorsed the authority of the VHA itself. White adults conferred authority on the VHA based on it being recommended directly by a medical doctor. For White adults, perceptions that a "real doctor" maintained authority was important. Potential communication strategies: Add an introduction from a medical doctor. Disseminate via a local, reputable health organization or a patient portal.	**BW**: When you look at the way she was dressed . . . you knew that she was a doctor or a nurse. Yeah, she was 100%. (P30) **BW**: I would definitely go for that 'cuz I like all that information coming in . . . basically be an expert authority on different things. (P10) **BM**: Being that he [the VHA] was a brother-doctor . . . it was more acceptable to listen to. (P150) **BM**: His voice was knowledgeable and patient, um, kind of, has some authority . . . but he wasn't judgmental. (P17) **WW**: I would say phooey, because if the doctor hasn't asked me to do an exam, the question is, then why are you asking me to do this? I don't have time to do this. (P80) **WW**: I know studies show that you put the white coat on and that's where people see authority, I see what I think you're trying to get at with like, a step down from a doctor, here, but still a medical person, and I do think that's probably a smart way to go. (P86) **WM**: I just think if you're going to do it [create a VHA], you might as well go all the way and have a medical doctor. (P97) **WM**: No, I'm just saying. It, he's not an authority. He's an authority on the subject, but he's not an authority as a doctor or a nurse or a policeman or something. He is helping us to make a decision, so does he really need our personal information to do that? (P95)
VHA Cue	Definition	Insights/Communication Strategies	Participant Quotes
Friendliness	The degree to which an individual feels an affective bond toward the VHA For example, people agree . . . with those they like based on the reasoning that "People I like usually have correct opinions on issues"	Similarities: Both Black and White participants desired a friendly and likable VHA. Adjusting VHA appearance (e.g., smiling) and voice cues improved perceptions of friendliness. Participants referenced the VHA acting like a "friend" or "best friend" when it comes to helping them navigate their health. Differences: None discerned. Potential communication strategies: Perceived friendliness of the message source was universally desired. In this context, friendliness may not require specific or extensive tailoring beyond a basic perception of an engaged, caring, and kind communicator.	**BW**: Make her a little more friendly. (P21) **BW**: The one they said sounded country sounded fun to me. She was like, "Alright y'all, let's get it" (laughter). (P19) **BM**: He look like he more could be a doctor or a friend or something. Somebody that's concerned about your problem with cancer – that you could trust, really trust. (P109) **BM**: You probably feel more comfortable with the – the virtual human walking you through it than sitting there listening to the doctor talking about it. (P107) **WW**: It would have been nice to be a little more human, a little bit warmer. I want to hear the smile. (P10) **WW**: I like more of a smile. . . . But more receptive look on the face, like they're hearing you and interacting, and something that's positive. (P76) **WM**: I like the woman's voice on my GPS, and I would like to have a VHA that was a nice friendly woman that was very knowledgeable, an artificial intelligence that when I ask it a question, it could become my best friend in terms of getting me the right answer. (P96) **WM**: You want your Virtual Human to be your more loving, affectionate friend. Your dear most friend. The one that's always going to be there for you, that's always trustworthy, that's always gonna support you when you're down. (P96)

BM = Black man, BW = Black woman, VHA = virtual health assistant, WM = White man, WW = White woman.

acknowledging that human expertise can be fallible and that the VHA could offer an alternative opinion to help fill a knowledge or access gap. In this way the VHA supplemented access to the expertise and knowledge of a real doctor. Black women, in particular, expanded on this concept. For example: "It's good to have different viewpoints of things, and different doctors have different feelings about procedures or what you should do next or how you should do it" (BW, P6).

Only among White participants did we hear comments linking the VHA's expertise to perceptions that information was from an external source. White participants perceived the VHA as an expert due to it being informed by the medical profession broadly or by evidence-based research specifically: "I would enjoy it – because the virtual human is backed by the research and profession, it's not just a website from some test mode, testimony?" (White woman [WW], P88). White participants' comments relied heavily on evaluating external sources, whereas Black participants did not use external sources as a way to appraise the VHA's expertise. In addition, only White men suggested that visual evidence of the VHA's expertise was needed: "If I can see his diploma, I will be like, where did he go to school for this?" (WM, P3), or "Some authorship of [university name] in the background would help" (WM, P84).

Friendliness

Participants wanted the VHA to be a friendly, understanding, caring entity to interact with. All groups desired to see the VHA as a "friend." The only identifiable difference in how groups discussed perceptions of friendliness was that the groups of Black women and White women, but not the men, critiqued aspects of the early VHA prototypes by identifying cues that hindered perceptions of friendliness. Sample comments include: "She forgot to say thank you"; "She looks angry like she doesn't want to be here"; and suggesting that the VHA looked "stressed" or "harsh" or like she had an "attitude." These critiques informed modifications to improve perceptions of friendliness in later prototypes.

The focus group participants wanted the VHA to project real concern when communicating CRC risk and prevention options. Voice attributes such as speed of speech, persuasive intent, and warmth of voice influenced participants' perceptions of friendliness. Appearing calm, smiling, and having an open and inviting face were described as likable, with all groups mentioning that they wanted the VHA to smile. Men described the VHA as "cool" and wanted the VHA to be a friend who could provide tangible guidance in a considerate way:

> I like—I like that virtual human also long as they just like maybe the GPS system. They're gonna make sure you're right. . . . And so that virtual human could be good if he's gonna make sure you stay on the path. (BM, P104)

Trustworthiness

The extent to which participants perceived the VHA as trustworthy was revealed by comments on the VHA's ability to be a reliable, truthful, fair, or unbiased source of information. While all participants demonstrated a capacity to trust the VHA, the comments indicated variations in perceptions of trust between Black and White adults.

For all participants, the local context influenced perceptions of trust. Both Black and White participants indicated that the intervention and VHA should appear affiliated with the local university hospital or a known reliable source, and that this affiliation conveyed trustworthiness. This finding was indicative of the location of the study activities in a place where the local hospital maintains a largely positive reputation within the community. Differences were seen in that White participants said they preferred the intervention to come directly from their own doctor: "He or she has to say, 'You need to look at this'" (WW, P11). Black adults did not explicitly state a need for the VHA to come from their own doctor as an essential component of trust.

Black adults (both men and women) discussed trust in terms of their perception of the VHA's voice and appearance and the extent to which the VHA could meet patient needs. This indicated that trust could be communicated through linguistic characteristics that cued competency: "I trusted what he said; it sounded real convincing to me" (BM, P14). When the voice sounded scripted, participants described this as reducing trust. Black men specifically perceived the VHA as trustworthy when they felt it could alleviate fear and uncertainty or "help me out." If the VHA was honest, logical, and could help them learn and "normalize fears and concerns," it was considered trustworthy. Homophily-the tendency to from connections with people who share similar characteristics-may also have been important for Black men when it came to trust: "Like I say, bein' as that he was a brother-doctor look, it was more acceptable to listen to it opposed to another type" (BM, P150). Also: "I like the aspect that he was a brother" (BM, P152). Another way appearance seemed to play a role in trust was when participants described the VHA as generally looking like a trustworthy person. Black men thought people would be more truthful with the VHA than with a real doctor. Black women described the VHA appearing knowledgeable as influencing trust.

For White men, a variety of things lowered trust, including typos within the intervention, perceptions that the VHA was misrepresenting itself as a human person, concerns about the intrusiveness of the app, and uncertainty about how much personal information the VHA could access. White men discussed a desire to interact with the VHA while remaining anonymous. Some also described the ability to link to anonymized medical history as a potential benefit that would increase trust and allow for tailored information to facilitate decision making. White women expressed concerns about the security of the personal information used within the intervention and questioned its potential to be hacked. They suggested that using MyChart, a patient portal, would be a way to deliver the VHA that would improve trust related to security. Additionally, White participants (both men and women) perceived any intention on the part of the VHA to sell a medical product or procedure, or any interaction that cost money, as a barrier to developing trust with the VHA. For example, one participant stated that to increase trust, you need to "have a comfort level with the source or the team. You don't want us to think it's a pharmaceutical company or some insurance company or some other type of issue where they're kind of cleaning information" (WM, P4).

Behavioral intentions

Our second research question explored intentions to engage in CRC prevention behaviors among the focus group participants who had engaged in informing the development of the VHA-delivered intervention. Our analysis found similarities and differences in three behavioral intentions related to CRC prevention: (a) information seeking, (b) information sharing, and (c) CRC screening. Nuanced differences between the Black and White participants' intentions to engage in cancer prevention behaviors emerged (Table 3).

Information seeking intentions

Information seeking behaviors among participants included wanting to learn more about CRC risk in general and wanting to talk to a doctor about screening. All participants expressed some extent of interest in learning more about CRC risk. They expressed a variety of intentions to search for more information about CRC. Among Black adults, there was a tangible interest in wanting to learn about risk from the VHA specifically. White adults expressed intentions to seek additional information from more familiar or traditional routes, including their own doctors or their own research efforts. While it was difficult to determine what drove these nuanced differences, Black participants' comments indicated that they were impressed with the option to obtain information about CRC and screening from a novel source. For example, one Black participant expressed an intention to forgo her regular information seeking behaviors and instead trust the VHA's information:

> I think being a computer, having all that information and everything, I would trust that doctor. I don't really trust doctors 'cuz they all, I mean they all have the knowledge, but they all have different opinions. I like to do my research because I don't always agree with some of them, so, but that doctor I would trust. (BW, P8)

The views expressed in this quote indicate that the VHA produced a sense of trust that made this participant feel she would agree with the information it delivered. The VHA allowed Black users to imagine how obtaining CRC risk information from someone other than a traditional doctor might affect them if it became an available option in the future: "It'll have a tremendous influence. I think – and I hate to segregate, but the Black community definitely because we don't do the doctor visits ... – that app would do a world of good" (BM, P106).

Information sharing intentions

All groups said they would feel comfortable and confident sharing the app that delivered the intervention, and that they would be interested in sharing content about CRC they learned from the VHA. However, Black adults wanted to share the content with their family members and in particular with young members of their social network:

> Yeah, because I wanna call them now and say, 'Look, they got this app out now.' See, they got boys, too. The boys are ages where around 10, 11. Get them involved, and then you can go there and get more information, too. It's stuff you might not get from your doctor. (BM, P126)

Only Black participants expressed interest in learning more about CRC risk at younger age than 45 or 50 years, which is when CRC screening is recommended to begin.

Among Black participants, a common motivation to share information was that it could save a life. Black participants were comfortable sharing the app with friends and family, specifically mentioning brothers, sisters, children, and boyfriends. Black women commented that they wanted to share the app because the VHA would communicate the information more efficiently than they would themselves.

White participants also wanted to share the app and discussed sharing the information with family and friends. In addition to sharing the app for its content on cancer prevention, White men said it could facilitate them sharing their own health information with others:

> You could save it and refer back to it or send it to somebody. So, you'd want to be able to do that. You want to capture the valuable information and almost always, you want to share these important things that are happening to you. (WM, P96)

White men provided several suggestions for how to share the app widely with others, recommending employees, American Association of Retired Persons (AARP), Veterans Affairs (VA), Facebook, advertising, celebrities, football, and word of mouth to "get it out to millions of people" (WM, P95).

CRC screening intentions

We found that many participants in the moderated focus groups already had experience with CRC screening in general. Their exposure to different screening modalities varied. Most were familiar with traditional colonoscopy. Some had heard about fecal or stool testing such as FIT (fecal immunochemical test), but Cologuard commercials were referenced most often. Some were even familiar with the details of FIT (e.g., how to use it, why and when to use it, and who can use it), but for many this was new information.

Comments indicated that the intervention's combination of novel technology (i.e., the VHA) and new screening options (i.e., FIT) provided opportunities for participants to access different experiences and choices within the healthcare system: "I didn't know I had a choice, I guess. I thought the app was very informing. I really like it" (BM, P16). Seeing the virtual demonstration of how to use the FIT had a positive effect on intentions to try it: "In the application, when you put the thing across the seat – 'cause I didn't know that. That's why I haven't really been botherin' with the thing. But now, I might try and put [it] across the seat" (BM, P152). FIT was also seen as an easy alternative to colonoscopy: "Yeah, no muss, no fuss, very, at home, not intrusive, you know. I was actually relating to that, because I've done that, you know. I was saying, this is really easy stuff" (WM, P3). Others joked, "I wish my doctor would say I could use the FIT (laughing)" (WW, P11).

Some comments suggested that Black adults may be likely to experience a lack of support in the process of CRC screening. One particularly vivid account demonstrated this:

Table 3. Intentions to engage in colorectal cancer prevention behaviors among black and white adults who tested a VHA-delivered intervention.

Intentions	Definition	Insights/Communication Strategies	Participant Quotes
Information seeking intentions	Wanting to talk to someone about screening or learn more about personal cancer risk from a trusted source	Similarities: All participants expressed interest in receiving CRC screening information from the VHA and responded positively to new information. Differences: Black adults liked the idea of receiving information from the novel source. White adults wanted to talk to a doctor, engage in additional research, or contact another source in addition to the VHA. Potential communication strategies: This novel source (e.g., a VHA) may have a specific appeal for Black adults. Framing a VHA as a new way to get information vs. as a way to connect you with existing resources may be useful to engage audiences with different information seeking orientations.	**BW**: It convinced me to go ahead and do this, to talk to my doctor about this. (P19) **BM**: On this little app thing, when can I contact you if me and brother-doctor [VHA] here clash on certain issues? (P152) **WW**: I don't think there's anything wrong with it, but I just think you really ultimately, you're gonna have to go to a doctor. (P77) **WM**: It was enough to make me wanna look further into it. (P131) **WM**: I think it would be really nice if this [app] actually gave you references for the studies that back up the thing this guy is saying, and actually gives you a link so you can actually read those. (P81)
Information sharing intentions	Wanting to share the information learned or share the intervention with friends and/or family members	Similarities: Most participants wanted to share content with friends, family, and others. Differences: Black participants expressed a strong desire for screening information to be shared with people at younger ages than the recommended age for CRC screening (e.g., children, grandchildren). Potential communication strategies: To enhance perceived utility, enable easy and secure platforms for users to share content with others.	**BW**: You've heard of the game "telephone"? By the time it gets back around to you it's different. It's the same thing. I would rather give them, from the horse's mouth [the VHA]. (P22) **BW**: It would help save somebody else also. If I can help save a life, or help prevent this from coming about? I would tell the world, you know? (P3) **BM**: I would definitely share it, even with the teenagers. I'd share it with them right now. (P126) **WW**: If I used it myself and liked it, I'd share it. (P78) **WM**: That's right! Get the football players to sign autographs, you get a free jersey if you watch it. Or a free ticket! (P98)
Intentions	Definition	Insights/Communication Strategies	Participant Quotes
CRC screening intentions	Discussing the intention to engage in CRC screening (includes expressing a desire to screen without explicit preference, expressing a desire to avoid screening)	Similarities: Participants were interested in pursuing CRC screening, saw it as important, and saw FIT as an easy way to screen. Differences: For Black adults' previous negative experiences with healthcare may affect screening decisions. White adults may be more influenced by perceptions of accuracy and process. Potential communication strategies: Visual demonstrations of the screening process may enhance screening intentions. Incorporate user preferences and lived experience. Address the user's feelings (e.g., what modalities do they trust and why).	**BW**: It's good that you do have a choice, that they're giving you a choice now, whether you can do it with the FIT or the old way. (P13) **BM**: I've been through the FIT test, and I can tell you most men of our age and our color, we have that feelin'. That's why I asked about, do they put you to sleep? I'm a do the FIT. (P154) **WW**: I actually might have that [FIT] done. (P8) **WM**: I guess I'm old-fashioned. I'd rather have a colonoscopy where they scope and they see what's up there. If somethin' there, they scrape it, take it, and biopsy it right then and there. (P131) **WM**: I kind of question whether it might be better to drop [the FIT sample] off in person, than to trust the US mail. Not that I don't trust . . . but that's a very unusual thing to put in the mail. It's the kind of thing that young people are going to make jokes about and that's gonna make me mad and that's gonna jack my blood pressure again. (P82)

BM = Black man, BW = Black woman, CRC = colorectal cancer, VHA = virtual health assistant, WM = White man, WW = White woman.

> Last time I went to my doctor, he did the finger and made me throw up. I threw up. The nurse just laughed at me. I didn't never go back there. I was scheduled to go get it done [colonoscopy] and didn't go 'cause I was scared. (BM, P154)

This account of the visceral negative experience of being laughed at by a healthcare provider during a vulnerable moment is important for understanding the emotional and lived experience of Black men engaging with the healthcare system. A healthcare provider, rather than addressing this man's fear and embarrassment, mocked him at a critical point. This behavior negatively affected the patient's motivation to complete future screening tests. In this example, we see a specific way that a patient's needs were not met at the point of care, as well as how the lack of care created a barrier to seeking recommended CRC screenings.

Most participants felt that screening was important and that FIT would be an easy way to complete the important task. FIT was described as offering increased control of the screening process plus the ability to avoid the hassles of colonoscopy prep. "In my experience, the biggest challenge for the colonoscopy is the preparation, not the actual process. So, with the FIT you don't have to go through that preparation, so, I found that attractive" (BM, P15).

For Black participants, the benefits of FIT compared to colonoscopy may be implicitly activated by previous poor experiences with the healthcare system. White adults may not access negative associations with the healthcare system as readily, either because they have no negative associations or because any such associations occurred in different contexts. When participants did express preferences for colonoscopy, their comments reflected concerns over the accuracy of FIT or a lack of clarity regarding the benefits of FIT over colonoscopy. Some preferred coloscopy because it could be done in a more formal setting and provide more information. Some mentioned that the FIT might be a strange item to put in the mail.

Discussion

In this study, we employed a subjective culture approach to understand and compare rural Black and White adults' perceptions of a VHA that promoted CRC screening. The analysis assumed that people's various experiences within, and perceptions of, the healthcare system are driven by dynamics of race. These healthcare experiences likely shape patient engagement in care and the pervasiveness of screening inequities. Our study provided an opportunity to use telemedicine, specifically through VHAs, to enhance healthcare access among Black and White adults. We identified a range of benefits of the VHA-delivered messages, including that the message recipients had the opportunity to learn about CRC screening without an in-person clinic visit and to formulate questions prior to talking to their doctor.

We also analyzed the participants' perceptions of the source of information – the VHA itself. All participants wanted the VHA to be a friendly authority with expertise on CRC screening. Across gender and race, participants reported that the VHA having a medical background, being informative, looking and sounding professional, and appearing to be the right age appeared to cue perceptions of credibility. While perceptions and desires for friendliness were consistent across participant groups, there were nuanced differences between Black and White participants in preferences for how authority and expertise was communicated. White participants, and White men in particular, reported reluctance to trust the VHA and often expressed a desire for a more formal authority to be visibly connected to the VHA.

A number of cues were found to calibrate trust of the VHA. However, we found that once the VHA was developed to the point where most participants expressed trust in it, they described wanting to engage fully with it. This is one reason why trust is so important: once gained, it can help participants use and engage with the content and benefit from its full potential. This finding regarding trust is in line with previous research. Positive source attribution has also been demonstrated as being associated with increased intentions to seek additional cancer information, to share information, and to intend to screen for cancer – all important cognitive precursors to actual cancer screening (Ruzek et al., 2016). In fact, Nivens et al. (2001) found that among a predominantly African American study population, receiving information from a trusted health source was more strongly associated with increased prostate screening than any other kind of predictor.

This study's findings offer multiple implications for effective health communication strategies. First, intervention dissemination and implementation strategies that build on knowledge of the local community context may yield better buy-in. In this study, all participants responded positively to the VHA being affiliated with the local university hospital, which is well known to the community. We also found perceptions of the source of the VHA are important. For White participants, it was important for the VHA to be delivered directly from doctors: they said they would use the VHA intervention fully if their doctor said they should, but if it was disseminated via other methods, they might look and listen but would not interact fully. This is an important implication given that more and more healthcare interventions are being developed with and disseminated via web-based platforms. It's important to understand how digital interventions should be disseminated during implementation phases to encourage full engagement. Learning the nuances of what drives certain patient populations to engage fully with recommendations, and recognizing that these drivers may vary across populations, is warranted.

Second, framing the VHA as a way to improve communication with an existing provider (i.e., a patient's real doctor) may be an important part of marketing an intervention to White adults. Black adults did not explicitly express the same need or desire for the VHA to connect them to "their own doctor," although they did find the VHA appealing in that it could provide a valuable second opinion on options for care. Thus, for Black adults, dissemination efforts that position the VHA as a trusted, reliable source who has access to diverse health information and can provide a second opinion may be particularly engaging. And while, previous literature indicates African Americans may be less likely to ask questions of medical professionals when getting a physical exam (Whetten et al., 2006), our data indicated a specific desire to ask questions of the VHA and concern over not being able to do so. While, we are not able to determine if a desire to ask questions would translate into the behavior of asking questions during either patient provider interactions or VHA-user interactions, this is an important point that could be tested in future research as a component of assessing the quality of VHA communication.

The use of VHA technology in healthcare also presents opportunities to explore how people's previous experiences of having a race-concordant doctor in real life may influence their perceptions of concordant or discordant VHAs. Black Americans receive poorer-quality healthcare than White Americans, even after controlling for various sociodemographic factors and ability to pay for care, and there is growing acknowledgment among health professionals that racial bias is a likely contributor to this disparity (Bailey et al., 2020; James, 2017). These well-documented biases may or may not affect clinical decision making. However, poor experiences with healthcare among Black adults likely contribute to a well-earned mistrust of medical systems going back to the infamous Tuskegee study (Dula, 1994). With the emergence of telehealth and remote access to healthcare, trust and experiences of racism remain important issues, with technology-supported solutions emerging that have the potential to shape patient engagement with healthcare.

Of particular importance, all men and women in our focus groups repeatedly expressed interest in sharing the intervention and the information learned with their networks, including family, friends, and others. A significant point of concern was the need to promote CRC screening and prevention at a younger age: participants said they wanted to share content with younger children or family members, well before the age of screening guidelines. The desire to disseminate CRC education to a range of network members may reflect the lived experiences of Black adults, who experience higher rates of morbidity and mortality at earlier ages compared to other groups. This finding – of the importance of CRC prevention and screening messages for younger populations in the Black community – has implications for healthcare policy and guidelines. It also raises questions about insurance and reimbursements for screening, as well as a number of other barriers to screening.

Finally, while all participants were open to CRC screening, Black adults were more expressive about the novelty of the FIT test. In comparison, White adults were positive about FIT but engaged in more discussion about concerns with its accuracy. It is possible that the convenience of FIT becomes more or less appealing as a function of previous healthcare experiences. The driving force behind CRC screening preferences should be further explored, and future research findings could facilitate the development of engaging, patient-centered messages to promote screening. While more research, and perhaps triangulation of different types of data, could enhance these insights regarding CRC screening preferences, we found our participants were open and responded positively to learning about alternatives to more well-known, and more invasive, screening tests such as colonoscopies.

Study limitations

One limitation of this study is that some of the differences and similarities described here as a function of race may be related to components of identity that the analysis did not account for. For example, all our participants lived in rural zip codes; however, the rurality of areas within the zip codes varies. Thus, rural identity may also have been a factor influencing both perceptions of healthcare access and previous experiences with the healthcare system. Study participants also represented a specific demographic of adults living in the southern United States, and results may not be transferable to those from different geographic and cultural backgrounds. In addition, our analysis did not link participant comments in focus groups to individuals' questionnaire responses. This limited our ability to infer how other demographic factors may shape perceptions. Finally, our stimuli (the VHA) were evolving from focus group to focus group as participants provided feedback and suggested changes to the intervention. These changes included adjustments to graphics, backgrounds, affordances within the digital interface, and the VHA's appearance. Findings reported here should be interpreted with consideration that different groups of study participants were exposed to different and evolving versions of the intervention.

Conclusions

Assessing perceptions of health interventions that deliver cancer prevention messages is becoming increasingly important, as this information can play a significant role in improving access to medical services. Professional and academic organizations working at the intersection of health and practice are formally identifying that racism is an intrinsic part of the healthcare experience for the Black community and that it is prudent for health communication scholars to understand this perspective and incorporate that knowledge into communication goals and strategies aimed at improving health outcomes (O'Reilly, 2020). Borrowing the assumptions of CRT, we defined race in the context of culture as shared experiences of the healthcare system. The tenets of CRT align well with the strategies used to develop culturally-informed health messages. Bridging theory, health communication, and technology can be a powerful tool for inclusive delivery of CRC prevention messages.

Disclosure of potential conflict of interest

The content is solely the responsibility of the authors and does not necessarily represent official views of the NIH.

Funding

This research was supported by the National Cancer Institute, National Institutes of Health, Award #R01CA207689.

ORCID

Melissa J. Vilaro http://orcid.org/0000-0003-3975-0274
Danyell S. Wilson-Howard http://orcid.org/0000-0002-5912-4097
Jordan M. Neil http://orcid.org/0000-0001-5769-4961
Fatemeh Tavassoli http://orcid.org/0000-0002-3769-7679
Mohan S. Zalake http://orcid.org/0000-0002-6799-6784
Benjamin C. Lok http://orcid.org/0000-0002-1190-3729
François P. Modave http://orcid.org/0000-0003-4366-0757
Thomas J. George http://orcid.org/0000-0002-6249-9180
Folakemi T. Odedina http://orcid.org/0000-0003-3796-1385

Peter J. Carek http://orcid.org/0000-0003-3937-1733
Aubrey M. Mys http://orcid.org/0000-0002-3664-3361
Janice L. Krieger http://orcid.org/0000-0001-9950-9170

Data availability statement

The data that support the findings of this study are available from the corresponding author upon reasonable request.

References

Bailey, Z. D., Feldman, J. M., & Bassett, M. T. (2020). How structural racism works—Racist policies as a root cause of U.S. racial health inequities. *The New England Journal of Medicine*, *384*(8), 768–773. https://doi.org/10.1056/NEJMms2025396

Chaiken, S. (1987). The heuristic model of persuasion. In P. Zanna, J. M. Olson, & C. P. Herman (Eds.), *Social influence: The Ontario symposium* (Vol. 5, pp. 3–39). Lawrence Erlbaum Associates, Inc.

Claypool, H. M., O'Mally, J., & DeCoster, J. (2012). Dual-process models of information processing. In N. M. Seel (Ed.), *Encyclopedia of the sciences of learning* (pp. 1046–1048). Springer. https://doi.org/10.1007/978-1-4419-1428-6_676

DeSantis, C. E., Miller, K. D., Goding Sauer, A., Jemal, A., & Siegel, R. L. (2019). Cancer statistics for African Americans, 2019. *CA: A Cancer Journal for Clinicians*, *69*(3), 211–233. https://doi.org/10.3322/caac.21555

Dula, A. (1994). African American suspicion of the healthcare system is justified: What do we do about it? *Cambridge Quarterly of Healthcare Ethics*, *3*(3), 347–357. https://doi.org/10.1017/S0963180100005168

Griffin, L., Lee, D., Jaisle, A., Carek, P., George, T., Laber, E., Lok, B., Modave, F., Paskett, E., & Krieger, J. (2019). Creating an mHealth app for colorectal cancer screening: User-centered design approach. *JMIR Human Factors*, *6*(2), e12700. https://doi.org/10.2196/12700

James, S. A. (2017). The strangest of all encounters: Racial and ethnic discrimination in US health care. *Cadernos de Saúde Pública*, *33*(Suppl. 1), e00104416. https://doi.org/10.1590/0102-311x00104416

Ladson-Billings, G. (2013). Critical race theory—What it is not! In M. Lynn & A. D. Dixon (Eds.), *Handbook of critical race theory in education* (1st ed., pp. 34–47). Routledge. https://doi.org/10.4324/9780203155721.ch3

LaVeist, T. A., Nuru-Jeter, A., & Jones, K. E. (2003). The association of doctor-patient race concordance with health services utilization. *Journal of Public Health Policy*, *24*(3/4), 312–323. https://doi.org/10.2307/3343378

Lin, J. S., Piper, M. A., Perdue, L. A., Rutter, C. M., Webber, E. M., O'Connor, E., Smith, N., & Whitlock, E. P. (2016). Screening for colorectal cancer: Updated evidence report and systematic review for the US preventive services task force. *JAMA: The Journal of the American Medical Association*, *315*(23), 2576–2594. https://doi.org/10.1001/jama.2016.3332

May, F. P., Yang, L., Corona, E., Glenn, B. A., & Bastani, R. (2020). Disparities in colorectal cancer screening in the United States before and after implementation of the Affordable Care Act. *Clinical Gastroenterology and Hepatology*, *18*(8), 1796.e2–1804.e2. https://doi.org/10.1016/j.cgh.2019.09.008

McCurdie, T., Taneva, S., Casselman, M., Yeung, M., McDaniel, C., Ho, W., & Cafazzo, J. (2012). mHealth consumer apps: The case for user-centered design. *Biomedical Instrumentation & Technology*, *46* (s2), 49–56. https://doi.org/10.2345/0899-8205-46.s2.49

Merriam-Webster. (n.d.). *Professional*. Merriam-Webster.com Dictionary. Retrieved September 1, 2020, from https://www.merriam-webster.com/dictionary/professional

Metzger, M. J., Flanagin, A. J., Eyal, K., Lemus, D. R., & Mccann, R. M. (2003). Credibility for the 21st century: Integrating perspectives on source, message, and media credibility in the contemporary media environment. *Annals of the International Communication Association*, *27*(1), 293–335. https://doi.org/10.1080/23808985.2003.11679029

Nivens, A. S., Herman, J., Pweinrich, S., & Weinrich, M. C. (2001). Cues to participation in prostate cancer screening: A theory for practice. *Oncology Nursing Forum*, *28*(9), 1449–1456.

O'Keefe, D. J. (2002). *Persuasion: Theory and research* (2nd ed.). Sage Publications.

O'Reilly, K. (2020). *AMA: Racism is a threat to public health*. American Medical Association. https://www.ama-assn.org/delivering-care/health-equity/ama-racism-threat-public-health

Oetzel, J., Devargas, F., Ginossar, T., & Sanchez, C. (2007). Hispanic women's preferences for breast health information: Subjective cultural influences on source, message, and channel. *Health Communication*, *21* (3), 223–233. https://doi.org/10.1080/10410230701307550

Pasick, R. J., D'Onofrio, C. N., & Otero-Sabogal, R. (1996). Similarities and differences across cultures: Questions to inform a third generation for health promotion research. *Health Education Quarterly*, *23*(1_suppl), S142–S161. https://doi.org/10.1177/10901981960230S101

QSR International. (2018) *NVivo qualitative data analysis software* (Version 12) [Computer software].

Resnicow, K., Baranowski, T., Ahluwalia, J. S., & Braithwaite, R. L. (1999). Cultural sensitivity in public health: Defined and demystified. *Ethnicity & Disease*, *9*(1), 10–21.

Ruzek, S. B., Bass, S. B., Greener, J., Wolak, C., & Gordon, T. F. (2016). Randomized trial of a computerized touch screen decision aid to increase acceptance of colonoscopy screening in an African American population with limited literacy. *Health Communication*, *31*(10), 1291–1300. https://doi.org/10.1080/10410236.2015.1069165

Shen, M. J., Peterson, E. B., Costas-Muñiz, R., Hernandez, M. H., Jewell, S. T., Matsoukas, K., & Bylund, C. L. (2018). The effects of race and racial concordance on patient-physician communication: A systematic review of the literature. *Journal of Racial and Ethnic Health Disparities*, *5*(1), 117–140. https://doi.org/10.1007/s40615-017-0350-4

Tseng, S., & Fogg, B. J. (1999). Credibility and computing technology. *Communications of the ACM*, *42*(5), 39–44. https://doi.org/10.1145/301353.301402

Vilaro, M. J., Wilson-Howard, D. S., Griffin, L. N., Tavassoli, F., Zalake, M. S., Lok, B. C., Modave, F. P., George, T. J., Carek, P. J., & Krieger, J. L. (2020). Tailoring virtual human-delivered interventions: A digital intervention promoting colorectal cancer screening for Black women. *Psycho-Oncology*, *29*(12), 2048–2056. https://doi.org/10.1002/pon.5538

Whelehan, P., Evans, A., & Ozakinci, G. (2017). Client and practitioner perspectives on the screening mammography experience. *European Journal of Cancer Care*, *26*(3), e12580. https://doi.org/10.1111/ecc.12580

Whetten, K., Leserman, J., Whetten, R., Ostermann, J., Thielman, N., Swartz, M., & Stangl, D. (2006). Exploring lack of trust in care providers and the government as a barrier to health service use. *American Journal of Public Health*, *96*(4), 716–721. https://doi.org/10.2105/AJPH.2005.063255

Zhou, S., Bickmore, T., Paasche-Orlow, M., & Jack, B. (2014). Agent-user concordance and satisfaction with a virtual hospital discharge nurse. In T. Bickmore, S. Marsella, & C. Sidner (Eds.), *Lecture notes in computer science: Vol. 8637. Intelligent virtual agents* (pp. 528–541). Springer. https://doi.org/10.1007/978-3-319-09767-1_63

African American Women's Maternal Healthcare Experiences: A Critical Race Theory Perspective

Comfort Tosin Adebayo, Erin Sahlstein Parcell, Lucy Mkandawire-Valhmu, and Oluwatoyin Olukotun

ABSTRACT

Black women are experiencing pregnancy-related complications at a significantly higher rate than women of other races in the U.S., as Black women are three to four times likely to die from pregnancy-related complications compared to non-Hispanic White women. Structural barriers and different forms of marginalization continue to limit Black women's access to quality healthcare services. Through critical race theory, we examine what structural barriers exist in the U.S. healthcare system, one that limits access to quality care during their prenatal and postnatal doctor's visits. Using qualitative in-depth interviews, 31 African American women, living in Milwaukee, WI, shared their pregnancy stories. The emergent themes include, institutionalized care – racially insensitive biomedical approach, race and class – unfair treatment based on health insurance, and race as a social concept – dismissed pain concerns because you are a strong Black woman. These themes reveal the experience of racial discrimination toward African American women through healthcare [communicative] practices that are often times seen as "standard" practices, albeit marginalizing minority populations. Findings from this study offer insights for healthcare providers on communicative practices that foster a racially-safe healthcare environment for African American women.

Racial disparities in healthcare delivery is well established in the literature [Centers for Disease Control and Prevention (CDC), 2019; Creanga et al. (2015); Mkandawire-Valhmu (2018)]. Numerous studies report that African Americans receive low-quality care and differential treatment when accessing healthcare services, as a result of their racial identity[1] (Cuevas et al., 2016; Dovidio & Fiske, 2012; Keith et al., 2010; Krieger et al., 2011). Disparities exist for African Americans and other minority populations, for example, in limited information disclosure by healthcare providers (Ryn & Burje, 2002), verbal dominance by healthcare providers (Ha & Longnecker, 2010), dismissive attitude of healthcare providers toward patients' concerns (National Public Radio, 2017), and ultimately, provision of low-quality care (Ward et al., 2013). Racism and racial discrimination are factors that have been linked to the delivery and experience of race-based care[2] in the U.S. healthcare system. From the historical events of slavery to the Tuskegee Syphilis study of 1932 (Scharff et al., 2010) and the ongoing socio-political discourses that reinforce racial discrimination in the U.S. (Williams & Wyatt, 2015), African Americans continue to report racial disparities that impact their health.

Maternal health disparities are a major health concern for African American women. According to the Centers for Disease Control and Prevention (CDC) (2019), the maternal healthcare crisis among African American women is evidence of health disparities in U.S. society. African American women, as well as American Indian and Alaska native women, are two to three times more likely to die from pregnancy-related complications when compared to White women. Sadly, for Black women, this disparity exists regardless of socio-economic status or determinants of health as "[t]he PRMR (the pregnancy-related mortality ratio) for Black women with at least a college degree was 5.2 times that of their white counterparts" (Centers for Disease Control and Prevention (CDC), 2019, para. 6). This provides strong evidence that the issue of health inequities for African American women is not solely of a function of social factors such as socioeconomic status, but rather, it is a complex problem reflective of structural factors that negatively and disproportionately impact African American women (Gee & Ford, 2011; Homan, 2019).

Given the complex nature of maternal health inequities in African American women, critical theoretical perspectives, such as the critical race theory, offer an appropriate analytical lens to deconstruct the unique experiences of African American women within the U.S. context. Employing a critical race theory perspective (Delgado et al., 2017) to the study of African American women's health is valuable in exploring and critiquing hegemonic ideologies and structures that impact the realities and health outcomes of African Americans. In this study, we sought to unravel how African-American women make sense of the influence of their racial identity during maternal healthcare encounters. Specifically, through their stories, we explored and critiqued manifestations of racial discrimination in communicative acts of healthcare providers when providing medical services, with the goal of understanding their participation in the maternal healthcare crisis in the United States. Further, a secondary objective was to illuminate how healthcare providers perpetuate institutionalized and structural practices that advance racial discrimination in the U.S. healthcare system. In the following sections, we conduct a review of previous studies that have revealed the myriad problems African American women experience in accessing the U.S. healthcare system, followed by a description of our study and findings.

Literature review

The problem–health disparities, race, and gender

Health disparities have garnered increased attention in the United States over the past twenty years. However, despite a significant comprehensive report on health inequities by the Institute of Medicine and the scholarly discussion that ensued, ethnic minority communities continue to experience a high burden of poor health outcomes across a number of health indicators (Baciu et al., 2017; Institute of Medicine, 2003; Noonan et al., 2016). For instance, African Americans continue to be disproportionately impacted by adverse maternal child health outcomes (Howland et al., 2019; Singh & Stella, 2019). Compared to White women, African American women are twice as likely to have a child with low birth weight and one-and-a-half times more likely to have a preterm birth (Martin et al., 2017). Similar patterns of disparities in African American women are seen across other reproductive health indicators including perinatal loss mortality (Koch & Geller, 2019), and maternal (Petersen et al., 2019) and infant mortality (Kitsantas & Gaffney, 2010).

While ongoing efforts are made to comprehensively delineate the causes of persistent health disparities, growing evidence points to the effects of a myriad of complex, multilevel factors rooted in institutionalized discrimination based on race and gender (Gee & Ford, 2011; Gollust et al., 2018; Shavers & Shavers, 2006). Their systematic marginalization, operationalized through policies, societal practices, and differential access to resources and power, has been cited as the distal cause of adverse health outcomes for African American women (Gee & Ford, 2011; Homan, 2019). Notably, for African American women, the marginalization they experience as a result of their racial and gender identities cannot be analyzed independently of each other. Strong evidence indicate that the combination of both racial and gender discrimination that African American women experience adversely impacts health through physiological and psychological stress pathways (Perry et al., 2013). Beyond the differential access to resources that results from institutionalized discrimination, understanding the experiences of marginalized communities during healthcare encounters are a critical component of unearthing how disparities in health outcomes are produced within the healthcare infrastructure (Penner et al., 2014), particularly for African American women who bear a disproportionate burden of adverse birth outcomes.

Provider-patient communication and the experience of racial discrimination

Communication occupies a central role in healthcare encounters (Adebayo et al., 2020). The sensemaking process of healthcare services is mostly interpreted from the perspective of communication. In reporting their experiences of racial discrimination when accessing healthcare services or low-quality care, patients (regardless of racial identity) have identified communication factors as key variables when examining experiences of racial discrimination during healthcare encounters (Cuevas et al., 2016; Ha & Longnecker, 2010; Raine et al., 2010). For instance, African Americans have reported poor communication and lack of expressed respect by healthcare workers (Cuevas et al., 2016). These findings are similar to many others that have examined the healthcare barriers of African Americans (Ha & Longnecker, 2010; Mazul et al., 2017).

As evidenced in previous studies (e.g., Cuevas et al., 2016; Raine et al., 2010), patients also often assess the quality of care received through the lens of communication; how the provider related to them, the clarity of the message, the depth of the message, the content of the message, and the display of interpersonal connection with the patient. Specifically, the quality of interpersonal communication between physicians and patients impacts health outcomes by influencing patient satisfaction, physician-patient trust, and rapport, willingness to disclose important health information (Arnold & Boggs, 2019). Communication functions as a significant tool in shaping the quality of healthcare services in any context (Abioye Kuteyi et al., 2010; Ha & Longnecker, 2010). Quality communication, or its lack thereof, influences patients' perceptions of the healthcare system and the services delivered during patient visits. More specifically, implicit and explicit racial biases thrive through verbal and non-verbal communication. Studies show that "Black patients feel less respected by the physician, like the physician less, and have less confidence in the physician regarding their medical encounters when the physician exhibits greater implicit racial bias" (Dovidio & Fiske, 2012, p. 948). Moreover, in the context of maternal healthcare visits, African American women have reported poor communication along the lines of rushed interactions, ambiguous word choices, and lack of affection or empathy (Raine et al., 2010). Evidently, healthcare experiences are communicatively interpreted; hence, analyzing women's maternal healthcare experiences as a communication phenomenon provides an important perspective.

Maternal mortality among African American women

Despite efforts made to unravel and ameliorate racial disparities in maternal mortality in the U.S., the persistent inequities in outcomes for African American women remains alarming. Specifically, non-Hispanic African American women have higher rates of maternal mortality compared to other ethnic and racial groups with a two to three-fold increased odds of dying from pregnancy-related complications when compared to non-Hispanic White women (Centers for Disease Control and Prevention (CDC), 2019). One study found that being a Black woman with a chronic illness was associated with a two to three-fold increased odd of maternal mortality in comparison to White women with the same chronic condition (Tucker et al., 2007).

Arguably, while some evidence exists for the clinical and pathological causes of maternal mortality in the U.S. (Centers for Disease Control and Prevention (CDC), 2019; Creanga et al., 2014), the prevalence of this health problem among African American women remains a puzzle. Previous studies have documented the existence of racial and health disparities in the quality of care received by African Americans when accessing healthcare services (Krieger et al., 2011). Consequently, to analyze the U.S. maternal health crisis from a biomedical perspective with inattention to race and racial discrimination, as often times reported by the CDC, presents an incomplete argument. The role of race as an integral factor in maternal health inequities is evident in extant literature (Mazul et al., 2017). Race, as a factor in healthcare experiences, is further illustrated by the reported experiences of prominent African American women like Shalon Irvings, an Epidemiologist at the Centers for Disease Control and Prevention, who passed away weeks after delivery in 2017 (National Public Radio, 2017). Irving's case was not one linked to poverty or low education, she had two doctoral degrees; rather it was linked to racial disparities in quality of healthcare she received as reports indicate that her health symptoms were repeatedly dismissed days before her demise (National Public Radio, 2017).

Similar to Dr. Irvings experience, the African American maternal health literature is replete with reports of health symptoms being trivialized or dismissed. Stemming from historical events of slavery, African American women are often perceived to be "strong" and able to go through hardships and withstand pain beyond what is considered "normal" (Davis, 2015; Watson-Singleton, 2017). This racial discourse of (perceived) strength negatively impacts African American women within the healthcare context. The perception of being strong has been reported to "force" African American women to internalize their pains and hardships, and healthcare providers often reinforce this discourse (Collins, 2000; Watson-Singleton, 2017). The foregoing review provides an overview of the African American women's interactions with the healthcare systems. However, beyond the problematic communication encounters there are structural barriers, otherwise labeled "standard practices," that propagate health inequities for African American women, which is the focus of our study.

Structural barriers in African American women's maternal healthcare experiences

In this study, we focus on two main structural barriers confronting African American women during prenatal and postnatal care: the institutionalized biomedical approach to maternal care and the structural barrier of public health insurance. The biomedical approach to maternal healthcare is notorious for its overt focus on Western medicine and procedures in attending to women's reproductive healthcare needs. Traditionally, the biomedical approach has been criticized for disempowering women, since women are the primary consumers of healthcare services in the United States and even other parts of the world (Willard, 2005). Particularly concerning women's reproductive health, the medical profession has been critiqued for the medicalization of women's experiences, including pregnancy. In this way, the woman's body is treated as a machine programmed to perform certain operations that can be managed when "faulty" to ensure its appropriate functioning (Andipatin et al., 2019). The dominance of the biomedical approach in healthcare has been found to result in "the medicalization of normal life events (e.g., giving birth, menopause) and an over-reliance on technological solutions" (Willard, 2005, p. 135). Consequently, within the U.S. healthcare system, pregnancy is primarily considered a medical condition, which needs medical intervention for its management and treatment.

Given the lived realities of African American women in U.S. society, the biomedical approach to maternal care further situates African American women as objects in a system that denigrates their racial identity and realities. It is important for healthcare providers to become aware of the reality that "pregnancy and its associated biological processes are complex and expressed in an assortment of ways, they are lived out in equally complicated sets of social and power relations" (Andipatin et al., 2019, p. e553). African American women have unique social and cultural milieu that position them on the margins of the society. Thus, it is important to understand how the biomedical approach works to usurp power and agency from these women based on institutional healthcare practices that likely do not put racial realities into perspective.

Another notable structural barrier in African American women's healthcare access is the type of insurance they carry. In the United States, an individual's socio-economic status can be accurately assessed based on the type of health insurance (that is, public versus private/employer-sponsored). Public (also known as state insurance or Medicaid) health insurance is provided to low-income individuals. For African American women, using the public insurance is often stigmatized (Allen et al., 2014; Taylor, 2019); it does not only label them as low-income, it goes further to limit the access they can have to healthcare. Studies have shown that one of the challenges that confront African Americans on public insurance is finding doctors who accept such insurance plans (Mazul et al., 2017). For those who are lucky enough to find doctors, they are treated with suboptimal care while also discriminated against based on their health insurance (Weech-Maldonado et al., 2012), including limited breastfeeding support (Thorburn & De Marco, 2010). These barriers, as they intersect with race and class, continue to limit African American women's access to quality care during this vulnerable time of their lives. Critically exploring these barriers and their manifestations from a critical race theoretical perspective provides a holistic understanding of health inequities common to these women, if we are to effectively address the U.S. maternal health crisis.

Theoretical framework: Critical race theory

Critical race theory (CRT) is an interdisciplinary theory that provides a framework for studying the experiences of racially marginalized populations in the U.S. society. It was developed by the collective work of scholars like Derrick Bell, Alan Freeman, and Richard Delgado (Delgado & Stefancic, 2012). Though developed by U.S. scholars, the application of the theory has extended to other parts of the world (Warmington, 2012). Three basic tenets guide the understanding and application of CRT as discussed by Delgado et al. (2017). First, CRT functions to critique the idea that racism is ordinary, that is, normal. This notion of the ordinariness and normality of racism in the society advances the "color-blind, or 'formal', conceptions of equality, expressed in rules that insist only on treatment that is the same across the board, can thus remedy the most extreme forms of discrimination" (Delgado et al., 2017, p. 8). This way, people of color are indiscriminately ignored or unaccounted for in social policies, "because an individual (white) person 'does not see race' and therefore 'is not racist" (Wesp et al., 2018, p. 321). Not only are people of color ignored in social policies that underserve them, they are also discriminated against given the hallmark of what is "good" only resides in whiteness. Second, CRT critiques "interest convergence" and material accumulation of wealth as a core manifestation of racism, one that predominantly serves whites in the U.S. society (Delgado et al., 2017, p. 8). In this regard, as whiteness is positioned as a property of interest (Ladson-Billings & Tate, 2006, p. 2006), CRT challenges the hegemonic functioning of social institutions that advance the interests of Whites, materially and otherwise. Third, CRT upholds the fact that race is socially constructed. In other words, ethnic minority populations are only relevant to the extent to which the society "endows them with pseudo-permanent characteristics," subjecting them to social and power hierarchies (Delgado et al., 2017, p. 9) where they are relegated to the lowest rungs.

CRT, in its usage, attends to issues of racism, which are believed to be ingrained in social institutions in the U.S., especially in the education sector (Ladson-Billings & Tate, 2006). In its scope, CRT identifies issues of racial injustices among ethnic minorities as well as unveils the impact of social, political, and philosophical structures in advancing different forms of marginalization and injustices toward members of minority racial groups (Hylton, 2012). Consequently, CRT allows for a holistic view of racial discrimination as it manifests systemically, leading to inequities in various sectors of society, including healthcare.

Within the context of healthcare scholarship, CRT "guides us in acknowledging the reality of inequality among these racialized groups and the racist ideology that informs healthcare interactions in our society" (Mkandawire-Valhmu, 2018, p. 50). It affords healthcare scholars a unique perspective for understanding the causes of racism in the healthcare system (Ford & Airhihenbuwa, 2010), as rooted in "standard practices and structures." CRT highlights systemic structures that underserve racial minorities, which in turn advance racism. Within health communication scholarship, CRT has been used to study the healthcare experiences of racial minorities like Hispanics, and African Americans (Vardeman-Winter, 2017). For instance, in the application of CRT to African American and Black Hispanics' healthcare experiences, Freeman et al. (2017) found that structural racism persists with institutionalized healthcare practices that might not represent the interest of minority groups. This includes lack of personalized care, as they reported being treated based on papers and numbers. One serious implication of these practices that perpetuate racist ideologies is a deeply-rooted, distrust of healthcare providers and healthcare practices. While studies like theirs have employed CRT to unveil how structural racism shape the experiences of ethnic minority groups within the healthcare system, there is a dearth of literature that utilizes a similar approach to analyze structural racism within the maternal healthcare context.

In this study, CRT provides a lens to critically analyze the interconnectedness of racial injustice and the maternal care experiences of African American women. Focusing on the experiences of African American women will center their voices while simultaneously recording how race and systemic racism construct their healthcare realities for Black women. We used the following question to guide our work:

RQ: How does racial discrimination manifest in the maternal healthcare narratives of African American women?

Method

Upon the approval of the study by the University of Wisconsin-Milwaukee IRB (UWM IRB # 19.A.238), the first author recruited women to participate in qualitative interviews through purposive and snowball sampling. Lindlof and Taylor (2019) argue that qualitative interviews are valuable in contexts where participants lived experience and worldview are central to the research questions. Purposive sampling involves the recruitment of research participants by directly asking members of groups or populations who fit the research criteria to participate in the study, while snowball sampling takes place when individuals are recruited through those who have participated in a study (Lindlof & Taylor, 2019; Tracy, 2012). In other words, it involves recruitment through referrals – asking research participants to encourage other individuals (e.g., friends, family members, etc.) who qualify for the study to participate (Lindlorf & Taylor, 2019). Announcements were made on Facebook groups and pages dedicated to moms (e.g., Milwaukee Moms, KidsCycle: NS Milwaukee area, and African American Breastfeeding network Milwaukee), and the one she created (Black Moms Maternal Health) for African American women living in the Milwaukee area.

Study site

Data collection for this study took place in Milwaukee county, Wisconsin, for close to a year, between March 2019 and February 2020. Milwaukee presently ranks as the most racially segregated metropolitan city in the U.S. (Frey, 2018). Milwaukee also has some of the highest rates of Black infant mortality (City of Milwaukee Health Department, 2018; Ward et al., 2013). According to the Wisconsin Department of Health Services (2019), for the most recent statistics on maternal health outcomes, maternal mortality rates were five times higher among African American women compared to non-Hispanic White women in the city of Milwaukee.

Participants

Thirty-one African American women participated in this study, which includes four women who participated in the pilot study[3] for this present research. Participants were African American women who were currently living in Milwaukee County and had maternal care experiences with healthcare providers in the city or surrounding area. Participants ranged from 20–44 years old and were either pregnant (n = 6) or had been pregnant within the previous year (n = 21). Participants also included women who were part of the pilot study and had been pregnant within the last ten years (n = 4). The majority of the women were either pregnant with their first child or had only one child (n = 16). Ten of the women reported having employer-sponsored insurance, eighteen reported having state insurance, one reported not having insurance, while the remaining three participants did not report their health insurance status. In reporting their marital relationship status, eight women reported being married while twenty-three reported being single or engaged. For participants who reported their annual income, ten did not report their income or were currently unemployed, thirteen had a household income of less than 35,000 USD per year, five reported an income between 36,000 USD and 70,000 USD per year, while three reported an annual household income between 71,000 USD and 120,000. USD

Semi-structured in-depth interviews

Participants who met the eligibility criteria were interviewed by the first author, either face-to-face (n= 6) or over the phone (n= 25). Before the commencement of each interview, the interviewer read the consent form to the participants, and consent was established through verbal affirmation for both face-to-face and virtual participants. Each interview was audio-recorded and lasted between 50 to 75 minutes.

Participants were asked to narrate their most recent pregnancy stories starting from the day they learned of their pregnancy until delivery or present (for those who are still currently pregnant; narrative interview format). Follow-up questions to clarify meanings and solicit other relevant information based on their stories and the focus of the study (respondent interview format) were asked. This included descriptive, experience, typology, and example questions (Spradley, 1979; Tracy, 2012). In the latter part of the interview, participants answered questions that solicited information about their perception of the maternal crisis among African American women. These include questions on their racial and pregnancy identities. Upon the completion of the interview, each participant received a 20 USD Walmart or Amazon gift card.

Reflexivity and positionality

As critical scholars, reflexivity and positionality are key to the unbiased interpretation of our data, especially when relating with members of marginalized groups (D'Silva et al.'s, 2016). Reflexivity focuses on how methodological choices impact the interpretation of the data (Corlett & Mavin, 2018). Knowing that truth is socially constructed, it is imperative for researchers to critically examine how our presence in this research process impacts the process and ultimately the outcome (Dutta, 2010). Our culturally diverse team is composed of Black (three) and White (one) women, from interdisciplinary fields of communication and nursing. We deliberately prioritized the contribution of our minority yet diverse voices to the ongoing discourse of maternal health crisis among African Americans. Our cultural and disciplinary diversity allowed for rigorous and critical analysis of our data-giving room for careful interpretation and report of our findings.

Through a pilot study, the first three authors rigorously assessed the research questions and the interpretation of the data refining it to remove possible biases in how participants respond to questions and how we ultimately analyzed the data. Regarding our positionality, we understand that our lived and ongoing experiences (via our social locations of race, class, education, and gender) are capable of influencing our interpretation of the data. As such we deliberately chose to analyze the data from a theoretical perspective without losing the diversity that our interdisciplinary and multicultural backgrounds contribute to the research.

Data analysis

The first three authors conducted the analysis of the data. The first author took the lead in this process. Data analysis commenced during data collection as the first author engaged in an iterative process of interviewing and reflection. Reflecting on interviews and reading notes during the process of data collection are useful practices in making sense of the data at the preliminary level (Saunders et al., 2018). Following the transcription of the interviews by a third-party service (Temi™ software) and a research assistant, the first author assessed the 554 pages of transcripts for accuracy. This process included removing any identifying information from the data while assigning pseudonyms to participants to further protect their confidentiality.

In the first stage of coding, we engaged in value coding, a type of descriptive coding that copiously accounts for participants' "values, attitudes, and beliefs" as it reflects their perspective to social issues (Miles et al., 2013, p. 75). This type of coding is useful for understanding and reporting issues of identity as it relates to social realities and issues. Since the study focuses on how the racial identity of Black women interfere with their healthcare experiences and outcomes, employing this kind of coding was valuable in unveiling the role race plays in this context. After identifying initial codes (e.g., biomedical approach to maternal care, women as machines), we merged similar codes by categorizing them into themes as they reflected the tenets of critical race theory issues of racial discrimination propagated by social structures in the U.S. society. The third author, given expertise in CRT carefully revised the themes to assess their representation and explanation of CRT. These include analyzing systemic issues, present in women's narratives, and their impact on healthcare encounters. At the end of this stage, we merged themes that were similar in the information they provided. In the end, the first author closely read through the findings again to identify and clarify any form of ambiguity.

Findings

In applying critical race theory to African American women's maternal healthcare narratives, we highlight dimensions of racial discrimination present in women's experiences during medical interactions and the healthcare practice for maternal care. One of the central arguments of CRT scholars is that racial issues and racism are so ingrained in our system and structures that we fail to perceive them as such-they have become "normal life" (Delgado & Stefancic, 2012; Ford & Airhihenbuwa, 2010). As a result of this, the current study employs CRT to uncover dimensions of racial discrimination and racism that are present in maternal healthcare "standard practices," while demystifying the ideology of color-blind healthcare system – "the notion of a racially neutral and democratic social order that works for all people" (López, 2003, p. 83). Using the three tenets of CRT as guiding lens, three themes emerged from the analysis: Institutionalized care – Racially insensitive biomedical approach, Race and class – Unfair treatment based on health insurance, and Race as a social concept – Dismissed pain concerns because you are a strong Black woman. A fourth theme emerged from the analysis outside of the of CRT's basic tenets, Distrust – African American women as charity case.

Institutionalized care – racially insensitive biomedical approach

One of the basic tenets of CRT is the notion that racism is so deeply embedded in the fabric of U.S. social and political institutions that its presence has been normalized and accepted as "standard practice". However, women in this study challenged these standard practices revealing their shortcomings in advancing a racially insensitive maternal healthcare. Centrally woven throughout the narratives of women in this study is the experience of a racially insensitive healthcare system – the supposed color-blind healthcare. In this context, the institutionalized biomedical approach was criticized for its dominance in maternal healthcare practice. African American women challenged this approach as racially denigrating as it has been structurally positioned as "the" way to provide maternal care while ignoring other health approaches to providing maternal care, especially the cultural dimension of health. The narratives of the women in this study pointed out the lack of consideration for women's preferences during pregnancy, speaking to how healthcare providers treated them based on what "textbooks" say, while taking away their racial and cultural presence in maternal care. They criticized it for its White-centric method in attending to women's needs; as the healthcare practices are mostly viewed from the hegemonic standpoint of White women, whose experiences mostly form the basis for healthcare practices during maternal care. When we asked Beth, a 21-year old mother, to narrate her maternal care story, she said:

> So, from the first time that I found out I was pregnant, I knew right away that I wanted to have my child at home or at a birthing center. I know that I wanted it to be as natural as possible and I knew that I did not really want to go the regular route of going to like the doctor checkups and stuff … ."I want to have this baby at home, I want to do a natural, I don't plan a birth in the hospital" … .So, I talked to my doctor about it and he became inconsistent. He said that I'm high risk and blah blah. And I feel like he started to say that because I told him about me wanting to birth at home. I feel like as soon as I told him about that, everything just changed. So, then they started telling me that I would have to come in every two weeks and monitor my baby's growth because I had IUGR, which is injuring growth restriction. So, they claimed, they told me I was really high risk. … I had told the doctor like, "Well, I'm still gonna have my baby at home." And the doctor walked out on me He never came back in the room … I'm like, "Y'all are treating me wrong. You're not listening to me. You're not respecting me. This is my body, my baby."

Beth's narrative shows a rigid biomedical approach to maternal care, one that subtly rejects other maternal care methods such as midwifery and home birthing – practices that are historically and traditionally upheld in the African American community (Dawley, 2003). Given this dominant biomedical maternal healthcare practice, African American women are indiscriminately treated based on a hegemonic model of care, one that inherently does not account for their unique realities, as with other social institutions.

The biomedical approach was not only criticized for its White-centric approach to maternal care, but also for its structured, one-size fits all approach for Black women. In this manner, Black women are treated as a monolith based on "what is generally known about Black health," rather than being treated as individuals, further reinforcing the ideology that they are mere statistics. Rachel, a 23-year-old first-time mother, shared:

> I was diagnosed with gestational diabetes … they also diagnosed me to take baby aspirin. Like no reason. They said that as Black people, it's more common to have that preeclampsia … I honestly don't see why I need to take this. Like I don't have a history of it. This is my first pregnancy. So, I'm like, "I'm not taking the baby aspirin," but me being me, when they asked me like, "Oh, are you taking your medicine?" "Yes," because I don't want to say no, and they'd try to diagnose me with something, like, "Well she's not taking her medicine, so she probably has this thing."

Rachel considered this medical push as a hegemonic and homogenous view about Black women's health, such that they are often perceived as having poor health, just as they are perceived in other contexts (Freeman et al., 2017). She explained that healthcare providers usually lump African American women together, without paying attention to each individual. She said, "Like I don't have a history of it. You can't like, um, basically stereotype me because I'm African American." This way, they believe an instance of illness or behavior in one African American is present with others. This institutionalized practice further led to the silencing of these women, which is a long-term effect of racism in our society. Telither, in a similar experience, also encountered the imposition of medicalized birth by her healthcare providers. She recalled the reaction of her nurses in the delivery room when she told them she wanted a natural birth:

> I think the staff pushed more for different directions for my choices. So, like if I said I want to do a natural birth, they were like, "Why? Why would you want to go natural? We got drug for that and you won't do this" … I think they have the assumption that we don't know what our bodies are capable of.

Telither considered her experience as one that invalidates her ability to make an informed decision about her maternal care. She attributed this experience to both her racial and gender identities.

Race and class – unfair treatment based on health insurance

The interest convergence tenet of CRT was foregrounded as women reported the influence of their racial identity, as it intersects with their socioeconomic status, in the quality of care they received. Unique, a 24-year old pregnant woman, in her narrative, said African American women begin to experience differential treatment not only in the quality of care given to them but even based on the type of insurance they have:

> Like when you're asked what type of insurance you have and you feel like, "Oh, I have government insurance" and they like look at you differently or they treat you differently, different from if you had like private insurance or insurance through an employer or something like that."

The fact that Medicaid is only accessible to low-income individuals, and in Wisconsin a majority of these recipients are African Americans (Kaiser Family Foundation, 2019), put these women in a situation where they are constantly disenfranchised because of the intersections of race and class. While Medicaid offers benefits for low income individuals, for African American women, it can function as a reminder of their disenfranchisement and institutionalized practices that foster racism. Rachel further evidenced this insurance-based discrimination in her narrative:

> So I feel like, yeah, I feel like this thing [race and class] is definitely real, they definitely judge you on that. They look at you and it's like, "Oh well we're not going to do much with them. We just gonna patch them up, get them okay, and throw them out of the door." … I feel like that's how they treat African-Americans. You don't have the best insurance. A lot of us, don't get me wrong, we're in all different ranks of course, but like I'm in lower class so I can't afford to, insurance puts us in different places.

Rachel's narrative shows both an expression of lament and distrust in the healthcare system that allows a supposed help for minority through the prism of Medicaid. The issue even becomes more complicated because of the racial climate of the city, where there is evident racial segregation. Shirval articulates how Milwaukee as a city naturally positions African American women as low class, public insurance patients, resulting in low quality of care:

> Ultimately [the way you are treated] I would say it depends on the type of insurance you have. And then we are talking about African American women a lot. And especially here is Milwaukee, if you're talking about this region, I feel like there is a lot of African American women or Black women that's in poverty and might need assistance, whether that's needed, state insurance or whatever that looks like. And I feel like they are treated differently than someone with employers insurance … they [healthcare providers] can see or read into my history and find out if you have some form of education, you know, I feel like that, that, that sometimes they could make that separation … Not to say that I couldn't be treated poorly just by looking at me and not knowing anything about me, but ultimately these people (healthcare provider)], I feel like, it definitely has a lot to do with, your insurance and what's the first thing they see from your records-your socioeconomic status, all of that.

Without mincing words, Shirval's narrative unveiled the workings of race and class in the type of treatment African American get when accessing maternal care. While this is not new (Allen et al., 2014; Taylor, 2019), women's narratives, here, show how covert racial discrimination in the healthcare system leads to mistrust, and poor treatment, which are factors consistently cited in women's maternal crisis narratives (National Public Radio, 2017). Kevris furthered this argument in her narrative by saying:

> I feel like it's because of our race and the things that we've gone through. In America, there's always been a difference in, you know, race, in the color of your skin. You know, it's always been that way. Like if you're white, you have more of a privilege and you are given more opportunities, you know, but if you're Black and if your skin color is Black, no matter if you're, you know, Black from Africa, like, have African roots, I feel like you're still seen as lesser.

Clearly, discourse of systemic racism and the historical events of slavery and colonization were evident in Shirval's narrative, as she attributed African American women's experiences to what is considered "normal" in America – the ordinariness of racism (Delgado & Stefancic, 2012). Consequently, African American women's experiences of discrimination in medical encounters are a reflection of the U.S.'s institutional practices that underserve racial minorities.

Race as a social concept – dismissed pain concerns because you are a strong Black woman

Being a Black woman did not only mean differential treatment for African Americans. For the women interviewed, it also meant that they had to endure pain beyond what they considered normal because they were "strong Black women." Delgado and Stefancic (2012) explained this ideology as the social construction of race, where African American women are not only treated based on science but also on how they have been historically constructed as strong. While this discourse of strength is traceable to the history of slavery, it has become a welcomed racial identity marker, even for African American women themselves. Yet, within the context of healthcare, this discourse leads to women's disadvantage (Abrams et al., 2014). In the current study, this stereotype resulted in the undermining or dismissing African American women's concerns, especially in relation to pain. Sadiat, a 23-year-old first-time mother, narrated her experience as follows:

> At about one in the morning … I was just like, I like, this is not feeling right. I am not comfortable. … We went to the ER and I don't know if it was because it was late that they just like were not taking their job seriously, but like the tone of voice, like I said, super nonchalant … disregarding my pain, and I remember one nurse is just like, "Well yeah, you're pregnant." … as a doctor, if I'm explaining my pain to you and the symptoms that I'm having, like I expect you to take me seriously. I don't expect you to tell me, "Well yeah you're pregnant." "I know I'm pregnant. That's why I'm here explaining my pain to you so I can make sure that my child is okay."

Similarly, during labor and delivery, Ebony spoke of experiencing excruciating pain that was repeatedly dismissed by her healthcare providers:

> She was like, "No, you're just being paranoid." And I was like, "I still don't feel well." She was like, "Oh, you're fine, you're fine." And I was like, "Something isn't right." And then I was telling her like, "I'm passing these, these chunks of blood clot." They were like … "You're fine … ." I'm still having problems and, in a strain, even after taking the narcotics, I'm still like damn pain, cramping bad. And she was like, "You're fine. You know, you're older. That's why you know, you're feeling like this." And I was like, "That's not what this is." And all I kept telling her, "Something is wrong with [the baby]. Something is wrong with me." She's like, "You're okay." So, two weeks after he was born, I decided to go to the ER, and they told me that I needed a D & C [Dilation and curettage] because I still had some of my placenta in me.

Tragically, Ebony lost her baby while also having to go through emergency surgery following complications post-delivery. Similarly, Tabithe, a 20-year old mother of one, explained how she felt healthcare providers perceived African American women as deceitful about their pain level. When asked about how healthcare providers perceived pregnant African American women, she said:

> African American woman are seen as lying about what type of pain we're in and how bad it hurts. "Don't tell me how bad I'm hurting. You are not inside of me." And that's how they always come at you … like you're lying or exaggerating … they treat you like you're lying or like it's not that serious.

Tabithe's story highlights how the dismissal of African American women's concerns on the part of healthcare providers', exacerbates women's lack of trust in healthcare providers and the healthcare system, leaving women feeling disempowered and less-valued.

Distrust – African American women as charity case

Under this theme, African American women expressed how they felt that their racial identity positioned them as a "charity case." Even when healthcare providers provided what they considered quality care, because of their overall experiences, they wondered whether healthcare providers genuinely cared about them and their healthcare needs. In this way, the women viewed the quality of care provided to them as a favor to help the "helpless." Consequently, these women reported that even "good" care provided to them was often accompanied with the notion of charity provided by whites to the helpless Blacks. In Unique's narrative she said:

> I think there's racism everywhere, but I think there's racism in the healthcare system … we're just looked at differently … I think African American women are more looked at as a charity case in a way. They looked at us like, "It looks better if I help this lady lift weights because I'm Caucasian and I'm helping somebody different than me, so it'll look better on my end if I help her."

Unique reasoned that the care delivered to African American women during pregnancy is not aimed at their best interest, rather as a way that doctors, whom she framed as Caucasians, foster a positive image for themselves, so as "to look better." Zee's story was similar as she agreed African American women are often treated as low-class patients:

> I just feel like people care about other races than our, than our own race. Uh, you know, they're just like, "Well, we don't care about the Blacks. Let's just make sure that other races are okay." Like, the Caucasian just make sure they're okay before we make sure the African Americans are okay. So, they basically like put us on the backburner.

Specifically, Zee believes that Caucasians get better treatment at the expense of African Americans, as African Americans are treated as inferior, thus, uncared for. In her narrative, Megan reasoned that African American women are treated poorly because whites have positioned them as inferior who should be "helped" When we asked Megan why she had this perception about doctors, she said:

> It's just, I don't know, like I never had that problem with a doctor, but it's just a thought that crosses my mind too as well. Like, you know, "You [whites] sit and help us, but you feel like we just beneath y'all, like we don't deserve it." Like they think, some not all, but some doctors could possibly think, "We shouldn't have to help because this money [for your healthcare] expenses is coming out of our pockets, we got to help y'all. We really don't want to.

Megan, similar to other women in this study, reasoned that the problem of maternal crisis among African American women is rooted in systemic racism, to control the Black population so that whites may continue to dominate them. While this perception may be subjective, it exemplifies a bigger issue of mistrust in the healthcare system.

The Study's findings show how racial identity impacts healthcare access and experiences for African American women during pregnancy, labor and delivery and in the postpartum period. Through implicit and explicit biases, healthcare providers' communicative acts were identified as racially denigrating and discriminatory toward women.

Discussion

Communication stands at the core of women's narratives when reporting their experiences of racism in the way maternal healthcare services were provided to them. Communication strategies, acts, and dynamics culminate to form the platform through which racial discrimination is enacted and perceived (Kreps, 2006). Studying maternal healthcare experiences from a communication perspective helps to center the voices of women, and CRT helps to uncover ways in which structural racism is communicatively enacted.

In revealing structural practices that inherently advance racial discrimination in the healthcare system, the biomedical approach was critiqued in women's narratives. The biomedical structure of the U.S. healthcare system, as an institutionalized form of racism, paves the way for the denigration and the dismissal of African American women's choices in maternal care. Ultimately, the biomedical approach, as a healthcare "standard" practice, creates a space that dehumanizes women, rendering them incapable of making decisions that concern their own health and the health of their babies. Functioning in a hegemonic healthcare system, positions healthcare providers as the only ones who can make decisions on behalf of women, through structured practices that are not tailored to meet women's unique needs, leaving African American women feeling incapacitated and dehumanized (Freeman et al., 2017).

Through the interest convergence tenet of CRT, our data reveals how the supposed help for the minority groups further places them on the margins of society for less than optimal care during pregnancy. Racial discrimination manifests through healthcare providers' disposition toward public insurance, that is, Medicaid, as women consistently reported discriminatory treatment based on their type of insurance. In some cases, they were denied care, when the care requested was deemed by a provider as being unnecessary. Again, CRT helps to uncover how systemic practices aimed at promoting health equities are disguised forms of racial discrimination because of the way they are enacted.

CRT further enabled us to see how dominant cultural norms, especially socially constructed racial and gender expectations, negatively impact African American women's maternal care (Freeman et al., 2017). The cultural notion of women as "natural endurers" of pain alongside the racial stereotype of Black women as extraordinarily strong impacted how African American women's pain was perceived and managed, especially during labor and delivery. African American women are indeed often perceived as possessing extraordinary ability for putting up with pain (Davis, 2015; Stewart, 2017; Watson-Singleton, 2017). The strong Black woman, a cultural discourse, evolved from the historical experiences of African American women as they assumed different roles (wives, mothers, breadwinners, activists; Parks, 2010; Woods-Giscombé, 2010) during the era of slavery, and was developed as a coping discourse to upend the notion of promiscuity or "baby mamas" ascribed to African American women (Parks, 2010). This discourse has been found to work to the disadvantage of African American women especially in the healthcare setting (Ashley, 2014; Woods-Giscombé, 2010). Perceived for their supernatural strength, African American women have continued to experience a disenfranchised form of healthcare, one that undermines or dismisses their concerns as patients within the healthcare setting. The dismissal of pain under the stereotype of being strong is a major theme of maternal crisis narratives from Black women in the United States (National Public Radio, 2017). Until healthcare providers begin to confront implicit biases toward African American women, women will continue to experience implicit racism in maternal care and poor maternal health outcomes for African American women will persist.

Distrust in the healthcare system has been a long-standing experience of African Americans, traceable to the Tuskegee study of 1932 and many more unethical treatment of Blacks in medical research (Scharff et al., 2010). As a result of this, women in this study also reported the same perception, albeit not because they were discriminated against. They already had an existing perception that the healthcare system, just like any other social institution in the U.S., is set up against them, and to their disadvantage. Consequently, even when healthcare providers are putting up their best practice, there is still some level of distrust in the way those services are perceived (Durant et al., 2011). This may lead to unwillingness to comply with healthcare providers' recommendations (Adebayo et al., 2020) This experience shows how damaging systemic racism can impact patient relationship with their healthcare providers.

Consistent with the argument of Kreps (2006), communication functions as the tool for uncovering racial disparities in the healthcare. Similarly, our study reveals that the enactment of structural racism and different institutional practices that marginalize minority groups are communicatively performed. For instance, the women who reported different forms of racial discrimination made sense of them through the way their healthcare providers communicated to them both verbally and nonverbally. Essentially, communication is not merely a way through which we make sense of healthcare practices, it is the primary platform of operation for provider-patient relationships in every form.

In identifying the role of communication in healthcare context, health communication scholars can be positioned to address these issues through communication concepts (Parker & Kreps, 2005). Our study has led to the development of important knowledge about healthcare practices that underserve African American women, which include ignoring women's concerns under the guise of standard practice and structural racism. As evidenced in our study, the continuation of these practices lead to medical mistrust and in some cases fatal complications, exacerbating poor maternal and infant health outcomes.

Study implications for healthcare providers and health communication scholars

Findings from this study show that healthcare providers may not be aware of some standard practices in the healthcare system that inherently underserve African American women. Thus, we suggest that policies that are developed by healthcare administrators should target the needs of African American women, as well as other minority populations. To create a healthcare system that serves African American women, healthcare providers and administrators should continuously receive training in intercultural awareness, addressing issues such as racism, health inequities among minority population, as may be manifested in healthcare institutional practices.

In communication scholarship, our study's findings contribute the body of knowledge confirming the central influence of communication in healthcare delivery, as women in this study identified their experience of racial discrimination in healthcare structures and practices, they made sense of them through communication. In reporting how healthcare providers perceive them, African American women consistently reported communicative acts, both verbal and nonverbal, as indicators of how they are perceived. Communication functions at the heart of healthcare delivery. Specifically, with the end goal of addressing maternal mortality crisis among African American women, communication scholars are better positioned to identify communication markers, discourses that may significantly affect healthcare processes, including the interpretation of healthcare providers' attitudes toward patients.

Racial discrimination is not only existent in the health system. It is everywhere; in universities, in workplaces, and in health care. As such, issues of racial disparities should be treated from an intersectional perspective, through active collaboration between individuals and groups from different sectors of society. Facilitating such intersectoral collaboration that will effectively address racial health inequities, is an important research focus for future community engagement research.

Notes

1. In this study, we do not use the terms "Black" and "African American" interchangeably. Whenever the term "Black" is used, we are referencing all people of African descent, including African Americans, while the use of African Americans specifically speaks to African Americans in the United States (See American Psychological Association, 2019, p. 143).
2. This is a type of healthcare delivery that displays healthcare disparities based on racial differences, especially between Black and white patients (Goodman et al., 2016).
3. We conducted a pilot study to explore if both Black immigrant women and African American women share similar maternal care experiences. The findings showed that African American women's experiences are different from that of Black immigrant women. We included the data of the African American women who participated in the pilot

Funding

This work was supported by the Department of Communication, University of Wisconsin-Milwaukee [N/A].

ORCID

Comfort Tosin Adebayo http://orcid.org/0000-0002-1288-2296
Erin Sahlstein Parcell http://orcid.org/0000-0001-6922-8108

References

Abioye Kuteyi, E., Bello, I., Olaleye, T., Ayeni, I., & Amedi, M. (2010). Determinants of patient satisfaction with physician interaction: A cross-sectional survey at the Obafemi Awolowo University Health Centre, Ile-Ife, Nigeria. *South African Family Practice, 52*(6), 557–562. https://doi.org/10.1080/20786204.2010.10874047

Abrams, J. A., Maxwell, M., Pope, M., & Belgrave, F. Z. (2014). Carrying the world with the grace of a lady and the grit of a warrior: Deepening our understanding of the "strong Black woman" schema. *Psychology of Women Quarterly, 38*(4), 503–518. https://doi.org/10.1177/0361684314541418

Adebayo, C. T., Walker, K., Hawkins, M., Olukotun, O., Shaw, L., Sahlstein Parcell, E., Dressel, A., Luft, H., & Mkandawire-Valhmu, L. (2020). Race and Blackness: A thematic review of communication challenges confronting the Black community within the U.S. health care system. *Journal of Transcultural Nursing: Official Journal of the Transcultural Nursing Society, 31*(4), 397–405. https://doi.org/10.1177/1043659619889111

Allen, H., Wright, B. J., Harding, K., & Broffman, L. (2014). The role of stigma in access to health care for the poor. *Milbank Quarterly, 92*(2), 289–318. https://doi.org/10.1111/1468-0009.12059

American Psychological Association. (2019). *Publication manual of the American Psychological Association* (7th ed.).

Andipatin, M. G., Naidoo, A. D., & Roomaney, R. (2019). The hegemonic role of biomedical discourses in the construction of pregnancy loss. *Women and Birth, 32*(6), e552–e559. https://doi.org/10.1016/j.wombi.2019.03.006

Arnold, E. C., & Boggs, K. U. (2019). *Interpersonal relationships e-book: Professional communication skills for nurses.* Elsevier Health Sciences.

Ashley, W. (2014). The angry Black woman: The impact of pejorative stereotypes on psychotherapy with Black women. *Social Work in Public Health, 29*(1), 27–34. https://doi.org/10.1080/19371918.2011.619449

Baciu, A., Negussie, Y., Geller, A., & Weinstein, J. N. (2017). The state of health disparities in the United States. In J. N. Weinstein, A. Geller, Y. Negussie, & A. Baciu, National Academies of Sciences, Engineering, and Medicine Eds., *Communities in action: Pathways to health equity* (pp. 57–98). National Academies Press (US).

Centers for Disease Control and Prevention (CDC). (2019). *Pregnancy mortality surveillance system.* https://www.cdc.gov/reproductivehealth/maternalinfanthealth/pregnancy-mortality-surveillance-system.htm

City of Milwaukee Health Department. (2018). *City of Milwaukee 2015–2017 infant mortality rate (IMR): Data brief.* https://city.milwaukee.gov/ImageLibrary/Groups/healthAuthors/ADMIN/PDFs/Reports/IMRDataBrief2015-2017.pdf

Collins, P. H. (2000). *Black feminist thought: Knowledge, consciousness, and the politics of empowerment* (2nd ed.). Routledge.

Corlett, S., & Mavin, S. (2018). Reflexivity and researcher positionality. In C. Cassell, A. L. Cunliffe, & G. Grandy (Eds.) *The Sage handbook of qualitative business and management research methods* (pp. 377–398). Sage. https://doi.org/10.4135/9781526430212

Creanga, A. A., Berg, C. J., Ko, J. Y., Farr, S. L., Tong, V. T., Bruce, F. C., & Callaghan, W. M. (2014). Maternal mortality and morbidity in the United States: Where are we now? Journal of Women's Health, 23(1), 3–9. https://doi.org/10.1089/jwh.2013.4617

Creanga, A. A., Berg, C. J., Syverson, C., Seed, K., Bruce, F. C., & Callaghan, W. M. (2015). Pregnancy-related mortality in the United States, 2006–2010. *Obstetrics & Gynecology, 125*(1), 5–12. https://doi.org/10.1097/AOG.0000000000000564

Cuevas, A. G., O'Brien, K., & Saha, S. (2016). African American experiences in healthcare: "I always feel like I'm getting skipped over. *Health Psychology, 35*(9), 987–995. https://doi.org/10.1037/hea0000368

D'Silva, M. U., Smith, S. E., Della, L. J., Potter, D. A., Rajack-Talley, T. A., & Best, L. (2016). Reflexivity and positionality in researching African-American communities: Lessons from the field. *Intercultural Communication Studies, 25*(1), 94–109. https://web.uri.edu/iaics/files/XXV1%E2%80%93D%E2%80%99SILVA-SMITH-DELLA.pdf

Davis, S. M. (2015). The "strong Black woman collective": A developing theoretical framework for understanding collective communication practices of Black women. *Women's Studies in Communication, 38*(1), 20–35. https://doi.org/10.1080/07491409.2014.953714

Dawley, K. (2003). Origins of nurse-midwifery in the United States and its expansion in the 1940s. *Journal of midwifery & women's health, 48*(2), 86–95. https://doi.org/10.1016/s1526-9523(03)00002-3

Delgado, R., & Stefancic, J. (2012). *Critical race theory: An introduction.* University Press.

Delgado, R., Stefancic, J., & Harris, A. (2017). Critical race theory: An introduction. New York University Press.

Dovidio, J. F., & Fiske, S. T. (2012). Under the radar: How unexamined biases in decision-making processes in clinical interactions can contribute to health care disparities. *American Journal of Public Health, 102* (5), 945–952. https://doi.org/10.2105/AJPH.2011.300601

Durant, R. W., Legedza, A. T., Marcantonio, E. R., Freeman, M. B., & Landon, B. E. (2011). Different types of distrust in clinical research among Whites and African Americans. *Journal of the National Medical Association, 103*(2), 123–130. http://dx.doi:10.1016/s0027-9684(15)30261-3

Dutta, M. J. (2010). The critical cultural turn in health communication: Reflexivity, solidarity, and praxis. *Health Communication, 25*(6–7), 534–539. https://doi.org/10.1080/10410236.2010.497995

Ford, C. L., & Airhihenbuwa, C. O. (2010). Critical race theory, race equity, and public health: Toward antiracism praxis. *American Journal of Public Health, 100*(1), S30–S35. https://dx.doi.org/10.2105/AJPH.2009.171058

Freeman, R., Gwadz, M. V., Silverman, E., Kutnick, A., Leonard, N. R., Ritchie, A. S., Reed, J., & Martinez, B. Y. (2017). Critical race theory as a tool for understanding poor engagement along the HIV care continuum among African American/Black and Hispanic persons living with HIV in the United States: A qualitative exploration. *International Journal for Equity in Health, 16*(54), 1–14. https://doi.org/10.1186/s12939-017-0549-3

Frey, W. (2018). *Black-White segregation edges downward since 2000, census shows.* https://www.brookings.edu/blog/the-avenue/2018/12/17/black-white-segregation-edges-downward-since-2000-census-shows/

Gee, G. C., & Ford, C. L. (2011). Structural racism and health inequities: Old issues, new directions. *Du Bois Review: Social Science Research on Race, 8*(1), 115–132. https://doi.org/10.1017/S1742058X11000130

Gollust, S. E., Cunningham, B. A., Bokhour, B. G., Gordon, H. S., Pope, C., Saha, S. S., Jones, D. M., Do, T., & Burgess, D. J. (2018). What causes racial health care disparities? A mixed-methods study reveals variability in how health care providers perceive causal attributions. *Inquiry: The Journal of Health Care Organization, Provision, and Financing, 55*, 1–11. https://doi.org/10.1177/0046958018762840

Goodman, M. S., Gilbert, K. L., Hudson, D., Milam, L., & Colditz, G. A. (2016). Descriptive analysis of the 2014 race-based healthcare disparities measurement literature. *Journal of Racial and Ethnic Health Disparities, 4*(5), 796–802. https://doi.org/10.1007/s40615-016-0281-5

Ha, J. F., & Longnecker, N. (2010). Doctor-patient communication: A review. *The Ochsner Journal, 10*(1), 38–43. https://doi.org/10.1043/TOJ-09-0040g.1

Homan, P. (2019). Structural sexism and health in the United States: A new perspective on health inequality and the gender system. *American Sociological Review, 84*(3), 486–516. https://doi.org/10.1177/0003122419848723

Howland, R. E., Angley, M., Won, S. H., Wilcox, W., Searing, H., Liu, S. Y., & Johansson, E. W. (2019). Determinants of severe maternal morbidity and its racial/ethnic disparities in New York City, 2008–2012. *Maternal and Child Health Journal, 23*(3), 346–355. https://doi.org/10.1007/s10995-018-2682-z

Hylton, K. (2012). Talk the talk, walk the walk: Defining critical race theory in research. *Race Ethnicity and Education, 15*(1), 23–24. https://doi.org/10.1080/13613324.2012.638862

Institute of Medicine. (2003). *Unequal treatment: Confronting racial and ethnic disparities in health care.* The National Academies Press. https://doi.org/10.17226/12875

Kaiser Family Foundation. (2019). *Medicaid coverage rates for the nonelderly by race/ethnicity.* https://www.kff.org/medicaid/state-indicator/nonelderly-medicaid-rate-by-raceethnicity/?currentTimeframe=0&sortModel=%7B%22colId%22:%22Location%22,%22sort%22:%22asc%22%7D

Keith, V. M., Lincoln, K. D., Taylor, R. J., & Jackson, J. S. (2010). Discriminatory experiences and depressive symptoms among African American women: Do skin tone and mastery matter? *Sex Roles, 62* (1–2), 48–59. https://doi.org/10.1007/s11199-009-9706-5

Kitsantas, P., & Gaffney, K. F. (2010). Racial/ethnic disparities in infant mortality. *Journal of Perinatal Medicine, 38*(1), 87–94. https://doi.org/10.1515/jpm.2010.014

Koch, A. R., & Geller, S. E. (2019). Racial and ethnic disparities in pregnancy-related mortality in Illinois, 2002–2015. *Journal of Women's Health, 28*(8), 1153–1160. https://doi.org/10.1089/jwh.2018.7557

Kreps, G. L. (2006). Communication and racial inequities in health care. *American Behavioral Scientist, 49*(6), 760–774. https://doi.org/10.1177/0002764205283800

Krieger, N., Kosheleva, A., Waterman, P. D., Chen, J. T., & Koenen, K. (2011). Racial discrimination, psychological distress, and self-rated health among us-born and foreign- born Black Americans. *American Journal of Public Health, 101*(9), 1704–1713. https://doi.org/10.2105/AJPH.2011.300168

Ladson-Billings, G., & Tate, W. F. (2006). Toward a critical race theory of education. In A. D. Dixson & C. K. Rousseau (Eds.), *Critical race theory in education: All God's children got a song* (pp. 11–31). Routledge.

López, G. R. (2003). The (racially neutral) politics of education: A critical race theory perspective. *Educational Administration Quarterly, 39*(1), 68–94. https://doi.org/10.1177/0013161X02239761

Martin, J. A., Hamilton, B. E., Osterman, M. J., Driscoll, A. K., & Mathews, T. J. (2017). *Births: Final data for 2015.* National vital statistics reports: From the Centers for Disease Control and Prevention, National Center for Health Statistics, National Vital Statistics System. https://stacks.cdc.gov/view/cdc/43595

Mazul, M. C., Ward, T. C., & Ngui, E. M. (2017). Anatomy of good prenatal care: Perspectives of low income African-American women on barriers and facilitators to prenatal care. *Journal of Racial and Ethnic Health Disparities, 4*(1), 79–86. https://doi.org/10.1007/s40615-015-0204-x

Miles, M. B., Huberman, A. M., & Saldaña, J. (2013). *Qualitative data analysis.* Sage.

Mkandawire-Valhmu, L. (2018). *Cultural safety, healthcare and vulnerable populations: A critical theoretical perspective* (1st ed.). Routledge. https://doi.org/10.4324/9781315708706

National Public Radio. (2017, December 7). *Black mothers keep dying after giving birth. Shalon Irving's story explains why.* https://www.npr.org/2017/12/07/568948782/black-mothers-keep-dying-after-giving-birth-shalon-irvings-story-explains-why

Noonan, A. S., Velasco-Mondragon, H. E., & Wagner, F. A. (2016). Improving the health of African Americans in the USA: An overdue opportunity for social justice. *Public Health Reviews, 37*(12), 1–20. https://doi.org/10.1186/s40985-016-0025-4

Parker, R., & Kreps, G. L. (2005). Library outreach: Overcoming health literacy challenges. *Journal of the Medical Library Association, 93*(S1), S81–S85. https://www.ncbi.nlm.nih.gov/pmc/articles/PMC1255757/pdf/i0025-7338-093-04S-0081.pdf

Parks, S. (2010). *Fierce angels: The strong Black woman in American life and culture.* One World.

Penner, L. A., Blair, I. V., Albrecht, T. L., & Dovidio, J. F. (2014). Reducing racial health care disparities: A social psychological analysis. *Policy Insights from the Behavioral and Brain Sciences, 1*(1), 204–212. https://doi.org/10.1177/2372732214548430

Perry, B. L., Harp, K. L., & Oser, C. B. (2013). Racial and gender discrimination in the stress process: Implications for African American women's health and well-being. *Sociological Perspectives, 56* (1), 25–48. https://www.ncbi.nlm.nih.gov/pmc/articles/PMC3783344/pdf/nihms492047.pdf.

Petersen, E. E., Davis, N. L., Goodman, D., Cox, S., Syverson, C., Seed, K., Shapiro Mendoza, C., Callaghan, W. M., & Barfield, W. (2019). Racial/ethnic disparities in pregnancy-related deaths—United States, 2007–2016. *Morbidity and Mortality Weekly Report, 68*(35), 762–765. http://dx.doi.org/10.15585/mmwr.mm6835a3externalicon

Raine, R., Cartwright, M., Richens, Y., Mahamed, Z., & Smith, D. (2010). A qualitative study of women's experiences of communication in antenatal care: Identifying areas for action. *Maternal Child Health Journal, 14*(4), 590–599. https://doi.org/10.1007/s10995-009-0489-7

Ryn, M. V., & Burje, J. (2002). The effect of patient race and socio-economic status on physicians' perceptions of patients. *Social Science & Medicine, 50*(6), 813–828. https://doi.org/10.1016/S0277-9536(99)00338-X

Saunders, B., Sim, J., Kingstone, T., Baker, S., Waterfield, J., Bartlam, B., Burroughs, H., & Jinks, C. (2018). Saturation in qualitative research: Exploring its conceptualization and operationalization. *Quality & Quantity, 52*, 1893–1907. https://doi.org/10.1007/s11135-017-05748

Scharff, D. P., Mathews, K. J., Jackson, P., Hoffsuemmer, J., Martin, E., & Edwards, D. (2010). More than Tuskegee: Understanding mistrust about research participation. *Journal of Health Care for the Poor and Underserved, 21*(3), 879–897. https://doi.org/10.1353/hpu.0.0323

Shavers, V. L., & Shavers, B. S. (2006). Racism and health inequity among Americans. *Journal of the National Medical Association, 98* (3), 386–396. https://www.ncbi.nlm.nih.gov/pmc/articles/PMC2576116/pdf/jnma00190-0078.pdf

Singh, G. K., & Stella, M. Y. (2019). Infant mortality in the United States, 1915–2017: Large social inequalities have persisted for over a century. *International Journal of MCH and AIDS, 8*(1), 19–31. https://doi.org/10.21106/ijma.271

Spradley, J. P. (1979). *The ethnographic interview.* Waveland Press.

Stewart, C. P. (2017). The mule of the world: The strong Black woman and the woes of being "independent". *Knots: An Undergraduate Journal of Disability Studies, 3*, 31–39. https://jps.library.utoronto.ca/index.php/knots/article/view/29187

Taylor, J. (2019). *Racism, inequality, and health care for African Americans.* The Century Foundation. Retrieved on August 27, 2020, from https://tcf.org/content/report/racism-inequality-health-care-african-americans/?session=1&session=1&agreed=1

Thorburn, S., & De Marco, M. (2010). Insurance-based discrimination during prenatal care, labor, and delivery: Perceptions of Oregon mothers. *Maternal Child Health Journal, 14*(6), 875–885. https://doi.org/10.1007/s10995-009-0533-7

Tracy, S. J. (2012). *Qualitative research methods: Collecting evidence, crafting analysis, communicating impact.* Wiley & Sons.

Tucker, M. J., Berg, C. J., Callaghan, W. M., & Hsia, J. (2007). The Black-White disparity in pregnancy-related mortality from 5 conditions: Differences in prevalence and case-fatality rates. *American Journal of Public Health, 97*(2), 247–251. https://doi.org/10.2105/AJPH.2005.072975

Vardeman-Winter, J. (2017). The framing of women and health disparities: A critical look at race, gender, and class from the perspectives of grassroots health communicators. *Health Communication, 32*(5), 629–638. https://doi.org/10.1080/10410236.2016.1160318

Ward, T. C., Mazul, M., Ngui, E. M., Bridgewater, F. D., & Harley, A. E. (2013). "You learn to go last": Perceptions of prenatal care experiences among African American women with limited incomes. *Maternal and Child Health Journal, 17*(10), 1753–1759. https://doi.org/10.1007/s10995-012-1194-5

Warmington, P. (2012). 'A tradition in ceaseless motion': Critical race theory and Black British intellectual spaces. *Race, Ethnicity and Education, 15*(1), 5–21. https://doi.org/10.1080/13613324.2012.638861

Watson-Singleton, N. N. (2017). Strong Black woman schema and psychological distress: The mediating role of perceived emotional support. *Journal of Black Psychology, 43*(8), 778–788. https://doi.org/10.1177/0095798417732414

Weech-Maldonado, R., Hall, A., Bryant, T., Jenkins, K. A., & Elliott, M. N. (2012). The relationship between perceived discrimination and patient experiences with health care. *Medical Care, 50*(9 Suppl 2), S62–S68. https://doi.org/10.1097/MLR.0b013e31825fb235

Wesp, L. M., Scheer, V., Ruiz, A., Walker, K., Weitzel, J., Shaw, L., Kako, P. M., & Mkandawire-Valhmu, L. (2018). An emancipatory approach to cultural competency: The application of critical race, postcolonial, and intersectionality theories. *ANS. Advances in Nursing Science, 41*(4), 316–326. https://doi.org/10.1097/ANS.0000000000000230

Willard, B. E. (2005). Feminist interventions in biomedical discourse: An analysis of the rhetoric of integrative medicine. *Women's Studies in Communication, 28*(1), 115–148. https://doi.org/10.1080/07491409.2005.10162486

Williams, D. R., & Wyatt, R. (2015). Racial bias in health care and health: Challenges and opportunities. *JAMA, 314*(6), 555–556. https://doi.org/10.1001/jama.2015.9260

Wisconsin Department of Health Services. (2019). *Maternal mortality and morbidity*. https://www.dhs.wisconsin.gov/mch/maternal-mortality-and-morbidity.htm

Woods-Giscombé, C. L. (2010). Superwoman schema: African American women's views on stress, strength, and health. *Qualitative Health Research, 20*(5), 668–683. https://doi.org/10.1177/1049732310361892

World Health Organization. (2014). *Global health expenditure database*. Retrieved March 5, 2020, from http://apps.who.int/nha/database/Country_Profile/Index/e

Individually Tailoring Messages to Promote African American Men's Health

Derek M. Griffith, Emily Cornish Jaeger, Andrea R. Semlow, Jennifer M. Ellison, Erin M. Bergner, and Elizabeth C. Stewart

ABSTRACT

In this paper, we describe our approach to individualizing messages to promote the health of middle-aged and older heterosexual, cisgender African American men. After arguing the importance of being population specific, we describe the process we use to increase the salience of health messages for this population by operationalizing the identity concepts of centrality and contextualization. We also present a measure of African American manhood and discuss how manhood is congruent with qualitative research that describes how African American men view their values, identities, goals, and aspirations in ways that can be utilized to create more meaningful and impactful messages to promote and maintain health behaviors. Our tailoring strategy uses an intersectional approach that considers how the centrality of racial identity and manhood and the salience of religiosity, spirituality, and role strains may help to increase the impact of health messages. We highlight the need to consider how the context of health behavior and the meaning ascribed to certain behaviors are gendered, not only from a man's perspective, but also how his social networks, behavioral context, and the dynamic sociopolitical climate may consider gendered ideals in ways that shape behavior. We close by discussing the need to apply this approach to other populations of men, women, and those who are non-gender binary because this strategy builds from the population of interest and incorporates factors that they deem central and salient to their identities and behaviors. These factors are important to consider in interventions using health messages to pursue health equity.

Over the last 30 years, individual tailoring has been used in myriad studies to increase recipient attention and perceived message salience and to decrease processing effort, thereby outperforming generic or group targeted messages in promoting health behavior change (Hawkins et al., 2008; Latimer et al., 2010). Tailored messages are customized to each individual (Noar et al., 2009) using strategies and information intended to reach a specific person, based on characteristics that are unique to that person (Kreuter et al., 1999) because these strategies for individualizing messages increase the likelihood that people will view the message as relevant to them and consciously choose to make and sustain healthy behavior changes. Over the last decade, faculty and staff of the Center for Research on Men's Health at Vanderbilt University have worked to achieve men's health equity by developing and testing an approach to individually-tailor behavioral weight loss interventions for middle-aged and older African American men (Griffith & Jaeger, 2020).

We begin this paper by describing the theory, approach, and conceptual foundation of how we tailor text messages to African American men. After describing the epidemiologic reasons we focus on middle-aged African American men, we detail how we individualize messages and what is unique about our tailoring approach. Then we illustrate how we use African American Manhood to tailor messages to this population in ways that consider the heterogeneity among African American men.

We recognize that our empirically derived framework and messages are heteronormative and designed primarily for cisgender African American men who are middle-aged or older. We view the specificity of the identities that our messages speak to as a strength of our tailoring methodology because it allows us to increase the salience and perhaps the impact of our messages for our population. The scope and focus of our messages are shaped by the qualitative data collected in a midsized Midwestern city and a midsized Southeastern city. As a result, there are a range of masculinities and identities for which our framework, messages and interventions may not be ideal. Yet, to our knowledge, we are the first to demonstrate that it is possible to use an intersectional approach to tailor individual health messages for a specific group whose experiences are shaped by their race, ethnicity, age, and gender. This approach, therefore, could be used to develop messages for populations that would not resonate with our messages as currently designed. We conclude this paper with a discussion of the future of intersectional, identity-based tailoring and how it may be a useful strategy to continue to use a strengths-based approach that is consistent with notions of promoting minority health (Duran & Pérez-Stable, 2019a) and men's health equity (Griffith, Bruce et al., 2019).

Background of tailoring strategy

Our approach to tailoring is unique in that it combines evidence-based behavior-change goal algorithms to produce weight loss (Greaney et al., 2009) with tailoring to African American manhood (Griffith, Pennings et al., 2019), but this paper focuses on the latter aspect of tailoring to the heterogeneity in manhood. The approach is an illustration of how tailoring can incorporate an intersectional approach that integrates age, race, ethnicity, and gender to increase the salience of health messages to a population for whom all of these factors are relevant to their identity and health behavior through the concept of African American manhood (Griffith, 2012, 2016; Griffith & Jaeger, 2020). Next, we will describe our tailoring approach and explain why and how we locate the lived experience of our population of interest in messages to promote their health and well-being.

Theoretical foundations

Our tailoring strategy combines Self-Determination Theory (Ryan & Deci, 2000) and self-efficacy (Bandura, 2004). A fundamental aspect of Self-Determination Theory, autonomous motivation is key because it is the primary factor that helps men overcome modifying factors that constrain opportunities and motivation to engage in healthier behaviors (Ryan & Deci, 2000). The autonomously motivated individuals not only see the importance of the behavior, but also connect change with their core values and beliefs. These individuals feel competent, are ready to take action and persist when faced with obstacles and have identified meaningful reasons for change (Ryan & Deci, 2000). In addition to autonomous motivation, the second key mediating mechanism is to increase self-efficacy, or the confidence one has in his ability to exert control over his own motivation, behavior, and social environment (Bandura, 2004). Social Cognitive Theory (Bandura, 2004) posits that self-efficacy affects health behavior directly and indirectly through its impact on goals, outcome expectations, and perceived facilitators and impediments. Thus, an important objective of health interventions is to increase the perceived ability to engage in healthier behavior despite environmental, social, and time pressures that may present barriers to healthy eating or physical activity. An intersectional approach that helps to capture the structural foundation of these factors and how they intersect in the lives of specific populations is critical to the process of developing messages for populations defined by the combination of age, race, gender, and other factors.

Intersectionality

Building on the work of Kimberlé Crenshaw and others (Bowleg, 2017b; Crenshaw, 1995), we use an intersectional approach as the foundation of our tailoring strategy. An intersectional approach suggests that socially defined and socially meaningful characteristics are inextricably intertwined and experienced simultaneously. Consideration of how the blending of identities and experiences creates a new understanding of these factors helps researchers understand the complex array of factors that affect men's health and well-being (Griffith, 2012; Ragonese et al., 2019). Men's health should consider how micro structures may relate to how men navigate the precarious, racialized, and class bound aspects of manhood (Griffith, 2015; Vandello & Bosson, 2013), and how macro-structures that may be related to the diverse and socially contingent nature of masculinities in their social and economic context (Griffith & Cornish, 2018; Robertson et al., 2016). Intersectionality provides a systematic way to explore how sex and gender affect men's health, yet these determinants of men's health also rely on other identities, characteristics and categories for meaning as determinants of health (Gilbert et al., 2016; Griffith, 2012). More specifically, we use an intersectional approach to capture aspects of a Social Ecological Framework of health behavior that define and influence the social, economic, built, and natural environment (McLeroy et al., 1988).

Observable (e.g., skin color, eye shape), psychosocial (e.g., sexual orientation, racial identity, ethnic identity, social class, economic position), and cultural (e.g., religion, Meritocracy, American Creed, homophobia) characteristics beyond sex, are necessary preconditions for understanding men's health and an intersectional approach provides a framework for considering these factors (Griffith, 2016). Intersectional approaches to men's health offer a way to examine why sex does not have the same meaning and influence within and across all men's lives or health outcomes (Griffith, 2012). Intersectional approaches help to highlight how dynamic cultural factors shape the norms, expectations, stressors, and practices in men's lives. An intersectional approach offers an important lens through which we may fine-tune intervention strategies (National Academies of Sciences, Engineering & Medicine, 2016) and health communication. The health communication messaging strategy that we have developed and described below does not seek to help men change these environmental factors; rather our goal is to use health messages to increase motivation, self-efficacy, and other psychosocial factors that can help men overcome structural and environmental constraints and limitations (Bandura, 2004; Griffith & Jaeger, 2020).

Manhood

Manhood is a social status and aspirational identity that perpetually needs to be proven; it reflects the embodiment of virtuous characteristics and traits, performance of social roles, and the fulfillment of gendered expectations associated with being an adult male that need to be proven continually (Vandello et al., 2019). Men need not engage in all masculine behaviors to be considered a man, but the more masculine behaviors men enact the greater likelihood that he will be respected as a man. One of the most enduring qualities of manhood is not its contents – stereotypically male qualities, behaviors, preferences, or tendencies – but the constant anxiety of its precariousness (Griffith, 2015; Griffith et al., 2015; Vandello et al., 2019). Manhood includes men's perceived ability to fulfill heteronormative social and cultural ideals and expectations beyond the achievement of age-related milestones or the presence of secondary sex characteristics (Griffith, 2015). A complex construct that is shaped by race/ethnicity, age, and other factors, manhood serves as a lens through which

African American men, in particular, see and identify themselves and are recognized by others as men (Griffith, 2015; Griffith & Cornish, 2018). Dimensions and ideals of manhood that shape how African American men see themselves and are viewed by others are shaped by race and class (Griffith, 2015; Kimmel, 2006).

Manhood is relationally constructed and reflects interconnections between self, family, and others; it is defined and exists in comparison with expectations of younger males and ideals and expectations of women and womanhood (Griffith, 2015). Among African American men, Whitehead and colleagues found that manhood status that comes from engaging in risky behavior may be associated with efforts to build a strong reputation, and that aspects of anti-femininity may be associated with efforts to achieve a level of respectability pursued through economic success, educational attainment, and upward social class mobility (Whitehead, 1997). Aspects of hegemonic ideals of masculinity have been associated with ideals that Whitehead (1997) characterizes as reputational aspects of demonstrating or performing masculinity (e.g., avoiding medical help-seeking, alcohol use, sexual risk taking, reckless driving) and that are associated with poor health outcomes (Ragonese et al., 2019). Caballerismo – the ideal of being a gentleman and one who may be more family oriented – is consistent with Whitehead's notion of the respectability aspect of masculinity (Whitehead, 1997). Conceptually, these strains and conflicts are rooted in the ideals of Caballerismo or the Victorian values that made one a virtuous member of a society who demonstrated character (e.g., self-control, honesty, thrift) (Summers, 2004).

Middle age

Middle age covers a large portion of an individual's lifespan from approximately age 30 to 64 (Lachman, 2015), but chronological age may not be the best anchor for identifying middle age (Lachman, 2015). Because the boundaries are not solidly defined by numerical age, middle age may be better considered in terms of or the assumption of certain social roles and responsibilities, the timing of events, and life experience (Lachman, 2015). Evidence exists that stresses involving multiple role demands or financial pressures may cluster in or take a greater toll in middle age (Lachman, 2015). In middle age, men often construct their identities in relation to the physicality of their work, the level of income or status that their labor produces, or both because work defines their status in the masculine hierarchy (Evans et al., 2011). Consistent with this focus on work and financial provision in midlife, role strain and adaptation theory suggests that during their middle-adult years, men's, particularly African American men's, evaluations of how well they feel they are fulfilling the roles of provider, husband, father, employee, and community member become fundamental aspects of their identities and a major focus of this phase of life (Bowman, 1989).

For these reasons, we focused on men in this phase of life because middle age is when African American men's efforts to fulfill the roles of provider, husband, father, and community member have been found to be key barriers to healthy eating and physical activity (Griffith et al., 2011; Griffith, Wooley et al., 2013). African American men's rates of physical activity tend to decline during middle age in part due to increasing responsibilities to fulfill social and cultural roles associated with work, family, and the community (Griffith et al., 2011). Particularly during this phase of life, men often define health by how they generally feel and whether they can complete activities of daily living (e.g., work, engage in sexual behavior) and function in roles (e.g., provider, father, spouse) that are important to them, their partners, and their families (Griffith, Ellis et al., 2013).

Middle-aged African American men's health

For more than 100 years the National Center for Health Statistics has documented that African American men in the US have had a shorter life expectancy than all other race by sex groups (National Center for Health Statistics (US), 2017). Last year, amid findings that life expectancy in the US declined three years in a row, Bilal and Diez-Roux attributed the national decline in life expectancy to non-Hispanic Black men, the only group whose mortality increased during that time (Bilal & Diez-Roux, 2018). African American men are the least likely race by gender group in the US to reach retirement age, and affluence, healthy lifestyles, and access to high-quality healthcare do not appear to be equally protective of these men when compared with other men or women (Gilbert et al., 2016).

Research on middle age has demonstrated for some time that disparities – particularly by race and sex – are greatest during middle age, and that is due primarily to the poor health and high mortality rates of middle-aged and older African American men (Griffith, Jaeger et al., 2019; Satcher et al., 2005). Whereas chronic diseases are often viewed as primarily an issue for older adults, globally, almost half of chronic disease deaths occur in people under 70 years old, and 25% of chronic disease deaths occur in people under 60 years old (Griffith, Jaeger et al., 2019; World Health Organization [WHO], 2018). Among racial/ethnic groups of men, African American men have the second highest rates of grade 2 obesity (BMI $\geq$ 35) and the highest rates of grade 3 obesity (BMI $\geq$ 40) (Flegal et al., 2010). Among African American men, those who are middle–aged (40–59 years old) have higher rates of obesity than African American men who are young adults (20–39 years old) or older adults (60 and older) (Flegal et al., 2010). Among men 40-59 years old with grade 3 obesity (BMI $\geq$ 40), rates for African American men are 50% higher than their White counterparts (Flegal et al., 2010).

Tailoring to middle–aged African American men

To increase the potential that messages will resonate with recipients, we use two levels of tailoring: one that focuses on the centrality of factors related to identity and a second that focuses on contextualizing messages to increasing their salience to men's foundational principles and sources of chronic stress and psychological strain (see Figure 1). This approach builds on the work of Ken Resnicow and colleagues (Davis et al., 2010; Resnicow et al., 2009). Figure 1 builds from a model developed by LaVeist that helps researchers studying race and

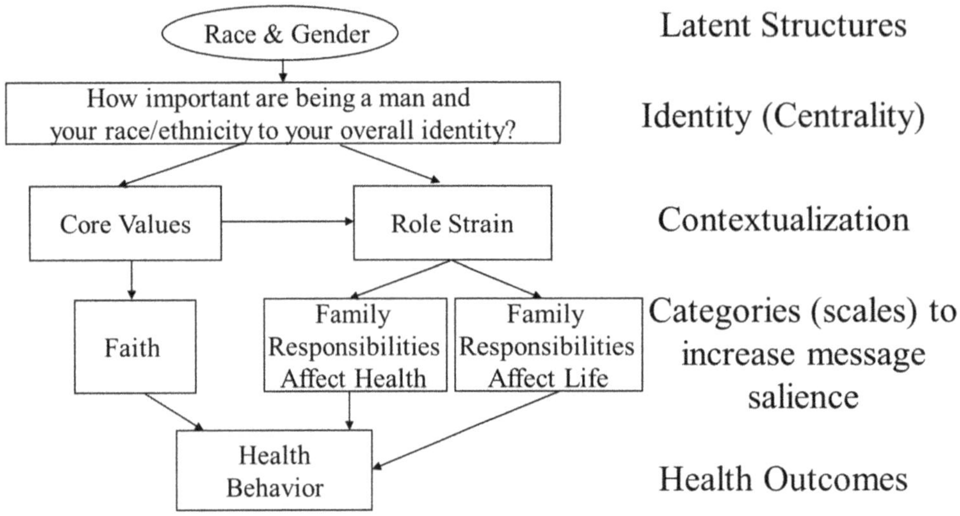

Figure 1. Framework for tailoring to African American manhood.

ethnicity to be more critical of the way they conceptualize, operationalize and utilize these terms in empirical research (La Veist, 1996). Griffith (2012) adapted this framework to highlight how race, ethnicity, gender, and age reflect pathways and determinants of men's health. Griffith's (2012) adaptation of the framework, is designed to move beyond identifying *which* social characteristics affect health to articulating *why* those factors affect health, and *how* they come together to influence a population's health. Structural factors, and the physical features (e.g., skin color, hair texture, facial hair) that serve as indicators of them, trigger physiological and behavioral responses that affect health outcomes (Griffith & Jaeger, 2020). These responses are shaped by how core certain aspects of identity are to how one sees themselves and how salient the aspects of identity are to a particular situation or context.

Tailoring based on the centrality of psychosocial identity

Centrality is the extent to which one typically defines himself with regard to race or some other aspect of his identity (Sellers et al., 1998). It is a relatively stable construct that is not likely to change by situation, context, or event, and centrality represents the most important ways of seeing oneself. Based on our formative research using an intersectional approach (Griffith & Cornish, 2018), we asked men about the centrality or importance of being a man to their overall identity and the importance of being Black or African American to their overall identity. The questions ask, "On a scale of 0–10 with 0 being 'not at all important' and 10 being 'very important', how important is [manhood or race] to your overall identity?" For both questions, a response of 0–5 was categorized as "low", and a response of 6-10 was categorized as "high".

Tailoring based on the contextualization of core values and the strain of social roles

Although centrality is considered stable, salience is contextually dependent. Salience has been described as the mechanism through which all other identities operate and as the mediating process between the more stable characteristics of identity and the way individuals construe and behave in specific situations (Sellers et al., 1998). Sellers et al. (1998) argue that salience refers to the extent to which the stable aspect of identity (i.e., centrality) is relevant to one's self-concept at a particular moment, in a particular situation, or in reference to a particular behavior. Salience is shaped by the context of the situation and one's proclivity to define oneself, and one's self-concept, in terms of that aspect of his identity.

Our formative research found that considering core values (i.e., religion and spirituality) and role strains (e.g., family responsibilities that affect health and family responsibilities that affect life) were important contextual factors that could be used to increase the salience of improving specific health behaviors for their lives and goals (see Figure 1). Griffith and Cornish (2018) found that religion and spirituality were fundamental to how middle-aged and older African American men defined manhood and their core values. African American men who were interviewed as part of the study described that their faith reshaped and redefined gendered roles (e.g., being a father) and helped them to find greater meaning and motivation to be better men through the integration of spirituality and manhood (Griffith & Cornish, 2018). Research has consistently shown that African Americans are more involved in religious practices and more consistently engage in prayer than White Americans (Gillum & Griffith, 2010). Even among African Americans who are not affiliated with a specific religious institution or those that do not attend services, prayer is often regarded as an important part of their lives (Gillum & Griffith, 2010).

In addition to the core value of faith (religiosity and spirituality), we focus on how men experience psychological strain from their perceived and actual ability to achieve life goals that may be associated with racialized and gendered social priorities (Bowman, 1989; Griffith et al., 2011). These psychological strains can be divided by how family roles, responsibilities, and priorities affect health (Family Responsibilities Affect Health – FRAH) and how these factors affect men's lives

Table 1. Centrality: Manhood and racial identity.

		Manhood	
		High	Low
Racial Identity	High	Black Man	African American
	Low	Man	'Me'/Person

more generally (Family Responsibilities Affect Life- FRAL). Role strains were critical factors that represented values and goals men perceived as most important to their identities and life goals (e.g., providing for their families, being a good spouse/partner). These values and goals were often more important to them and their loved ones than focusing on health behaviors like healthy eating and physical activity (Griffith et al., 2011; Griffith, Wooley et al., 2013).

Operationalizing centrality using African American manhood as an example

Combined responses from the two centrality items (manhood and race) resulted in a 2 × 2 table (Table 1) that determined the stem of each tailored message. The relationship between the constructs of interest and items on the centrality of identities reinforces the importance of utilizing an intersectional approach to understanding African American men's identities. This is because African American men's identities are an amalgamation of race and gender in a way that creates something distinct from racial or ethnic identity and gender identity alone (Bowleg et al., 2017; Griffith, 2012, 2015).

The four resulting categories, which we refer to as *buckets*, represent the first level of tailoring: *Man, Black Man, African American, and Me or Person*. These buckets provide a level of segmentation and heterogeneity in how African American men may consider how important race and manhood are to how they see themselves. For example, an individual who rated both manhood and race high would receive messages from the *Black Man* bucket. An individual who rated both manhood and race low would receive messages from the *Me or Person* bucket.

Operationalizing salience using African American manhood as an example

The variables within the second level of tailoring are designed to increase the salience of the messages to middle-aged and older African American men's lives and health. The questions that make up each variable within both levels of tailoring are listed within Table 2. This level of tailoring is designed to tap into men's core values and life goals in ways that will be memorable (Cooke-Jackson & Rubinsky, 2018) and in ways that tap into autonomous sources of motivation (Ryan & Deci, 2000).

Illustrating how we tailor to African American manhood

Let's consider four illustrative examples of African American men (Figure 2). Each man is unique, and each has different goals, values, beliefs, and perceptions related to manhood. Differences in perceptions of manhood have an impact on individual, interpersonal, community, and societal factors that are dynamic and change over time (Bronfenbrenner, 1994). Societal-level factors like racism, gendered norms and values, social expectations of men across the lifespan (i.e., young adult vs. middle-aged vs. older adulthood) may further contextualize perceptions of manhood and health. In addition to those unique goals and values, each man also has distinctive demographic characteristics that shape and inform his interactions with others and frame his understanding and experiences related to health.

A is a single, 36-year-old man with no children living close to downtown, which allows him to bike to work. *B* is a married 41-year-old man and a father of two young children. His family recently moved further outside the city to be closer to the children's school and activities. *C* is a married 53-year-old with three children, two of which are in college and one still living at home. He will soon be an "empty nester" and is interested in re-discovering new hobbies and interests. *D* is a divorced 64-year-old man who has two grown children and three young grandchildren. He recently downsized to a home that requires less upkeep and is closer to his grandchildren. This group of men is heterogeneous, with individual experiences that are reflective of age intersecting with gendered perceptions and ideals, which are key factors that distinguish manhood from masculinity. As these men age, gain new experiences, reflect, improve, and navigate challenges, their perceptions of manhood change.

Additionally, each man in our illustration has different psychosocial priorities and faces different role strains, some of which are anchored in his phase of life, that shape how he actively engages in health promoting behavior (Bowman, 1989; Griffith et al., 2011). Young man *A* is not currently experiencing health difficulties. He is generally aware of things he can do to prevent later-in-life disease and he is mindful of a family history of breast cancer and aggressive prostate cancer. However, his own health and the impact it may have on his friends and family is not yet an immediate concern. He supports his friends' attempts at healthier living, but considers his bike ride to and from work sufficient physical activity for the day. Young father, *B*, tries to set a healthy example for his family but struggles to make time for a regular workout regimen around busy schedules. Family is a priority right now, and often times other things, such as health, sleep, and self-care activities get pushed to the side. He and his wife are mindful of nutrition for the kids, but healthy meals for themselves can sometimes be a challenge when the easier option is a fast-food drive-thru or takeout from a restaurant. He is active at church and is trying to establish a social network of other dads in the congregation to help learn more about how to teach his children about faith. *C* is starting to experience symptoms of age-related conditions and has friends and family who are beginning to develop hypertension, type 2 diabetes and colon cancer. This has added some strain in that he worries more about his family and their overall health but does not feel that this affects other larger aspects of his life as a whole. Now that he has time, he dedicates

Table 2. Survey questions for each tailoring variable.

Variable	Source of Item	Survey questions for each variable	Tailoring Outcome
First Level of Tailoring: Racial & Gender Centrality			
Manhood x Race: (Scale of 0 = Not at all important to 10 = Very important)	Sellers et al. (1998) – Scoring instructions for the Multidimensional Inventory of Black Identity (MIBI), Sellers – Multidimensional model of racial identity	• How important is being African American to your overall identity? • How important is being a man to your overall identity?	High/Low score for each question places men into one of four 'buckets': • Black Man (High Manhood/ High Race) • Man (High Manhood/Low Race) • African American (Low Manhood/High Race) • Me/Person (Low Manhood/ Low Race)
Second level of Tailoring: Salience			
Family Responsibilities Affect Health (FRAH): (Scale of 1 = Strongly disagree to 5 = Strongly agree)	Gender Role Conflict Scale – Factor 4 – conflicts between work and family relations (O'Neil et al., 1986) and additional CRMH adapted items	• I feel torn between my family responsibilities and caring for my health. • My family responsibilities affect the amount of time I spend on my health. • Finding time to exercise is difficult for me because of family obligations.	Sum of scale produces High (7-15)/Low (0–6) score for FRAH variable.
Family Responsibilities Affect Life (FRAL): (Scale of 1 = Strongly disagree to 5 = Strongly agree)	Gender Role Conflict Scale – Factor 4 – conflicts between work and family relations (O'Neil et al., 1986) and additional CRMH adapted items	• My family responsibilities keep me from pursuing other leisure time physical activities (going on walks, playing sports with friends, etc.) • My family responsibilities often disrupt other parts of my life (health or leisure). • The stress I feel from a need to fulfill family responsibility affects/hurts my life.	Sum of scale produces High (7–15)/Low (0–6) score for FRAL variable.
Faith: (Scale of 0 = Never to 5 = Many times a day)	Daily Spiritual Experiences Scale – 6 item version of the scale used in the Brief Multidimensional Measure of Religiosity and Spirituality developed by selection of items from the Daily Spiritual Experiences scale (Underwood & Teresi, 2002)	• I feel God's presence • I feel strength and comfort in my religious or spiritual tradition • I feel deep inner peace and harmony • I desire to be closer to or in union with God • I am spiritually touched by the beauty of creation • I feel God's love for me, directly or through others	Sum of scale produces High (25–30)/Low (0–24) score for Faith variable.

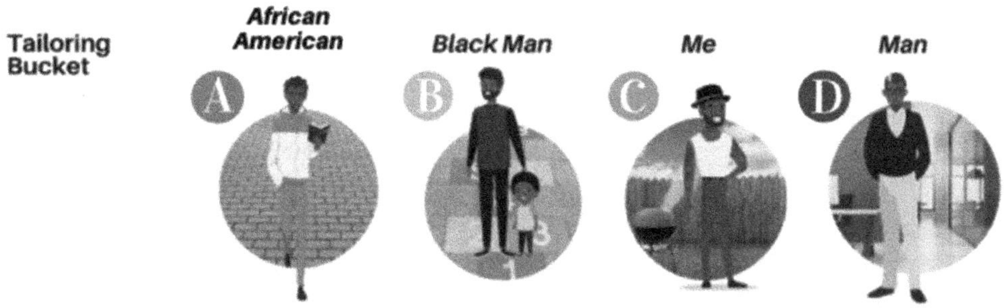

Manhood Salience	4 Low	9 High	5 Low	7 High
Racial Salience	9 High	8 High	5 Low	4 Low
FRAL	6 Low	14 High	6 Low	11 High
FRAH	5 Low	8 High	12 High	6 Low
Faith	16 Low	24 High	26 High	20 Low

Figure 2. Illustrative examples of how the tailoring framework would be applied to four African American men with different tailoring bucket and variable scores.

himself to a fitness regimen and is more involved in the men's ministry at his church. Retired grandfather, *D*, is experiencing symptoms of aging and age-related conditions. With changing family roles of being a grandfather, he feels that family time and strain plays more of an impact in his overall life and has little impact on his health. His doctor has prescribed a healthy diet and exercise regimen which he does his best to follow carefully. While each of these men have different experiences with health and health promoting behavior, they also have different motivations to strive to become healthier.

Each secondary tailoring variable from Table 2 received a *high/low* categorization option based on survey factor scoring and informed which message within an individual's designated *bucket* he would receive. Each of our men represent a different tailoring *bucket* with individual scores for each tailoring variable that makes him unique (Figure 2).

The resulting messages incorporated key goals, values, and important traits and characteristics of the individuals, and utilized language used by men themselves. While the messages had a stronger focus on centrality, they began to focus on message salience for each individual man. Figure 3 presents sample messages for each man based on his unique bucket and tailoring variable scores. Subtle differences in how each message was framed sought to highlight the differences in centrality and the content of each message aimed to increase the salience of the message for health. In Figure 3, family responsibilities are highlighted for those who indicated that they felt strongly that family responsibilities affect their life, in addition to the differing message

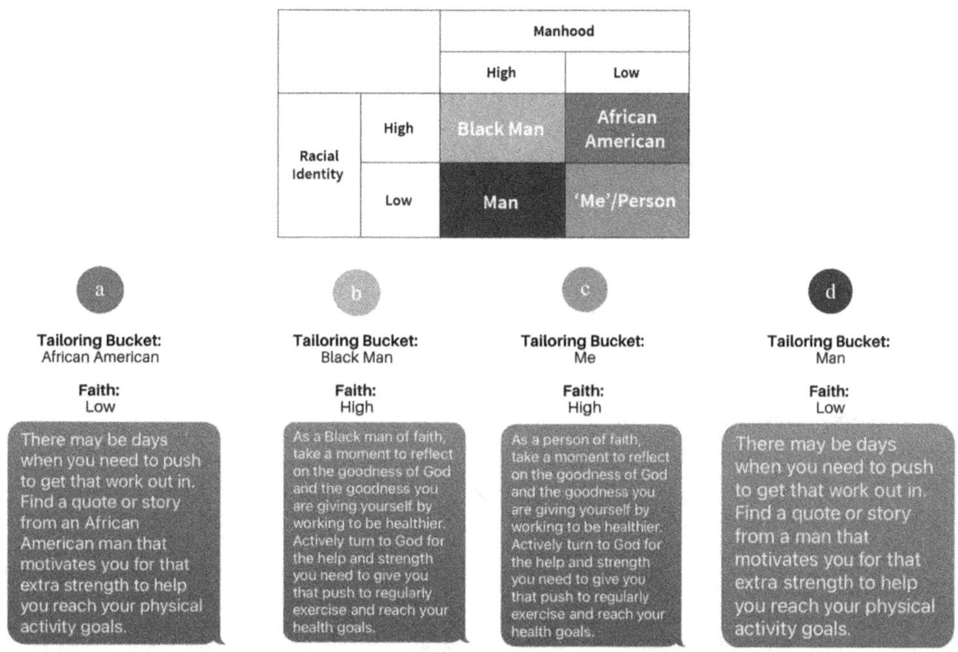

Figure 3. Examples of sample messages for each man based on his unique bucket and tailoring variable scores.

stem for each bucket. The addition of the mention of family increases the salience of the message by acknowledging that importance of the role that individual perceives he plays as a member of that family and often times as a man, and the head of the household.

Discussion

While there is a large body of research that has demonstrated the benefits of individually tailored health messages over messages that are not individualized (Kreuter et al., 1999; Noar et al., 2009), research considering the centrality and salience of identity-based factors remains limited. While there have been efforts to target and tailor health messages to African Americans (Davis et al., 2010; Kreuter et al., 1999; Resnicow et al., 2009), more research is needed to advance efforts to utilize individually-tailored health messages in minority health research. While tailoring to racial or ethnic identity has shown some benefits (Resnicow et al., 2009), using an intersectional approach is one of the next steps to embrace and advance if the goal is to improve minority health and to achieve health equity (Duran & Pérez-Stable, 2019a, 2019b).

In this paper, we argued for and sought to operationalize a strategy to utilize an intersectional approach to use health messages in a minority health intervention. We acknowledge that we have only scratched the surface of this approach and there are numerous other ways that the effectiveness of identity-based tailoring and using an intersectional approach may be used in pursuit of health equity. Additional formative research is needed to further identify candidate constructs that can be used in future health messages interventions with African American men, but hopefully our framework will be useful fodder for future efforts to improve the health of this and other populations.

We believe the focus on the centrality and salience of identity may be particularly important for other populations. As we illustrated with four examples of middle-aged or older African American men, there is considerable heterogeneity in a group that is often thought to be homogenous. Determining what aspects of identity and experience are most central to how people see themselves is an important foundational principle on which to build future intervention strategies (Davis et al., 2010). Building on the pioneering work of Ken Resnicow and colleagues (Davis et al., 2010; Resnicow et al., 2009), we believe our efforts to add to their approach by considering not only ethnic/racial identity but also gender is novel and consistent with the work on intersectionality in health equity research that has been led by Lisa Bowleg and others in recent years (Bauer & Scheim, 2019; Bowleg, 2017a, 2017b; Bowleg et al., 2017). We recognize that our approach only begins to touch on how men might see themselves and what might motivate them to engage in healthier behavior, but we also believe that we have outlined and advanced strategies and principles that may be a foundation for others.

One of the obvious next directions for this work would be to explore the centrality and salience of sexual orientation and non-binary gender identity for tailoring health messages (Fields et al., 2014; Ramos et al., 2019). Sexual and gender identity may be relevant aspects of identity centrality but perhaps less germane or salient to health behaviors like eating practices, physical activity, or sedentary behavior. Furthermore, it will be critical to consider how factors associated with sexual orientation and non-binary gender identity relate to the faith and role strain salience factors that are present in our current model. We recognize that sexual and gender identity are central and salient to men's identities and health behaviors in ways that may intersect with, expand and fundamentally reimagine how we conceptualize and tailor to African American manhood (Griffith, Pennings et al., 2019) and other identity-based constructs.

Conclusion

Individual tailoring of health messages may be a particularly important strategy for promoting minority health and achieving health equity, but this approach may be more effective if it incorporates an intersectional approach. Research on minority health and health equity should consider not only the factors that are most important in defining people's sense of self and the factors that may be most relevant to the health behaviors of interest. Researchers should continue to systematically consider what factors are candidate tailoring variables while critically analyzing why those factors may be more or less important in promoting the health and well-being of specific populations.

Funding

This paper has been supported in part by the American Cancer Society [RSG-15-223-01-CPPB] and NIMHD and NHGRI of the National Institutes of Health under award number U54MD010722.

ORCID

Derek M. Griffith http://orcid.org/0000-0003-0018-9176

References

Bandura, A. (2004). Health promotion by social cognitive means. *Health Education & Behavior*, *31*(2), 143–164. https://doi.org/10.1177/1090198104263660

Bauer, G. R., & Scheim, A. I. (2019, April). Advancing quantitative intersectionality research methods: Intracategorical and intercategorical approaches to shared and differential constructs. *Social Science & Medicine*, *226*, 260–262. https://doi.org/10.1016/j.socscimed.2019.03.018

Bilal, U., & Diez-Roux, A. V. (2018). Troubling trends in health disparities. *New England Journal of Medicine*, *378*(16), 1557–1558. https://doi.org/10.1056/NEJMc1800328

Bowleg, L. (2017a). Intersectionality: An underutilized but essential theoretical framework for social psychology. In B. Gough (Ed.), *The Palgrave handbook of critical social psychology* (pp. 507–529). Springer.

Bowleg, L. (2017b). Towards a critical health equity research stance: Why epistemology and methodology matter more than qualitative methods.

Health Education & Behavior, *44*(5), 677–684. https://doi.org/10.1177/1090198117728760

Bowleg, L., Del Río-gonzález, A. M., Holt, S. L., Pérez, C., Massie, J. S., Mandell, J. E., & Boone, C. A. (2017). Intersectional epistemologies of ignorance: How behavioral and social science research shapes what we know, think we know, and don't know about U.S. Black men's sexualities. *The Journal of Sex Research*, *54*(4–5), 577–603. https://doi.org/10.1080/00224499.2017.1295300

Bowman, P. J. (1989). Research perspectives on Black men: Role strain and adaptation across the adult life cycle. In R. L. Jones (Ed.), *Black adult development and aging* (pp. 117–150). Cobb & Henry Publishers.

Bronfenbrenner, U. (1994). Ecological models of human development. Reprinted in M. Gauvain & M. Cole (Eds.), *Readings on the development of children* (2nd ed., pp. 37–43). Freeman.

Cooke-Jackson, A., & Rubinsky, V. (2018). Deeply rooted in memories: Toward a comprehensive overview of 30 years of memorable message literature. *Health Communication*, *33*(4), 409–422. https://doi.org/10.1080/10410236.2016.1278491

Crenshaw, K. (1995). *Critical race theory: The key writings that formed the movement*. The New Press: Distributed by W.W. Norton & Co.

Davis, R., Alexander, G., Calvi, J., Wiese, C., Greene, S., Nowak, M., Cross, W. E., Jr, & Resnicow, K. (2010). A new audience segmentation tool for African Americans: The Black identity classification scale. *Journal of Health Communication*, *15*(5), 532. https://doi.org/10.1080/10810730.2010.492563

Duran, D. G., & Pérez-Stable, E. J. (2019a). Novel approaches to advance minority health and health disparities research. *American Journal of Public Health*, *109*(S1), S8–S10. https://doi.org/10.2105/AJPH.2018.304931

Duran, D. G., & Pérez-Stable, E. J. (2019b). Science visioning to advance the next generation of health disparities research. *American Journal of Public Health*, *109*(S1), S11–S13. https://doi.org/10.2105/AJPH.2018.304944

Evans, J., Frank, B., Oliffe, J. L., & Gregory, D. (2011). Health, illness, men and masculinities (HIMM): A theoretical framework for understanding men and their health. *Journal of Men's Health*, *8*(1), 7–15. https://doi.org/10.1016/j.jomh.2010.09.227

Fields, E. L., Bogart, L. M., Smith, K. C., Malebranche, D. J., Ellen, J., & Schuster, M. A. (2014). "I always felt I had to prove my manhood": Homosexuality, masculinity, gender role strain, and HIV risk among young Black men who have sex with men. *American Journal of Public Health*, *105*(1), 122–131. https://doi.org/10.2105/AJPH.2013.301866

Flegal, K. M., Carroll, M. D., Ogden, C. L., & Curtin, L. R. (2010). Prevalence and trends in obesity among US adults, 1999–2008. *Journal of the American Medical Association*, *303*(3), 235–241. https://doi.org/10.1001/jama.2009.2014

Gilbert, K. L., Ray, R., Siddiqi, A. A., Shetty, S., Baker, E. A., Elder, K., & Griffith, D. M. (2016). Visible and invisible trends in African American men's health: Pitfalls and promises for addressing racial, ethnic and gender health inequities. *Annual Review of Public Health*, *37*(1), 219–311. https://doi.org/10.1146/annurev-publhealth-032315-021556

Gillum, F., & Griffith, D. M. (2010). Prayer and spiritual practices for health reasons among American adults: The role of race and ethnicity. *Journal of Religion and Health*, *49*(3), 283–295. https://doi.org/10.1007/s10943-009-9249-7

Greaney, M., Quintiliani, L., Warner, E., King, D., Emmons, K., Colditz, G., Glasgow, R. E., & Bennett, G. (2009). Weight management among patients at community health centers: The "Be Fit, Be Well" study. *Obesity and Weight Management*, *5*(5), 222–228. http://dx.doi.org/10.1089/obe.2009.0507

Griffith, D. M. (2012). An intersectional approach to men's health. *Journal of Men's Health*, *9*(2), 106–112. https://doi.org/10.1016/j.jomh.2012.03.003

Griffith, D. M. (2015). "I am a man": Manhood, minority men's health and health equity. *Ethnicity and Disease*, *25*(3), 287–293. https://dx.doi.org/10.18865/ed.25.3.287

Griffith, D. M. (2016). Biopsychosocial approaches to men's health disparities research and policy. *Behavioral Medicine*, *42*(3), 211–215. https://doi.org/10.1080/08964289.2016.1194158

Griffith, D. M., Bruce, M. A., & Thorpe, R. J., Jr. (2019). Introduction. In D. M. Griffith, M. A. Bruce, & R. J. Thorpe, Jr (Eds.), *Men's health equity: A handbook* (pp. 3–9). Routledge.

Griffith, D. M., Pennings, J. S., Bruce, M. A., & Ayers, G. D. (2019). Measuring the dimensions of African American manhood: A factor analysis. In D. M. Griffith, M. A. Bruce, & R. J. Thorpe Jr (Eds.), *Men's health equity: A handbook* (pp. 101–126). Routledge.

Griffith, D. M., Jaeger, E. C., Sherman, L. D., & Moore, H. J. (2019). Middle-aged men's health. In D. M. Griffith, M. A. Bruce, & R. J. Thorpe Jr (Eds.), *Men's health equity: A handbook* (pp. 72–85). Routledge.

Griffith, D. M., & Jaeger, E. C. (2020). Chapter nine - Mighty men: A faith-based weight loss intervention to reduce cancer risk in African American men. In M. E. Ford, N. F. Esnaola, & J. D. Salley (Eds.), *Advances in cancer research* (Vol. 146, pp. 189–217). Academic Press.

Griffith, D. M., Brinkley-Rubinstein, L., Bruce, M. A., Thorpe, R. J., Jr, & Metzl, J. M. (2015). The interdependence of African American men's definitions of manhood and health. *Family and Community Health*, *38*(4), 284–296. https://doi.org/10.1097/FCH.0000000000000079

Griffith, D. M., & Cornish, E. K. (2018). "What defines a man?": Perspectives of African American men on the components and consequences of manhood. *Psychology of Men & Masculinity*, *19*(1), 78–88. http://doi.org/10.1037/men0000083

Griffith, D. M., Ellis, K. R., & Allen, J. O. (2013). An intersectional approach to social determinants of stress for African American men: Men's and women's perspectives. *American Journal of Men's Health*, *7*(4S), 16–27. https://doi.org/10.1177/1557988313480227

Griffith, D. M., Gunter, K., & Allen, J. O. (2011). Male gender role strain as a barrier to African American men's physical activity. *Health Education & Behavior*, *38*(5), 482–491. https://doi.org/10.1177/1090198110383660

Griffith, D. M., Wooley, A., & Allen, J. O. (2013). "I'm ready to eat and grab whatever I can get." Determinants and patterns of African American men's eating practices. *Health Promotion Practice*, *14*(2), 181–188. https://doi.org/10.1177/1524839912437789

Hawkins, R. P., Kreuter, M., Resnicow, K., Fishbein, M., & Dijkstra, A. (2008). Understanding tailoring in communicating about health. *Health Education Research*, *23*(3), 454. https://doi.org/10.1093/her/cyn004

Kimmel, M. S. (2006). *Manhood in America: A cultural history*. Oxford University Press.

Kreuter, M. W., Strecher, V. J., & Glassman, B. (1999). One size does not fit all: The case for tailoring print materials. *Annals of Behavioral Medicine*, *21*(4), 276. https://doi.org/10.1007/BF02895958

La Veist, T. A. (1996). Why we should continue to study race … but do a better job: An essay on race, racism and health. *Ethnicity & Disease*, *6*(1–2), 21–29. https://pubmed.ncbi.nlm.nih.gov/8882833/

Lachman, M. E. (2015). Mind the gap in the middle: A call to study midlife. *Research in Human Development*, *12*(3–4), 327–334. https://doi.org/10.1080/15427609.2015.1068048

Latimer, A. E., Brawley, L. R., & Bassett, R. L. (2010). A systematic review of three approaches for constructing physical activity messages: What messages work and what improvements are needed? *International Journal of Behavioral Nutrition and Physical Activity*, *7*(1), 36. https://doi.org/10.1186/1479-5868-7-36

McLeroy, K. R., Bibeau, D., Steckler, A., & Glanz, K. (1988). An ecological perspective on health promotion programs. *Health Education Quarterly*, *15*(4), 351–377. https://doi.org/10.1177/109019818801500401

National Academies of Sciences, Engineering, & Medicine. (2016). *The promises and perils of digital strategies in achieving health equity: Workshop summary*. The National Academies Press.

National Center for Health Statistics (US). (2017). *Health, United States, 2016: With chartbook on long-term trends in health* (Report No.: 2017-1232). PMID: 28910066.

Noar, S. M., Harrington, N. G., & Aldrich, R. S. (2009). The role of message tailoring in the development of persuasive health communication messages. *Annals of the International Communication Association*, *33*(1), 73–133. https://doi.org/10.1080/23808985.2009.11679085

O'Neil, J., Helms, B., Gable, R., David, L., & Wrightsman, L. (1986). Gender-role conflict scale: College men's fear of femininity. *Sex Roles, 14*(5), 335–350. https://doi.org/10.1007/bf00287583

Ragonese, C., Shand, T., & Barker, G. (2019). *Masculine norms and men's health: Making the connections.* Promundo-US.

Ramos, S. R., Warren, R., Shedlin, M., Melkus, G., Kershaw, T., & Vorderstrasse, A. (2019). A framework for using ehealth interventions to overcome medical mistrust among sexual minority men of color living with chronic conditions. *Behavioral Medicine, 45*(2), 166–176. https://doi.org/10.1080/08964289.2019.1570074

Resnicow, K., Davis, R., Zhang, N., Strecher, V., Tolsma, D., Calvi, J., Alexander, G., Anderson, J., Wiese, P., & Cross, W. E., Jr. (2009). Tailoring a fruit and vegetable intervention on ethnic identity: Results of a randomized study. *Health Psychology, 28*(4), 394. https://doi.org/10.1037/a0015217

Robertson, S., Williams, B., & Oliffe, J. (2016). The case for retaining a focus on "masculinities" in men's health research. *International Journal of Men's Health, 15*(1), 52–67. https://doi.org/10.3149/jmh.1501.52

Ryan, R. M., & Deci, E. L. (2000). Self-determination theory and the facilitation of intrinsic motivation, social development, and well-being. *American Psychologist, 55*(1), 68–78. https://doi.org/10.1037/0003-066X.55.1.68

Satcher, D., Fryer, G. E., Jr., McCann, J., Troutman, A., Woolf, S. H., & Rust, G. (2005). What if we were equal? A comparison of the black-white mortality gap in 1960 and 2000. *Health Affairs, 24*(2), 459–464. https://doi.org/10.1377/hlthaff.24.2.459

Sellers, R., Smith, M., Shelton, N., Rowley, S., & Chavous, T. (1998). Multidimensional model of racial identity: A reconceptualization of African American racial identity. *Personality and Social Psychology Review, 2*(1), 18–39. https://doi.org/10.1207/s15327957pspr0201_2

Summers, M. A. (2004). *Manliness and its discontents: The Black middle-class and the transformation of masculinity, 1900–1930.* University of North Carolina Press.

Underwood, L. G., & Teresi, J. A. (2002). The daily spiritual experience scale: Development, theoretical description, reliability, exploratory factor analysis, and preliminary construct validity using health-related data. *Annals of Behavioral Medicine, 24*(1), 22–33. https://doi.org/10.1207/S15324796ABM2401_04

Vandello, J. A., Bosson, J. K., & Lawler, J. R. (2019). Precarious manhood and men's health disparities. In D. M. Griffith, M. A. Bruce, & R. J. Thorpe Jr (Eds.), *Men's health equity: A handbook* (pp. 27–41). Routledge.

Vandello, J. A., & Bosson, J. K. (2013). Hard won and easily lost: A review and synthesis of theory and research on precarious manhood. *Psychology of Men & Masculinity, 14*(2), 101–113. https://doi.org/10.1037/a0029826

Whitehead, T. L. (1997). Urban low-income African American men, HIV/AIDS, and gender identity. *Medical Anthropology Quarterly, 11*(4), 411–447. https://doi.org/10.1525/maq.1997.11.4.411

World Health Organization. (2018). *Noncommunicable diseases country profiles 2018.* https://www.who.int/nmh/publications/ncd-profiles-2018/en/

The Influence of Memorable Message Receipt on Dietary and Exercise Behavior among Self-Identified Black Women

Natasha R. Brown and La'Marcus T. Wingate

ABSTRACT

Guided by Control Theory and the memorable messages framework, the current investigation examined the relationship between receipt of a health-related memorable message and self-reported diet and exercise behavior. A cross-sectional survey methodology was utilized to evaluate the relationship between receipt of a memorable message and dietary and exercise behaviors in a sample of Black women. Over 80% of the research sample (N = 121) reported receiving a memorable health message regarding diet and/or exercise. Women receiving a memorable message reported a significantly higher number of days engaging in healthy eating and exercise behaviors each week. Messages from medical professionals had the greatest impact on healthy dietary practices, while media-based messages were most influential on the enactment of exercise behavior. Additional research is warranted to determine how the utilization and reinforcement of memorable messages impacts health outcomes among Black women.

The investigation of factors associated with overweight and obesity among Black women living in the United States is a controversial topic. Body Mass Index (BMI; calculated as a person's weight in kilograms divided by the square of their height in meters) is often utilized to estimate a healthy adult weight. Although BMI is widely used, many argue this metric may not be the most accurate assessment of healthy weight for Black women (Katzmarzyk et al., 2011; Rahman & Berenson, 2010; Vaughn et al., 2014). Moreover, historical accounts of the development and usefulness of BMI have revealed this measurement is rooted in socio-economic and racist ideologies (Strings, 2019). Given these factors, we initially summarize the obesity-related health outcomes of Black women identified in the existing literature. We then highlight the existence of other under-researched factors, including messages received over their lifespan, that could influence the health behavior and outcomes of this group.

Non-Hispanic Black women have the highest prevalence of obesity (56.9%) when compared to all other groups (Hales et al., 2020). Higher rates of obesity among Black women have been linked to exposure to discrimination, racism and other stressful encounters (Cozier et al., 2014; Curry, 2020; Guyll et al., 2001). Black women also usually gain and retain more weight in adulthood (Agyemang & Powell-Wiley, 2013; Headen et al., 2012) and tend to have higher waist circumference measurements (Ford et al., 2012; Warren et al., 2012) when compared to other groups. Moreover, obesity is cited as an attributable cause of death for almost a quarter (24.3%) of Black women in the United States (Masters et al., 2013).

Given the context of how a healthy weight is estimated as well as other cultural and historical factors, it is not surprising that Black women are generally more accepting of a heavier weight (Lynch & Kane, 2014), particularly when compared to other groups (Himmelstein et al., 2017). A recent review noted factors associated with the body image perceptions of Black women are more complicated than once thought as members of this group are often inundated with media and interpersonal messages regarding needs to conform to both Black and white beauty ideals (Watson et al., 2019). Although acceptance of one's body is important, it is imperative to note that regardless of body size, taking to steps to maintain and improve Black women's health is critical. Prior research has linked a heavier weight to comorbidities including hypertension (Howard et al., 2018) and diabetes (Barnes, 2011) among Black women. There is also a disparity in the prevalence of coronary heart disease among Black women when compared to other groups, including Black men (Carnethon et al., 2017). In light of these observations, we focused on the experiences of dietary choice and exercise among Black women.

Intervention efforts for Black women are believed to achieve their greatest effect in promoting healthy behavior when they are culturally sensitive and tailored to the population (Agyemang & Powell-Wiley, 2013). To facilitate future intervention research, emphasis must be centered on personal health behaviors, which are identified as key factors responsible for up to an estimated 40% of premature deaths in the United States (Kino & Kawachi, 2020; Schroeder, 2007). Dietary choice and exercise specifically are integral factors to consider as Black women, when compared to other groups, consume fewer servings of fruits and vegetables (Gans et al., 2009; Webb et al., 2014) and report lower levels of physical activity (Ainsworth et al., 2003; Williams et al., 2018). We focused on the experiences of Black women to uncover information that may assist this group with the initiation, continuation, and/or maintenance of health promoting behavior to reduce coronary heart disease risk.

In the current study, we operationalized healthy eating as dietary habits associated with decreased morbidity and mortality. More specifically, healthy eating involves consumption of nutrient-dense foods (i.e. fruits, vegetables, whole grains, and lean protein) while limiting red meats and foods with high amounts of sugar, saturated fat, and sodium (U.S. Department of Agriculture and U.S. Department of Health and Human Services, 2020). The Dietary Approaches to Stop Hypertension (DASH) diet, which includes many of these components, is associated with lower mortality levels in Black women (Boggs et al., 2014).

In the context of this study, we operationalized healthy exercise habits as physical activity that may lead to demonstrable benefits such as decreased mortality. Current guidelines recommend that U.S. adults engage in at least 150 minutes of moderate intensity each week (U.S. Department of Health and Human Services, 2018). Among Black women specifically, consistent engagement in less than one hour per week of moderate intensity exercise confers a significant benefit of a 17% reduction in mortality, and even greater benefits are observed with more frequent and higher intensity exercise (Sheehy et al., 2020). Within this study, even one additional day of exercise, whether it be moderate or high intensity, is considered to contribute to better health outcomes.

Messages regarding health and wellness are normally embedded in everyday communication (Cline, 2003, 2011). Previous work has suggested these frequent interactions influence messages shared between peers regarding health promotion (Reno & McNamee, 2014). Recent research also suggests everyday communication influences the conversations individuals have within medical encounters (Head & Bute, 2018). One framework often utilized to examine health messages within the communication literature is Control Theory (Carver & Scheier, 1981, 1982) which has consequentially influenced much of the research associated with the memorable message framework (Knapp et al., 1981; Smith & Ellis, 2001).

Control theory

Heavily influenced by Self-Regulation Theory (Powers, 1973a, 1973b), Control Theory (Carver & Scheier, 1981, 1982) explains how the actions of others within a system can influence behavior. One of the key features of the theory is the negative feedback loop, a mechanism that motivates an individual to take steps to achieve their goals by minimizing the difference between their current and ideal states (Cooke-Jackson & Rubinsky, 2018). Goal achievement incorporates input, analysis (which involves a comparison of a person's current state and their idealized state), and consequential behavior. If there is a discrepancy perceived between an individual's current and idealized states, a behavior is performed to reduce this difference (Carver & Scheier, 1982, p. 112). The negative feedback loop explains how factors such as interpersonal communication influence decisions regarding whether to engage in health promoting behaviors.

Control Theory (Carver & Scheier, 1981, 1982) posits several levels of goal achievement, the most referenced include systems, principle, and program. The systems level is based upon the "idealized self-image" an individual seeks to attain (Carver & Scheier, 1982, p. 114). The principle level involves how people self-regulate their behavior over time. The program level focuses on the behavior enacted within the principle level (Carver & Scheier, 1982, p. 116). Control Theory has been utilized as a guiding framework for many studies investigating the influence of memorable messages on health promoting behavior.

Memorable messages framework

Knapp et al. (1981) define memorable messages as "verbal messages which may be remembered for extremely long periods of time and which people perceived as a major influence on the course of their lives" (p. 27). Memorable messages are typically brief; perceived as important; and usually articulated by a respected source (Nazione et al., 2011). Thus, memorable messages are easy to remember and may be referenced later to assess behavior (Butler Ellis & Smith, 2004; Cornacchione et al., 2016; Smith & Ellis, 2001). Seminal memorable messages research focused on the topics (Lauckner et al., 2012; Smith et al., 2009, 2011), sources (Smith et al., 2009, 2011), and framing of cancer detection messages and their relationship to the execution of cancer detection behaviors (Lauckner et al., 2012; Smith et al., 2010).

There has been an increased interest in memorable messages regarding body image, diet, and exercise in recent years (Anderson et al., 2014; Baiocchi-Wagner & Talley, 2013; Lambert, 2012; Reno & McNamee, 2014). The existing literature has focused on the sources, content, and influence of receipt of memorable messages on healthy behavior. Family members (Drummond, 2005; Hall et al., 2016; Rubinsky et al., 2019; Russell & Smith, 2017; Thompson & Zaitchik, 2012), friends (Rubinsky et al., 2019; Russell & Smith, 2017), the media (Russell & Smith, 2017), and medical professionals (Drummond, 2005; Russell & Smith, 2017) have been frequently identified as memorable message sources. Mutual contacts (including roommates, sorority/fraternity and other peers that may not be considered friends; Dunleavy & Yang, 2015; Lambert, 2012; Rubinsky et al., 2019) have also been identified as message sources regarding these topics.

Existing research has revealed the content of memorable messages regarding body image, diet, and exercise can differ. Memorable body image messages tend to promote a body size that is not too big or too small (Rubinsky et al., 2019; Thompson & Zaitchik, 2012). Parents and college peers have been noted to criticize weight gain and a larger body size (Reno & McNamee, 2014; Rubinsky et al., 2019; Thompson & Zaitchik, 2012). In regard to diet and exercise behavior, message content has focused on behavioral changes, sometimes asserting that weight control is easy, especially if the message recipient is younger (Thompson & Zaitchik, 2012). Messages regarding healthy behavior included suggestions regarding what the message recipients should or should not eat (Dunleavy & Yang, 2015; Lambert, 2012). Medical professionals were encouraging in their messages regarding exercise and healthy eating and noted these behaviors help with chronic disease management (Drummond, 2005).

The outcomes related to memorable message receipt vary based upon perceived intention, message valence, and family communication orientation. Receipt of negatively-valenced memorable messages negatively impact women's perceptions of their body (Anderson et al., 2014; Hall et al., 2016). Less frequently cited positively-valenced messages were mentioned in qualitative study focusing on health promotion (Lambert, 2012). Memorable messages perceived as helpful have been associated with healthier dietary behaviors (Russell & Smith, 2017) and greater satisfaction with one's body (Rubinsky et al., 2019). Communication in families with a high conversation orientation tended to emphasize more positive views of diet and exercise behavior (Baiocchi-Wagner & Talley, 2013) in comparison to familial conversations that involved criticism of the message recipient's choices (Hall et al., 2016; Ndiaye et al., 2013). In addition to the memorable messages literature, there is also a segment of the existing literature examining factors related to body image/weight perception among Black women.

Black women and body image/weight

Body image is a complicated topic among Black women as their perceptions in this area are influenced by conflicting social-cultural factors, some expressing acceptance/appreciation of a larger body size and others supporting a smaller one (Lynch & Kane, 2014). Black women have been exposed to various messages regarding body image and body weight via media sources, with the existing literature reporting mixed results regarding the influence of such messages. A comprehensive literature review regarding body image and healthy eating concluded that greater media use (particularly magazines and music videos) was positively correlated with body dissatisfaction and higher scores on disordered eating scales (López-Guimerà et al., 2010). Another study with young adults noted that individuals who engaged with an attractive peer on social media experienced an increase in negative body image versus those who interacted with a family member (Hogue & Mills, 2019). A recent content analysis revealed Black women on TV are typically portrayed as darker skinned and thin (Cox & Ward, 2019). These TV portrayals differ from those presented in prior research wherein Black women considered a curvaceous body shape as the most attractive more often than white women (Overstreet et al., 2010). Research with Black undergraduates has revealed that exposure to music videos and the content of Black magazines was related to the labeling of Black women as sexual objects (Jerald et al., 2017). Simply put, media outlets tend to disseminate and reinforce perceptions that a thinner body appearance is ideal (López-Guimerà et al., 2010).

Although Black women appear to resist adoption of the thin ideal as presented in the media, members of this group do report body dissatisfaction related to personal factors including quality of life, potential romantic partners, and family interactions. Prior research has noted body image dissatisfaction as well as the degree to which a Black woman wants to be smaller can influence their perceived quality of life (Cox et al., 2011). Some Black women also report maintaining or modifying their appearance (including their weight) to be perceived as attractive to Black men (Capodilupo & Kim, 2014). Body image perceptions are also influenced by communication with family members, with some Black women maintaining a particular body size to avoid familial criticism, including being described as "too big" (Capodilupo & Kim, 2014).

Within the current study, the memorable message framework provides guidance regarding the relationship between time since message receipt, message source, and self-reported diet and exercise practices. While the memorable message framework focuses on the message itself, Control Theory (Carver & Scheier, 1981, 1982) helps to explain the behavioral responses to memorable message receipt (Smith & Ellis, 2001). In line with previous research incorporating memorable messages, this study utilizes Control Theory as a framework to examine the behaviors associated with receipt of a memorable message. The literature regarding media consumption and body image provides insight regarding the source and content of messages to be reported.

While the work of Smith and Ellis (2001) set the foundation for the widespread application of Control Theory (Carver & Scheier, 1981, 1982) to the memorable messages literature, the theory has also been frequently used as a guiding framework for other studies assessing the influence of memorable messages on the promotion of healthy behavior (Miczo et al., 2013; Smith et al., 2011). The current study focuses on frequently enacted behavior (diet and exercise) instead of behavior in response to a pandemic (Miczo et al., 2013) or less frequent enacted behavior associated with cancer detection such as self-exams or mammograms (Smith et al., 2011).

We extend the existing memorable message literature in two ways. First, the work further explores the influence of memorable message timing on the enactment of health promoting behavior such as fruit and vegetable consumption and exercise frequency/intensity (Davis et al., 2016; Hall et al., 2016). Second, we examine messages targeting a segment of the population that has received little attention in the memorable message's literature, a nonwhite, adult research sample (Cooke-Jackson & Rubinsky, 2018). We focused on exploring the relationship between memorable message receipt and dietary and exercise patterns among a sample of Black women, a segment of the U.S. population with high rates of coronary heart disease (Carnethon et al., 2017). Nearly half of U.S. adults (49.1%) have initiated weight loss efforts in the last year (National Center for Health Statistics, 2019). Such weight loss attempts have included modifications to diet and exercise behavior (National Center for Health Statistics, 2019), two factors that, when enacted regularly, can reduce coronary heart disease risk (Buttar et al., 2005). The following hypotheses and research questions are addressed in this study:

H1: Receipt of a memorable message is associated with more exercise in the last 7 days.

H2: Receipt of a memorable message is associated with eating a healthier diet (operationalized as eating more fruits and vegetables and limiting the consumption of high fat foods such as red meat and full fat dairy products) in the last 7 days.

RQ: What is the relationship between the source of a memorable message and dietary and exercise practices in the last 7 days?

Materials and methods

The study procedures outlined here were approved by the first author's Institutional Review Board (IRB; Protocol #2014-037). To address the hypotheses and research questions posed, a cross-sectional methodology was utilized to gather survey data at one time to facilitate an efficient research process (White, 2020). In a fashion similar to other memorable messages studies (Dunleavy & Yang, 2015; Reno & McNamee, 2014; Russell & Smith, 2017; Thompson & Zaitchik, 2012), surveys were administered online. Participant recruitment incorporated methods utilized by King et al. (2010) wherein Black women were recruited via a multimodal approach involving community outreach, fliers/brochures, and media-based advertisements. Recruitment materials were distributed to and/or posted in places, groups, and organizations Black women have been known to visit or have membership including churches, hair salons, shopping centers, schools, and civic organizations. Fitness groups (face-to-face and virtual) were also contacted for participant recruitment. Participant recruitment flyers featured images of fruits and vegetables as well as Black women engaging in exercise. The flyers also included a brief description of the project (without identifying research hypotheses), the time required to complete the survey and incentives (the opportunity to be entered into a drawing to win one of ten $50 gift certificates) for survey completion.

After providing informed consent, respondents were asked "Have you ever received a memorable message regarding diet and/or exercise." If participants reported receiving a memorable message, they were prompted to provide more information regarding the content of the message. Survey respondents were also asked to indicate the time elapsed since receiving the message. In addition, respondents were prompted to select from five message source choices: family member, media, medical professional, friend or other.

Additionally, participants were asked to recall their recent dietary and exercise behaviors as elicited from responses to a modified version of the validated Summary of Diabetes Self-Care Activities Scale (Toobert et al., 2000). Most questions on this scale focused on a seven-day recall of dietary and exercise behavior as this was found to represent a suitable time frame for assessment of these behaviors. Data analysis was conducted in a fashion similar to previous research using a modified version of the Summary of Diabetes Self-Care Activities Scale to characterize respondent's health behaviors (Mogre et al., 2017). More specifically, the total diet score was operationalized as a composite variable by deriving the mean score of four questions. Two of the questions in the total diet score ascertained how often a healthy eating plan was followed, one question elicited how frequently at least five servings of fruits and vegetables were consumed, and one question evaluated how often respondents ate high fat foods such as red meat or high fat dairy foods. Responses to how often high fat foods were consumed were reverse coded. The frequency of exercise per week was derived as the mean to two questions, one of which elicited how often respondents participated in at least 30 minutes of physical activity and another which asked how often they engaged in a specific exercise session. Respondents were asked to provide basic demographic information including age and marital status as previous research suggests that married women may have higher weights when compared to women who are single (Averett et al., 2008).

SPSS version 24 (Armonk, NY) was utilized to conduct data analyses. Descriptive statistics were employed to summarize the demographic characteristics of the sample by using frequencies to describe how many individuals received a memorable message, the timing of the messages received, and the message source. The independent samples t-test was used to determine whether there was a significant difference in the mean number of days respondents followed a healthy eating plan and exercised among those that received a memorable message and those who did not receive a message. A one-way ANOVA was utilized to determine if there were any significant differences between the mean number of days following a healthy eating plan (e.g., eating more fruits and vegetables and consuming less high fat foods) and exercising for other categorical variables including message timing, message source, respondent age, and marital status. The Bonferonni test was used in post hoc testing to assess statistical significance. Separate multivariate linear regression models were utilized to evaluate the effects of the timing of memorable message and the source of the memorable message on 1) the frequency of healthy eating and 2) frequency of engaging in exercise while controlling for other factors. The alpha value was set a priori at 0.05 for all statistical analyses. A sample size of at least 77 respondents was needed to accommodate a desired power level of 0.80 to detect a moderate effect size of $f = 0.15$ in a linear regression model with three predictor variables (Faul et al., 2009).

Description of study sample

The final analytic sample was comprised of 121 women as seen in Table 1. All women self-identified as Black. The study sample ranged from 18 to 64 years old ($M = 37.04$, $SD = 9.10$). Nearly 60% of the sample (58.2%) was between the ages of 31 to 40. Approximately half (52.9%) of respondents were single or had never been married while more than a third (34.5%) were currently married. Most respondents (82.6%) reported receiving a memorable message related to diet and/or exercise.

The time elapsed since receipt of a memorable message varied across the sample. Approximately 40% of the research sample reported receiving a memorable message more than a year ago. A smaller percentage of respondents (28.9%) reported receiving a memorable message within the past year. The remaining respondents (12.4%) could not identify the timeframe in which the message was received.

Table 1. Sample characteristics of Black women responding to survey about memorable messages and diet and exercise habits (N = 121).

Variable	N (%)
Age	
18 to 30	18 (16.4)
31 to 40	64 (58.2)
Over 40	28 (25.5)
Marital Status	
Single	63 (52.1)
Married	41 (33.9)
Divorced	12 (9.9)
Other	5 (4.1)
Received memorable message regarding diet and/or exercise	
Yes	100 (82.6)
No	21 (17.4)
Length since memorable message received	
Message not received	22 (18.2)
One year or less	35 (28.9)
More than year ago	49 (40.5)
Do not remember	15 (12.4)
Nature of relationship with message source	
Message not received	22 (18.2)
Family member	24 (19.8)
Media (TV, radio, internet)	28 (23.1)
Medical professional	16 (13.2)
Friend	18 (14.9)
Other	13 (10.7)

Table 2. Bivariate analysis of impact of respondent characteristics on health promoting behaviors in Black women.

	Impact of memorable messages on health promoting behaviors			
	Reported days per week eating healthy (n = 119)		Days per week engaging in exercise (n = 121)	
	Mean±SD	p-value	Mean±SD	p-value
Received memorable message		.004		.005
Yes	3.68 ± 1.74*		3.25 + 2.17*	
No	2.65 ± 1.28		1.81 + 1.81	
Length since message received		.021		.004
Not received	2.67 ± 1.25		1.86 ± 1.78	
One year or less	3.77 ± 1.70		3.94 ± 2.04*	
More than year ago	4.02 ± 1.86*		2.90 ± 2.04	
Do not remember	3.52 ± 1.48		2.77 ± 2.63	
Source of message		.006		.009
Not received	2.67 ± 1.25		1.86 ± 1.78	
Family member or friend	3.42 ± 1.65		2.65 ± 2.05	
Media (TV, radio, internet)	4.01 ± 1.78		3.82 ± 2.17*	
Medical professional	4.41 ± 1.60*		3.47 ± 2.29	
Other	4.29 ± 1.97		3.65 ± 2.23	
Marital Status		.329		.592
Single	3.42 ± 1.71		2.99 ± 2.33	
Married	3.93 ± 1.61		3.21 ± 2.02	
No longer married	3.80 ± 2.03		2.53 ± 1.95	
Age		.017		.429
18 to 30	3.22 + 1.85#		3.11 ± 2.46	
31 to 40	3.46 + 1.63#		2.74 ± 2.13	
Over 40	4.48 + 1.71		3.38 ± 2.20	

* indicates significantly greater participation in health promoting behavior compared to those not receiving memorable message; # indicates significantly lower frequency of eating healthy in the week compared to those at least 40 years of age.

Memorable message source responses also varied considerably amongst the sample. Twenty-three percent (23.1%) of respondents indicated receiving a memorable message via a media-based source. Almost half of the memorable messages identified were received from interpersonal sources including family members (19.8%), medical professionals (13.2%), and friends (14.9%). The remaining percentage of respondents (10.7%) could not identify a memorable message source.

Results

Bivariate analysis: Receipt of a memorable message and diet and exercise

Table 2 summarizes results from a bivariate analysis performed to examine the influence of memorable message receipt on healthy behavior. The health behavior (as measured by the report of dietary and exercise practices in the last seven days) of individuals receiving a memorable message were compared to the health behavior of individuals who did not report receiving a memorable message. Women receiving a memorable message reported a significantly higher number of mean days following a healthy eating plan in the last week ($p = .004$). Women receiving a memorable message also reported a significantly higher number of mean days engaging in exercise in the past week ($p = .005$).

Post-hoc tests of the ANOVA examined the relationship between time since memorable message receipt and the enactment of health promoting behaviors. With regards to the number of days eating more fruits and vegetables and consuming less red meat and high fat dairy, memorable messages received more than one year ago were the only ones that had a significantly greater impact than not having received a message at all. When evaluating the days per week engaging in exercise, memorable messages received less than one year ago were the only ones that had a significant impact in comparison to not receiving a message at all.

Additional bivariate analyses examined the relationship between memorable message source and health promoting behavior. Messages received from a medical professional had a significant impact on the frequency of eating more fruits and vegetables and consuming less red meat and high fat dairy. When evaluating the days per week engaged in exercise, media-based sources were the only ones that had a significant impact. Age was the only other factor that had a significant influence on the frequency of healthy behaviors. Individuals over 40 followed a healthy eating plan in comparison to other groups (18 to 30 years old and 31 to 40 years old).

Multivariate analysis: Receipt of a memorable message and time since message receipt

Table 3 provides a summary of the multivariate linear regression analysis regarding whether the timing of memorable message receipt is predictive of greater engagement in certain dietary choices and exercise. After adjusting for other factors, receiving a memorable message less than one year ago or more than one year ago were both predictive of individuals consuming more fruits and vegetables and less high fat foods ($p = .004$ and 0.001 respectively). Black women over age 40 who received a memorable message reported consuming more fruits and vegetables and less high fat foods when compared to women between 18–30 years of age after adjusting for other factors ($p = .010$). Participants who received a message less than one year ago ($p = .001$) or more than one year ago ($p = .034$) exercised more frequently

Table 3. Multivariate linear regression analysis of time since memorable message on health promoting behaviors in Black women.

	Impact of time since memorable messages on health promoting behaviors					
	Reported days per week eating healthy (n = 119)			Days per week engaging in exercise (n = 121)		
	β-coefficient	SE	p-value	β-coefficient	SE	p-value
Intercept	2.15	0.44	<0.001	1.98	0.56	<.001
Length since message received						
Not received	Reference			Reference		
One year or less	1.31	0.44	.004	2.21	0.56	<.001
More than year ago	1.41	0.42	.001	1.14	0.53	.034
Do not remember	0.89	0.54	.101	0.90	0.69	.195
Marital Status						
Single	Reference			Reference		
Married	0.50	0.33	.142	0.38	0.42	.369
No longer married	−0.11	0.49	831	− 0.68	0.63	286
Age						
18 to 30	Reference			Reference		
31 to 40	0.01	0.37	.970	−0.62	0.48	.195
Over 40	1.20	0.46	.010	0.39	0.58	.505

compared to those who did not receive a memorable message after controlling for other factors.

Multivariate analysis: Receipt of a memorable message and source of message

Table 4 summarizes results from a multivariate linear regression analysis assessing whether memorable message source is predictive of greater frequency of healthy diet and exercise. In this model, memorable messages from all sources (family members or friends, media sources, medical professionals, and others) were predictive of healthier dietary practices as well as more exercise after controlling for other variables. In addition, women over the age of 40 consumed more fruits and vegetables and less high fat foods in comparison to those age 18 to 30 when controlling for other factors.

Table 4. Multivariate linear regression analysis of source of memorable message on health promoting behaviors in Black women.

	Impact memorable message source on health promoting behaviors					
	Reported days per week eating healthy (n = 119)			Days per week engaging in exercise (n = 121)		
	β-coefficient	SE	p-value	β-coefficient	SE	p-value
Intercept	2.12	0.43	<.001	1.98	0.57	.001
Source of message						
Not received	Reference			Reference		
Family member or friend	0.91	0.42	.034	0.94	0.55	.09
Media (TV radio, internet)	1.46	0.46	.002	2.00	0.60	.001
Medical professional	1.77	0.53	.001	1.64	0.69	.019
Other	1.59	0.57	.007	1.83	0.73	.014
Marital Status						
Single	Reference			Reference		
Married	0.52	0.33	.13	0.37	0.43	.39
No longer married	0.04	0.50	.94	− 0.46	0.65	.48
Age						
18 to 30	Reference			Reference		
31 to 40	0.06	0.37	862	−0.58	0.48	.23
Over 40	1.10	0.46	.018	0.19	0.60	.75

Discussion

The results of this study suggest that receipt of a memorable message is associated with dietary choice in Black women. Memorable messages received more than a year ago and those coming from health professionals had a stronger impact on this behavior. The research findings also demonstrate that receipt of a memorable message is associated with greater frequency of exercise in Black women, particularly if the message is derived from a multimedia source and if receipt has occurred within the past year. Black women over the age of 40 in the study sample exhibited better dietary and exercise behaviors in comparison to those that were younger. The study sample was unique in that it focused on memorable messages within Black women, one of the least researched demographic groups in the memorable messages literature. The project also included respondents from a broad age range, particularly beyond the traditional college student.

These results provide insight into the influence of memorable message receipt on health behavior beyond the cancer messages that have received most of the memorable message research attention (Lauckner et al., 2012; Smith et al., 2011, 2009). We examined the influence of memorable message receipt in a Black sample that has not been a demonstrated focus of the existing memorable messages literature (Cooke-Jackson & Rubinsky, 2018; Johnson et al., 2014). Most importantly, the study provides additional insight regarding the influence of memorable message receipt and their relationship to diet and exercise behavior (Davis et al., 2016; Hall et al., 2016; Reno & McNamee, 2014) as a potential area to investigate when designing future studies to reduce cardiovascular disease risk among Black women. These results are encouraging as previous research has indicated many Black women do not meet U.S. recommended diet and exercise guidelines (Gans et al., 2009; Webb et al., 2014). These results regarding memorable health message receipt provide further justification for the inclusion of a social support component within interventions focusing on dietary choice and exercise among Black women (Bland & Sharma, 2017).

Theoretical contributions

Results of the current study add to our understanding of the influence of timing, message source, and age on the enaction of healthy behavior as explained via Control Theory and the memorable messages framework. Study results suggest time since memorable message receipt has different implications for diet and exercise behavior. Messages regarding dietary choices appeared to have a longer lasting impact than those regarding exercise. Such differential influence is potentially explained via Control Theory's (Carver & Scheier, 1981, 1982) negative feedback loop. Dietary practices are choices an individual must incorporate into their everyday lives while exercise is typically enacted less frequently. Thus, the behavior that occurs more frequently (dietary choices) may be judged more critically to ensure an individual's ideal dietary composition corresponds with their food consumption. In addition, it appears that memorable messages focusing on regulation of an everyday behavior such as dietary choice could address issues impacting principle-regulation such as social undermining from family members and friends regarding healthy eating (Drummond, 2005). This finding also aligns with the existing literature suggesting younger Black women do not value exercise as much as other groups and are satisfied with a larger body size (Sanderson et al., 2013).

The source of a memorable message also appears to have different implications for diet and exercise behavior. Message sources with specialized expertise, such as medical professionals, had the largest impact on dietary behaviors. As emphasized in a review of the memorable messages literature (Cooke-Jackson & Rubinsky, 2018), these results have implications for medical professionals and how they could provide advice/guidance to Black women regarding healthy eating practices. More specifically, these messages should encourage Black women to engage in behavioral practices to reduce coronary heart disease risk rather than weight loss, which could be a secondary goal (Lynch & Kane, 2014). Alternatively, media-based messages influenced enactment of exercise behavior the most. Previous memorable message research has also identified the media as a key source of memorable messages (Smith et al., 2009). Future research should seek to examine how media-based messages work in the initiation or the maintenance of health promoting behavior in underserved populations such as Black women.

Age was also a factor influencing engagement in recent diet and exercise behaviors. Women aged 40 and above engaged in healthy dietary behavior more than younger women. This finding aligns with prior research indicating women seem to adopt healthier behaviors and have a higher quality diet as they age (Hiza et al., 2013; Imamura et al., 2015). Younger women may be less motivated to change their dietary choices and/or exercise partly due to the fact they are less likely to have chronic diseases such as diabetes that would prompt them to adopt healthier behaviors (Fang, 2018). More research is needed regarding the factors influencing diet quality among Black women across the lifespan, especially concerning dietary quality and mortality as prior research has shown that following the DASH eating style (which encourages lower red meat consumption and an increased amount of whole grains) is associated with a lower mortality rate for Black women (Boggs et al., 2014).

Results regarding age differences in dietary quality also align with Control Theory's (Carver & Scheier, 1982) negative feedback loop. There are likely different idealized states regarding dietary quality for those under 40 compared to those above 40 years of age. Moreover, Black women typically have lower metabolism rates (Sharp et al., 2002) that are likely to continue to decrease over time, especially if they embrace a sedentary lifestyle (Shook et al., 2014).

Limitations

As with all research, this project has limitations. Some limitations of this project are associated with the composition of the research sample and survey administration. First, the research sample appeared to engage in exercise and healthy eating more than Black women in the general U.S. population (Williams et al., 2018). Second, due to the nature of the study and participant recruitment methods, health-conscious Black women were more likely to complete the survey. Future studies should take steps to recruit both physically active and sedentary women to provide a more inclusive perspective of the influence of memorable message receipt on diet and exercise practices. The cross-sectional nature of the study also precludes causal inference. Research studies providing a longitudinal analysis of the influence of memorable messages on the initiation and/or maintenance of health promoting behaviors would be beneficial to examine long-term influence of memorable message receipt.

In addition, because questions regarding history of disordered eating and sexual orientation were not included as a part of the survey instrument, we cannot determine how those factors are associated with health-related memorable message receipt and the outcome variables measured in this study. We acknowledge that disordered eating is an understudied area in Black women's health that has primarily focused on the experiences of young women (Kelly et al., 2012). Future research in this area should focus on how messages received from various sources may contribute to disordered eating among Black women (López-Guimerà et al., 2010). Moreover, since information regarding sexual orientation was not collected as part of the study, we cannot determine the influence of this factor on the research results. Thus, future studies with larger study samples of Black women of varied sexual orientations can add to the existing literature as prior research focusing on the experiences of lesbian, bisexual, and queer (LBQ) women has noted these groups have had varied experiences with communication regarding body image (M. L. Smith et al., 2019) with bisexual women being more susceptible to the thinness ideal (Burnette et al., 2019).

Another study limitation is that data regarding the respondent's health status as relates to chronic diseases such as hypertension, diabetes and coronary heart disease was not collected. As such, we cannot ascertain if the presence of these chronic diseases may have impacted participant's health behaviors. Future research should seek to obtain this information as certain ailments, including chronic disease may influence health behavior of this group.

Contribution to the existing literature and future directions

The current project sought to examine the influence of memorable message receipt on health promoting behavior among Black women. Research results expand the existing literature regarding the impact of memorable messages on health promoting behavior in an underserved population that has received little attention in the memorable message literature. Future research should examine how additional factors, including memorable message content, are associated with the differential influence of such messages on the enactment of diet and exercise behavior. Additional inquiry regarding memorable message receipt should incorporate relational and environmental factors influencing the impact of memorable message receipt on the enactment of health promoting behavior (Agyemang & Powell-Wiley, 2013). With the emergence of scholarship theorizing memorable messages, future research must acknowledge the implications of conflicting messages over a lifespan as it relates to Black women's health and the ways in which messages this group have (historically) received might complicate or compete with initial messages (Cooke-Jackson & Rubinsky, 2021, p. 94). Identifying these pathways could assist in the development of additional tailored, culturally sensitive interventions to foster the initiation and/or maintenance of healthy behaviors (Michie et al., 2009) to reduce coronary heart disease risk among Black women.

Disclosure of potential conflict of interest

The authors declare there is no conflict of interest.

Funding

This work was supported in part by a grant from the National Heart, Lung, and Blood Institute to the University of Mississippi Medical Center [Grant #2R25HL126145 - MPIs Beech and Norris].

ORCID

Natasha R. Brown http://orcid.org/0000-0003-1467-237X

References

Agyemang, P., & Powell-Wiley, T. M. (2013). Obesity and Black women: Special considerations related to genesis and therapeutic approaches. *Current Cardiovascular Risk Reports*, *7*(5), 378–386. https://doi.org/10.1007/s12170-013-0328-7

Ainsworth, B. E., Wilcox, S., Thompson, W. W., Richter, D. L., & Henderson, K. A. (2003). Personal, social, and physical environmental correlates of physical activity in African-American women in South Carolina. *American Journal of Preventive Medicine*, *25*(3 Suppl 1), 23–29. https://doi.org/10.1016/s0749-3797(03)00161-2

Anderson, J., Bresnahan, M. J., & DeAngelis, B. N. (2014). The impact of personal metaphors and memorable interpersonal communication on body satisfaction. *Qualitative Health Research*, *24*(6), 727–737. https://doi.org/10.1177/1049732314529665

Averett, S. L., Sikora, A., & Argys, L. M. (2008). For better or worse: Relationship status and body mass index. *Economics & Human Biology*, *6*(3), 330–349. https://doi.org/10.1016/j.ehb.2008.07.003

Baiocchi-Wagner, E. A., & Talley, A. E. (2013). The role of family communication in individual health attitudes and behaviors concerning diet and physical activity. *Health Communication*, *28*(2), 193–205. https://doi.org/10.1080/10410236.2012.674911

Barnes, A. S. (2011). The epidemic of obesity and diabetes: Trends and treatments. *Texas Heart Institute Journal*, *38*(2), 142–144.

Bland, V., & Sharma, M. (2017). Physical activity interventions in African American women: A systematic review. *Health Promotion Perspectives*, *7*(2), 52–59. https://doi.org/10.15171/hpp.2017.11

Boggs, D. A., Ban, Y., Palmer, J. R., & Rosenberg, L. (2014). Higher diet quality is inversely associated with mortality in African-American women. *The Journal of Nutrition*, *145*(3), 547–554. https://doi.org/10.3945/jn.114.195735

Burnette, C. B., Kwitowski, M. A., Trujillo, M. A., & Perrin, P. B. (2019). Body appreciation in lesbian, bisexual, and queer women: Examining a model of social support, resilience, and self-esteem. *Health Equity*, *3*(1), 238–245. https://doi.org/10.1089/heq.2019.0003

Butler Ellis, J., & Smith, S. W. (2004). Memorable messages as guides to self-assessment of behavior: A replication and extension diary study. *Communication Monographs*, *71*(1), 97–119. https://doi.org/10.1080/0363452041000l691456

Buttar, H. S., Li, T., & Ravi, N. (2005). Prevention of cardiovascular diseases: Role of exercise, dietary interventions, obesity and smoking cessation. *Experimental and Clinical Cardiology*, *10*(4), 229–249.

Capodilupo, C. M., & Kim, S. (2014). Gender and race matter: The importance of considering intersections in Black women's body image. *Journal of Counseling Psychology*, *61*(1), 37–49. https://doi.org/10.1037/a0034597

Carnethon, M. R., Pu, J., Howard, G., Albert, M. A., Anderson, C., Bertoni, A. G., Mujahid, M. S., Palaniappan, L., Taylor, H. A., Jr, Willis, M., & Yancy, C. W., & American Heart Association Council on Epidemiology and Prevention; Council on Cardiovascular Disease in the Young; Council on Cardiovascular and Stroke Nursing; Council on Clinical Cardiology; Council on Functional Genomics and Translational Biology; and Stroke Council. (2017). Cardiovascular health in African Americans: A scientific statement from the American Heart Association. *Circulation*, *136*(21), e393–e423. https://doi.org/10.1161/CIR.0000000000000534

Carver, C. S., & Scheier, M. F. (1981). *Attention and self-regulation: A control-theory approach to human behavior*. Springer-Verlag.

Carver, C. S., & Scheier, M. F. (1982). Control theory: A useful conceptual framework for personality, social, clinical, and health psychology. *Psychological Bulletin*, *92*(1), 111–135. https://doi.org/10.1037/0033-2909.92.1.111

Cline, R. J. W. (2003). Everyday interpersonal communication and health. In T. L. Thompson, A. M. Dorsey, K. I. Miller, & R. Parrott (Eds.), *Handbook of health communication* (pp. 285–313). Lawrence Erlbaum Associates.

Cline, R. J. W. (2011). Everyday interpersonal communication and health. In T. L. Thompson, R. Parrott, & J. F. Nussbaum (Eds.), *Handbook of health communication* (2nd ed., pp. 377–398). Routledge/Taylor & Francis.

Cooke-Jackson, A., & Rubinsky, V. (2018). Deeply rooted in memories: Toward a comprehensive overview of 30 years of memorable message literature. *Health Communication*, *33*(4), 409–422. https://doi.org/10.1080/10410236.2016.1278491

Cooke-Jackson, A., & Rubinsky, V. (2021). Theory of memorable messages: Theorizing message disruption. In A. Cooke-Jackson & V. Rubinsky (Eds.), *Communicating intimate health* (pp. 89–98). Rowman & Littlefield.

Cornacchione, J., Smith, S. W., Morash, M., Bohmert, M. N., Cobbina, J. E., & Kashy, D. A. (2016). An exploration of female offenders' memorable messages from probation and parole officers on the self-assessment of behavior from a control theory perspective. *Journal of Applied Communication Research*, *44*(1), 60–77. https://doi.org/10.1080/00909882.2015.1116705

Cox, T. L., Ard, J. D., Beasley, T. M., Fernandez, J. R., Howard, V. J., & Affuso, O. (2011). Body image as a mediator of the relationship between body mass index and weight related quality of life in Black women. *Journal of Women's Health*, *20*(10), 1573–1578. https://doi.org/10.1089/jwh.2010.2637

Cox, V., & Ward, L. M. (2019). A wholistic view of Black women on scripted TV: A content analysis. *Journal of Black Psychology*, *45*(6–7), 540–570. https://doi.org/10.1177/0095798419887072

Cozier, Y., Yu, J., Coogan, P., Bethea, T., Rosenberg, L, & Palmer, J. (2014). Racism, segregation, and risk of obesity in the Black Women's Health Study. *American Journal of Epidemiology*, *179*(7), 875–883. https://doi.org/10.1093/aje/kwu004

Curry, G. D. (2020). The impact of educational attainment on Black women's obesity rate in the United States. *Journal of Racial and Ethnic Health Disparities*, *7*(2), 345–354. https://doi.org/10.1007/s40615-019-00663-z

Davis, L. A., Morgan, S. E., & Mobley, A. R. (2016). The utility of the memorable messages framework as an intermediary evaluation tool for fruit and vegetable consumption in a nutrition education program. *Health Education & Behavior: The Official Publication of the Society for Public Health Education*, *43*(3), 321–327. https://doi.org/10.1177/1090198115599987

Drummond, D. K. (2005). Diabetes management: An exploration into the verbal support attempts of relational others. *Qualitative Research Reports in Communication*, *6*(1), 60–76. https://doi.org/10.1080/17459430500262216

Dunleavy, V. O., & Yang, Q. (2015). Memorable messages and newcomer socialization on campus: Messages about body image among student athletes, sorority members, and freshmen. *Communication Research Reports*, *32*(3), 225–238. https://doi.org/10.1080/08824096.2015.1052902

Fang, M. (2018). Trends in the prevalence of diabetes among U.S. adults: 1999-2016. *American Journal of Preventive Medicine*, *55*(4), 497–505. https://doi.org/10.1016/j.amepre.2018.05.018

Faul, F., Erdfelder, E., Buchner, A., & Lang, A. (2009). Statistical power analyses using G*Power 3.1: Tests for correlation and regression analyses. *Behavior Research Methods*, *41*(4), 1149–1160. https://doi.org/10.3758/BRM.41.4.1149

Ford, E. S., Mokdad, A. H., & Giles, W. H. (2012). Trends in waist circumference among U.S. adults. *Obesity*, *11*(10), 1223–1231. https://doi.org/10.1038/oby.2003.168

Gans, K. M., Risica, P. M., Kirtania, U., Jennings, A., Strolla, L. O., Steiner-Asiedu, M., Hardy, N., & Lasater, T. M. (2009). Dietary behaviors and portion sizes of black women who enrolled in SisterTalk and variation by demographic characteristics. *Journal of Nutrition Education and Behavior*, *41*(1), 32–40. https://doi.org/10.1016/j.jneb.2008.05.013

Guyll, M., Matthews, K. A., & Bromberger, J. T. (2001). Discrimination and unfair treatment: Relationship to cardiovascular reactivity among African American and European American women. *Health Psychology*, *20*(5), 315–325. https://doi.org/10.1037/0278-6133.20.5.315

Hales, C. M., Carroll, M. D., Fryar, C. D., & Ogden, C. L. (2020). *Prevalence of obesity and severe obesity among adults: United States, 2017-2018. NCHS data brief, no 360.* National Center for Health Statistics.

Hall, E. D., Ruth-McSwain, A., & Ferrara, M. (2016). Models of health: Exploring memorable messages received from parents about diet and exercise. *Journal of Communication in Healthcare*, *9*(4), 247–255. https://doi.org/10.1080/17538068.2016.1187892

Head, K. J., & Bute, J. J. (2018). The influence of everyday interpersonal communication on the medical encounter: An extension of Street's ecological model. *Health Communication*, *33*(6), 786–792. https://doi.org/10.1080/10410236.2017.1306474

Headen, I. E., Davis, E. M., Mujahid, M. S., & Abrams, B. (2012). Racial-ethnic differences in pregnancy-related weight. *Advances in Nutrition*, *3*(1), 83–94. https://doi.org/10.3945/an.111.000984

Himmelstein, M. S., Puhl, R. M., & Quinn, D. M. (2017). Intersectionality: An understudied framework for addressing weight stigma. *American Journal of Preventive Medicine*, *53*(4), 421–431. https://doi.org/10.1016/j.amepre.2017.04.003

Hiza, H. A., Casavale, K. O., Guenther, P. M., & Davis, C. A. (2013). Diet quality of Americans differs by age, sex, race/ethnicity, income, and education level. *Journal of the Academy of Nutrition and Dietetics*, *113*(2), 297–306. https://doi.org/10.1016/j.jand.2012.08.011

Hogue, J. V., & Mills, J. S. (2019). The effects of active social media engagement with peers on body image in young women. *Body Image*, *28*, 1–5. https://doi.org/10.1016/j.bodyim.2018.11.002

Howard, G., Cushman, M., Moy, C. S., Oparil, S., Muntner, P., Lackland, D. T., Manly, J. J., Flaherty, M. L., Judd, S. E., Wadley, V. G., Long, D. L., & Howard, V. J. (2018). Association of clinical and social factors with excess hypertension risk in Black compared with white US adults. *JAMA*, *320*(13), 1338–1348. https://doi.org/10.1001/jama.2018.13467

Imamura, F., Micha, R., Khatibzadeh, S., Fahimi, S., Shi, P., Powles, J., & Mozaffarian, D., & Global Burden of Diseases Nutrition and Chronic Diseases Expert Group (NutriCoDE). (2015). Dietary quality among men and women in 187 countries in 1990 and 2010: A systematic assessment. *The Lancet: Global Health*, *3*(3), e132–e142. https://doi.org/10.1016/S2214-109X(14)70381-X

Jerald, M. C., Ward, L. M., Moss, L., Thomas, K., & Fletcher, K. D. (2017). Subordinates, sex objects, or sapphires? Investigating contributions of media use to Black students' femininity ideologies and stereotypes about Black women. *Journal of Black Psychology*, *43*(6), 608–635. https://doi.org/10.1177/0095798416665967

Johnson, A. L., Orbe, M. P., & Cooke-Jackson, A. (2014). "Let's talk about sex": Exploring HBCU student memorable message narratives. *Howard Journal of Communications*, *25*(3), 303–323. https://doi.org/10.1080/10646175.2014.925309

Katzmarzyk, P. T., Bray, G. A., Greenway, F. L., Johnson, W. D., Newton, R. L., Jr, Ravussin, E., Ryan, D. H., & Bouchard, C. (2011). Ethnic-specific BMI and Waist Circumference Thresholds. *Obesity. 19*(6), 1272–1278. https://doi.org/10.1038/oby.2010.319

Kelly, N. R., Cotter, E. W., & Mazzeo, S. E. (2012). Eating Disorder Examination Questionnaire (EDE-Q): Norms for black women. *Eating Behaviors*, *13*(4), 429–432. https://doi.org/10.1016/j.eatbeh.2012.09.001

King, D. W., Duello, T. M., Miranda, P. Y., Hodges, K. P., Shelton, A. J., Chukelu, P., & Jones, L. A. (2010). Strategies for recruitment of healthy premenopausal women into the African American Nutrition for Life (A NULIFE) Study. *Journal of Women's Health*, *19*(5), 855–862. https://doi.org/10.1089/jwh.2009.1682

Kino, S., & Kawachi, I. (2020). How much do preventive health behaviors explain education- and income-related inequalities in health? Results of Oaxaca-Blinder decomposition analysis. *Annals of Epidemiology*, *43*, 44–50. https://doi.org/10.1016/j.annepidem.2020.01.008

Knapp, M. L., Stohl, C., & Reardon, K. K. (1981). "Memorable" messages. *Journal of Communication*, *31*(4), 27–41. https://doi.org/10.1111/j.1460-2466.1981.tb00448.x

Lambert, C. A. (2012). Memorable health messages embrace student perspectives. *Public Relations Journal*, *6*(5), 1–23. https://prjournal.instituteforpr.org/wp-content/uploads/2012Lambert.pdf

Lauckner, C., Smith, S., Kotowski, M., Nazione, S., Stohl, C., Prestin, A., So, J., & Nabi, R. (2012). An initial investigation into naturally occurring loss- and gain-framed memorable breast cancer messages. *Communication Quarterly*, *60*(1), 1–16. https://doi.org/10.1080/01463373.2012.642269

López-Guimerà, G., Levine, M., Sánchez-Carracedo, D., & Fauquet, J. (2010). Influence of mass media on body image and eating disordered attitudes and behaviors in females: A review of effects and processes. *Media Psychology*, *13*(4), 387–416. https://doi.org/10.1080/15213269.2010.525737

Lynch, E. B., & Kane, J. (2014). Body size perception among African American women. *Journal of Nutrition Education and Behavior*, *46*(5), 412–417. https://doi.org/10.1016/j.jneb.2014.03.002

Masters, R. K., Reither, E. N., Powers, D. A., Yang, Y. C., Burger, A. E., & Link, B. G. (2013). The impact of obesity on US mortality levels: The importance of age and cohort factors in population estimates. *American Journal of Public Health*, *103*(10), 1895–1901. https://doi.org/10.2105/AJPH.2013.301379

Michie, S., Abraham, C., Whittington, C., McAteer, J., & Gupta, S. (2009). Effective techniques in healthy eating and physical activity interventions: A metaregression. *Health Psychology*, *28*(6), 690–701. https://doi.org/10.1037/a0016136

Miczo, N., Danhour, E., Lester, K. E., & Bryant, J. (2013). Memorable Messages and the H1N1 Flu Virus. *Western Journal of Communication. 77*(5), 625–644. https://doi.org/10.1080/10570314.2013.776099

Mogre, V., Abanga, Z. O., Tzelepis, F., Johnson, N. A., & Paul, C. (2017). Adherence to and factors associated with self-care behaviours in type 2 diabetes patients in Ghana. *BMC Endocrine Disorders*, *17*(1), 20. https://doi.org/10.1186/s12902-017-0169-3

National Center for Health Statistics (2019). *NCHS nutrition data [fact sheet]*. https://www.cdc.gov/nchs/about/factsheets/factsheet_nutrition.htm

Nazione, S., Laplante, C., Smith, S. W., Cornacchione, J., Russell, J., & Stohl, C. (2011). Memorable messages for navigating college life. *Journal of Applied Communication Research*, *39*(2), 123–143. https://doi.org/10.1080/00909882.2011.556138

Ndiaye, K., Silk, K. J., Anderson, J., Horstman, H. K., Carpenter, A., Hurley, A., & Proulx, J. (2013). Using an ecological framework to understand parent-child communication about nutritional decision-making and behavior. *Journal of Applied Communication Research*, *41*(3), 253–274. https://doi.org/10.1080/00909882.2013.792434

Overstreet, N. M., Quinn, D. M., & Agocha, V. B. (2010). Beyond thinness: The influence of a curvaceous body ideal on body dissatisfaction in Black and white women. *Sex Roles*, *63*(1–2), 91–103. https://doi.org/10.1007/s11199-010-9792-4

Powers, W. T. (1973a). *Behavior: The control of perception*. Aldine.

Powers, W. T. (1973b). Feedback: Beyond behaviorism. *Science, 179* (4071), 351–356. https://doi.org/10.1126/science.179.4071.351

Rahman, M., & Berenson, A. B. (2010). Accuracy of current body mass index obesity classification for white, Black and Hispanic reproductive-age women. *Obstetrics and Gynecology, 115*(5), 982–988. https://doi.org/10.1097/AOG.0b013e3181da9423

Reno, J. E., & McNamee, L. G. (2014). Do sororities promote members' health? A study of memorable messages regarding weight and appearance. *Health Communication, 30*(4), 385–397. https://doi.org/10.1080/10410236.2013.863702

Rubinsky, V., Hosek, A. M., & Hudak, N. (2019). "It's better to be depressed skinny than happy fat": College women's memorable body messages and their impact on body image, self-esteem, and rape myth acceptance. *Health Communication, 34*(13), 1555–1563. https://doi.org/10.1080/10410236.2018.1504659

Russell, J., & Smith, S. W. (2017). An examination of weight-associated memorable messages, sources, and outcomes. *Atlantic Journal of Communication, 25*(5), 263–279. https://doi.org/10.1080/15456870.2017.1377045

Sanderson, S., Lupinski, K., & Moch, P. (2013). Is big really beautiful? Understanding body image perceptions of African American females. *Journal of Black Studies, 44*(5), 496–507. https://doi.org/10.1177/0021934713497059

Schroeder, S. A. (2007). Shattuck Lecture. We can do better–improving the health of the American people. *New England Journal of Medicine, 357*(12), 1221-1228. https://doi.org/10.1056/NEJMsa073350

Sharp, T. A., Bell, M. L., Grunwald, G. K., Schmitz, K. H., Sidney, S., Lewis, C. E., Tolan, K., & Hill, J. O. (2002). Differences in resting metabolic rate between white and African American young adults. *Obesity Research, 10*(8), 726–732. https://doi.org/10.1038/oby.2002.99

Sheehy, S., Palmer, J. R., & Rosenberg, L. (2020). Leisure time physical activity in relation to mortality among African American women. *American Journal of Preventive Medicine, 59*(5), 704–713. https://doi.org/10.1016/j.amepre.2020.05.013

Shook, R. P., Hand, G. A., Wang, X., Paluch, A. E., Moran, R., Hébert, J. R., Swift, D. L., Lavie, C. J., & Blair, S. N. (2014). Low fitness partially explains resting metabolic rate differences between African American and white women. *The American Journal of Medicine, 127*(5), 436–442. https://doi.org/10.1016/j.amjmed.2014.02.003

Smith, M. L., Telford, E., & Tree, J. J. (2019). Body image and sexual orientation: The experiences of lesbian and bisexual women. *Journal of Health Psychology, 24*(9), 1178–1190. https://doi.org/10.1177/1359105317694486

Smith, S. W., & Ellis, J. B. (2001). Memorable messages as guides to self-assessment of behavior: An initial investigation. *Communication Monographs, 68*(2), 154–168. https://doi.org/10.1080/03637750128058

Smith, S. W., Hamel, L. M., Kotowski, M. R., Nazione, S., LaPlante, C., Atkin, C. K., Stohl, C., & Skubisz, C. (2011). Action tendency emotions evoked by memorable breast cancer messages and their association with prevention and detection behaviors. *Health Communication, 25* (8), 737–746. https://doi.org/10.1080/10410236.2010.521916

Smith, S. W., Nazione, S., Laplante, C., Kotowski, M. R., Atkin, C., Skubisz, C. M., & Stohl, C. (2009). Topics and sources of memorable breast cancer messages and their impact on prevention and detection behaviors. *Journal of Health Communication, 14*(3), 293–307. https://doi.org/10.1080/10810730902805903

Strings, S. (2019). *Fearing the black body: The racial origins of fat phobia*. New York University Press.

Thompson, C. M., & Zaitchik, S. T. (2012). Struggling with the freshman fifteen: College students' recollections of parents' memorable messages about weight. *Kaleidoscope, 11*, 39–58. https://opensiuc.lib.siu.edu/kaleidoscope/vol11/iss1/4

Toobert, D. J., Hampson, S. E., & Glasgow, R. E. (2000). The summary of diabetes self-care activities measure: Results from 7 studies and a revised scale. *Diabetes Care, 23*(7), 943–950. https://doi.org/10.2337/diacare.23.7.943

U.S. Department of Agriculture and U.S. Department of Health and Human Services. (2020, December). *Dietary guidelines for Americans, 2020-2025, 9th Edition*. DietaryGuidelines.gov.

U.S. Department of Health and Human Services. (2018). *Physical activity guidelines for Americans* (*2nd* ed.).

Vaughn, W., Baruth, M., Beets, M. W., Durstine, J. L., Liu, J., & Blair, S. N. (2014). Fitness vs. fatness on all-cause mortality: A meta-analysis. *Progress in Cardiovascular Disease, 56*(4), 382–390. https://doi.org/10.1016/j.pcad.2013.09.002

Warren, T. Y., Wilcox, S., Dowda, M., & Baruth, M. (2012). Independent association of waist circumference with hypertension and diabetes in African American women, South Carolina, 2007–2009. *Preventing Chronic Disease, 9*, E105. https://doi.org/10.5888/pcd9.110170

Watson, L. B., Lewis, J. A., & Moody, T. (2019). A sociocultural examination of body image among Black women. *Body Image, 31*, 280–287. https://doi.org/10.1016/j.bodyim.2019.03.008

Webb, F. J., Khubchandani, J., Doldren, M., Balls-Berry, J., Blanchard, S., Hannah, L., Stanford, J., & Webster-Bass, S. (2014). African-American womens' eating habits and intention to change: A pilot study. *Journal of Racial and Ethnic Health Disparities, 1*, 199–206. https://doi.org/10.1007/s40615-014-0026-2

White, S. (2020). *Basic and clinical biostatistics* (5th ed.). McGraw-Hill Education.

Williams, W. M., Yore, M. M., & Whitt-Glover, M. C. (2018). Estimating physical activity trends among blacks in the United States through examination of four national surveys. *AIMS Public Health, 5*(2), 144–157. https://doi.org/10.3934/publichealth.2018.2.144

Count Me Out: Perceptions of Black Patients Who are on Dialysis but Who are Not on a Transplant Waitlist

Charles R. Senteio and Matthew K. Ackerman

ABSTRACT

End-stage renal disease (ESRD) is characterized by racial inequity; Blacks are 3 times more likely to develop ESRD than Whites. Transplant is the preferred treatment option since transplanted patients experience better clinical outcomes. Racial inequities persist at each of the steps required for transplantation. Despite the vast literature describing these racial inequities, it does not include dialysis patients' awareness and understanding of treatment options, specifically for transplant. To address this gap, we purposely sampled Blacks in Detroit who were receiving dialysis and who were not active on any transplant waitlist to investigate their understanding and perceptions of transplants. We used uncertainty management theory (UMT) to better understand perceived barriers to getting and remaining on a transplant waitlist. We aimed to address a critical gap in the literature to inform approaches addressing this enduring inequity. For this qualitative study, we conducted individual, semi-structured interviews with 24 Black ESRD patients, aged 34–73 years: 9 male and 15 female. Participants shared their experiences of being on dialysis, perceptions, and understanding of transplants. We describe two key findings: 1) uncertainty for these patients is prevalent and multi-layered and 2) social support can both dissuade an individual from pursuing transplant (i.e., reluctance to ask family members to be donors) and it can result in decreasing uncertainty (e.g., participants wanting to pursue transplant to be with family). We highlight the specific need to improve patient education regarding treatment options and enhancing how relevant health information can be communicated.

Chronic kidney disease (CKD) is a prevalent condition in which the kidneys are damaged and cannot appropriately filter excess fluid and waste from the body; 37 million people, approximately 15% of the U.S. adult population, may have varying degrees of CKD, and one of three adults with diabetes and one in five adults with hypertension have CKD (Centers for Disease Control and Prevention [CDC], 2019). End-stage renal disease (ESRD), CKD that has progressed to a low level of kidney function and is being treated with dialysis or kidney transplant, is characterized by striking racial disparities. Blacks are three times more likely to develop ESRD than Whites and one-third of all ESRD patients are Black (CDC, 2019; Patzer et al., 2019). These racial disparities are driven by social factors (e.g., socioeconomic disparities), biological factors (e.g., higher prevalence of hypertension and diabetes in minority populations), and genetic factors (Crews et al., 2019).

In addition to racial disparities in ESRD prevalence, disparities are also observed in the transplant treatment option. Early stage CKD may be asymptomatic, though once detected, can be treated with dietary and other health behavioral changes to stave off disease progression. But CKD patients who develop ESRD need either renal replacement therapy (RRT), or a kidney transplant to survive. There are 500,000 individuals in the U.S. who are receiving renal replacement therapy (RRT), and the vast majority (90%) receive hemodialysis, a dialysis done multiple times a week at a dialysis center, versus peritoneal dialysis (10%), a dialysis done every day without the aid of a dialysis center (Jagdale et al., 2019). Transplant is the preferred treatment regimen over RRT when the patient is within specific clinical and psychosocial criteria because transplant patients experience better clinical outcomes, have a longer life expectancy, report higher quality of life, and incur a lower cost of care to the healthcare system (Axelrod et al., 2018). Despite these differences in both human and financial outcomes, there are only approximately 90,000 patients on waitlists for kidney transplantation, or less than 20% of all individuals receiving RRT (Kilambi et al., 2019). Consequently, a small proportion (3.0%) of ESRD patients receive a transplant (United States Renal Data System [USRDS], 2019). Racial disparities also characterize the proportions of ESRD patients who receive a transplant. Only 1.0% of Black ESRD patients receive a transplant, compared to 3.2% of White ESRD patients (Morgan, 2006). The percentage of Black ESRD patients who receive a transplant is lower than any other racial/ethnic group: Native Hawaiian or Pacific Islander (1.2%), Hispanic (1.8%), American Indian or Alaska Native (3.6%), and Asian (6.6%) (USRDS, 2019).

Transplant eligibility

Transplant eligibility is predicated on the patient indicating their desire to pursue a transplant. If the patient does not have a living donor, they can be evaluated for placement on a waitlist (Purnell et al., 2018). There are five steps to being placed on a waitlist; they include: (Step 1) patient expresses interest to receive a transplant to clinicians at their dialysis center (e.g., social worker, nephrologist), (Step 2) patient gets a referral from dialysis facility for evaluation, (Step 3) start evaluation, (Step 4) complete evaluation, and (Step 5) placed on and remain on a waitlist (Traino et al., 2015).

Completing the steps for transplant evaluation requires that the patient attend multiple clinical appointments for medical and psychosocial evaluations to assess and confirm that the patient does not have various other disqualifying health conditions (e.g., cardiovascular disease, active cancer, and obesity) nor psychosocial contraindications as determined by various members of the care team. This evaluation process can take over a year to complete and it must be performed periodically in order to remain on a waitlist (Kazley et al., 2012).

Also, a patient may remain on a waitlist but have inactive status (i.e., "status 7"). In 2003 the Organ Procurement and Transplantation Network (OPTN) policy was amended to enable kidney transplant candidates to accumulate time on the waitlist with inactive status. This waitlist status is used as a placeholder for patients who may not be eligible for transplant due to provisional reasons (e.g., incomplete transplant workup, beyond body mass index (BMI) threshold) (Grams et al., 2013). This status assumes that the transplant candidate will eventually move from inactive to active status. Approximately 30% of all patients on the OPTN waitlist are listed as inactive (Talamantes et al., 2017).

Racial disparities have been detailed at each step of the process to be placed on a waitlist. Black ESRD patients experience barriers at the patient, provider, and system level. For instance, Black patients are less likely to have access to transplant information and they are less likely to complete the transplant evaluation (Patzer et al., 2019). . However, the perceptions of Black ESRD patients concerning the waitlist have not been described. Understanding patient perspectives would enable improving access to information which would help patients make more informed treatment decisions.

Theoretical framework

Various theories and frameworks describe the perceptions of individuals who may be contemplating transplantation. Uncertainty Management and Social Support are appropriate frameworks for understanding Black patients' perspectives of the transplantation process.

Uncertainty management

A considerable level of uncertainty is deeply rooted in the ESRD treatment experience, especially for patients who may be eligible for transplantation. Uncertainty management theory has been used to both explain patient perspectives at the various stages in the transplantation process and to describe the steps individuals may take to manage uncertainty (Brashers, 2007; Scott et al., 2011).

Uncertainty is multi-layered, interconnected, and temporal (Brashers, 2001). And varying levels of uncertainty can result in conflicting emotions and motivations. The layers can include the self (e.g., individual may not want to undergo another operation/procedure), others (e.g., individual may perceive that they will not be treated fairly by clinical staff), social and/or familial relationships (e.g., individual may not want to receive a kidney from a family member), or other contextual factors (e.g., individual may be unsure of requirements of them in the process of getting a transplant). Uncertainties can also be interconnected. They may involve one topic (e.g., perceptions of clinical factors, like age, which determine eligibility) which can be connected to another (e.g., the likelihood of languishing on a waitlist). Last, uncertainties can be fleeting (e.g., on certain days an individual may not want to put themselves through another operation) or more sustained (e.g., an individual may be consistent in their preference to continue with the dialysis treatment option) because dimensions of uncertainty can change over time (Scott et al., 2011).

Individuals may reduce uncertainty by seeking health information. They may seek information directly from members of the healthcare team (e.g., dialysis nurses, social workers) (Bonner & Lloyd, 2012), from other individuals in similar clinical circumstances (e.g., dialysis peer mentoring/support) (Veinot, 2010; Zheng et al., 2010), or via others' behaviors or actions (e.g., seeking online information) (Costello & Murillo, 2014). Information seeking behavior, which includes avoiding information, can be influenced by the objectives of the individual, and their family, friends, or extended network which may include peer mentors who are also receiving dialysis. These objectives may not be consistent across these groups. For example, an individual may not be certain that they want to receive a transplant, but a family member may be convinced that they should (Brashers et al., 2002).

Social support

In a health context, social support is vital to an individual's ability to manage the stress of both physical and mental illnesses. Social support is defined as the network of personal ties that provide aid, also referred to as "emotional caring," which enable the individual (patient) to enhance or establish personal agency; there are four types 1) emotional support (e.g., esteem, affect, trust), 2) appraisal support (e.g., affirmation, positive feedback), 3) providing health information (e.g., advice, suggestions), and 4) instrumental support (e.g., financial support, time, caregiving) (Albrecht & Adelman, 1984). Social support can be provided through both face-to-face and indirect modalities (e.g., technology/computer) (Robinson & Tian, 2009).

Despite extensive research describing the racial and other demographic characteristics of ESRD patients who do not progress to transplantation, little is known of Black patients' perception of barriers, or other factors which may influence them not being placed on, or remain on, a waitlist (Crews et al., 2019; Patzer et al., 2019). Further, the literature does not describe the perceptions of Black ESRD patients, who happen to experience inequity at each stage of the transplant process. In fact, investigations of perceptions of dialysis staff concerning these persistent racial inequities have detailed low socioeconomic status as a primary driver, as staff perceive that Black patients are unable to develop a feasible financial plan to cover pre- and post-transplant costs. Dialysis staff also believe that Black patients do not pursue the transplant treatment option in order to keep disability income (Lipford et al., 2018). Staff perceptions are vital because clinical practices commonly rely on clinical staff to initiate referral to determine transplant eligibility (Step 2) (Yuan et al., 2012). Although previous studies have examined ESRD patients' experiences of being on a waitlist (Tong et al., 2015), no investigations have examined the perceptions of Black patients, specifically those who are on dialysis but who are not active on a waitlist. Given persistent racial disparities at each stage of the transplant referral and evaluation process, it is vital to understand Black patients' perceptions of the transplantation process and transplant waitlists.

Study hypotheses and research question

To address this gap in the literature we designed and completed an investigation to understand Black ESRD patients' perceptions of transplant waitlists. We posited that their perceptions would be characterized by high levels of uncertainty. We also posited that social support, across the four types, may affect their perceptions of transplantation.

A fuller understanding of Black ESRD patients' awareness and opinions will enable healthcare teams and equity researchers to design interventions to help address a persistent racial inequity that drives both human and financial costs. Thus, our primary research question is: what are the perceptions of transplantation of Black ESRD patients' who are on dialysis but not on a waitlist?

Materials and methods

Overall study design

Semi-structured interviews were used to investigate dialysis patients' perspectives and understandings of ESRD treatment options, transplants, and transplant waitlists. Purposive sampling was conducted in collaboration with the National Kidney Foundation (NKF) of Michigan who provided us with contacts to help to recruit Blacks in the Detroit area who were receiving dialysis. We purposely sampled in Detroit because according to the 2010 U.S. Census, it has the highest percentage of Black residents of any major city in the U.S. (82.7%) and has one of the largest number of Black residents (670,226). The Michigan State University Institutional Review Board approved the study protocol on February 11, 2016 (IRB# x16-133e). The study protocol included participant informed consent forms which were reviewed with each participant, who signed and dated the forms.

Inclusion criteria

Eligibility included self-identifying as Black or African American. Also, the participant could not be active on any transplant waitlist, but they may be inactive on a waitlist (status 7 or "on hold") (Grams et al., 2013). Participants may have had a prior transplant; however, they must be receiving dialysis at the time of the interview.

Data collection process and instruments

The first author conducted each of the individual, in-person interviews, from March 4th through April 20th, 2016. All interviews were conducted in the participant's home except for two, which were conducted in public locations of the participant's choosing, one in a restaurant and the other in a coffee shop. Each participant was compensated 50 USD for their time. The interview guide included open-ended, main questions based on our hypotheses and research questions and follow-up probes. Participants were asked to share their experiences of being on dialysis, perceptions, and understanding of kidney transplants, and, for some, experiences with previous transplants and reasons why the graft failed. The semi-structured interview format remained consistent; however, insights gleaned from the initial interviews helped guide probes in subsequent interviews. Each interview was digitally recorded, and the audio recordings of the interviews were transcribed verbatim. Interviews lasted an average of approximately one hour for a total 24 hours and 47 minutes. To maintain anonymity, all identifying information was removed from each of the transcripts.

Data analysis

The grounded theory approach was used to code, summarize, and condense the data. This approach is well-suited for the analysis of the interview data because it is conducive to understanding phenomena which is not well-described in the literature – Black dialysis patients' perceptions of transplants, and their understanding of waitlists (Creswell, 2006). The constant comparative method was used to analyze the interview data (Glaser, 1965). NVivo software (Version 12.0) was used to code the transcripts. Coding is a cyclical process, enabling the refinement and highlighting of patterns to generate categories and concepts. Line-by-line coding in the initial coding phase was completed, using in vivo codes to capture the participant meanings (Glaser, 1978). In the second coding cycle, axial coding was used to define conditions and actions (Corbin & Strauss, 2007). Consistent with grounded theory, in this second cycle, categories were developed for the first cycle codes, an approach well-suited to apply meaning to the data (Miles et al., 2014; Saldaña, 2009). Initial codes were analyzed to develop preliminary themes which were reviewed iteratively and discussed among the two authors, then they were refined by referring to the transcript data.

Results

All 24 participants except one received dialysis treatments at the same dialysis center in Detroit which is part of a large healthcare system. The other participant received dialysis at a center about 3 miles away from where the other participants received dialysis, which is part of a large, private series of dialysis centers. (See Table 1)

Participants range in age from 37– 71, 9 are male and 15 are female, all are Black and all have spent most of their lives in Detroit. All have received dialysis for more than three years, and three had already had a transplant, from a live donor who was a family member. They were receiving dialysis due to

Table 1. Participant demographics (n = 24).

Characteristics		
Median age (years)		55
18–34	8%	2 Participants
35–49	25%	6 Participants
50–64	46%	11 Participants
>65	21%	5 Participants
Sex		
Male	37.5%	9 Males
Female	62.5%	15 Females
Referred to dialysis by		
Emergency Department	58%	14 Participants
Clinic/Ambulatory Care		10 Participants
Previous kidney transplant	13%	3 Participants
Comorbidity		
Hypertension	92%	22 Participants
Diabetes	54%	13 Participants
3 or more comorbidities	46%	11 Participants
Kidney transplant waitlist[a]		
On a waitlist, inactive ("on hold")		
Wants to receive a kidney	37.5%	9 Participants
May not want a kidney	12.5%	3 Participants
Not on a waitlist		
Wants to be on a waitlist	37.5%	9 Participants
Does not want to be on a waitlist	12.5%	3 Participants

Categories listed are based on self-reporting by participants and were not verified by the transplant team as to whether the participant was on a waitlist, inactive on a waitlist, or off of a waitlist.

failure of the graft, which they indicated was due to their medication behavior which was inconsistent with clinical recommendations. Twenty-two participants indicate that they were living with hypertension and 13 participants indicate that they have been diagnosed with diabetes. Fourteen participants were referred to dialysis from the Emergency Room, while 10 were referred from a clinic or ambulatory care facility. Twelve participants are on a waitlist but are inactive ("on hold"), and 3 of the 12 were unsure if they would even accept a kidney at this point if they were transferred to active status. Participants refer to inactive status on the waitlist as "on hold." No participants referred to this status as "inactive." Participants understand being "on hold" to mean that they do not meet the necessary criteria for transplant, but they can remain on a waitlist.

There are two overall findings. First, Black ESRD patients' perspectives on transplantation and waitlists are characterized by high levels of uncertainty. Second, social support is a factor in these perceptions.

Uncertainty is prevalent

Uncertainty was prevalent among participants and sources of uncertainty were multi-layered, interconnected, and temporal. Participants expressed uncertainty regarding their current circumstances and about a future which may include a waitlist and/or transplant. Uncertainty about the self was reflected in lacking information about treatment options and the dismay that resulted in hearing the diagnosis. Some participants also perceived that their prognosis was better remaining on dialysis, rather than receiving a transplant.

Uncertainty at the layer of the self

Lack of information about waitlists and transplant option – I didn't even know. Information barriers to kidney transplant stem from a lack of information, incomplete information, or misconceptions concerning the assessment and transplant process. For example, P14 indicated that he was receiving dialysis for five years before ever being approached by dialysis center staff to inform him of the transplant option. He indicated his reaction when the social worker shared information with him about the transplant process, "I didn't even know that you had to go up and talk to the people and meet with the transplant team and stuff. I thought it was all automatic. I asked her 'why am I not on the list?.'" Another participant shared her experience with not knowing that the patient must initiate the evaluation process to be placed on a waitlist, "I thought that you just get on the list. They find your kidney and that was it. But it's more than that. No one actually told me I was supposed to go there [to the transplant team]." (P15) Several participants reported similar anecdotes in describing how they learned that the patient must indicate interest in a transplant to initiate the evaluation process. One participant expressed specifically that the onus was on the patient to be informed about the transplant process, "you gotta look into it. You gotta do some research yourself." (P02)

In addition to the waitlists, participants shared how other treatment-related information was conveyed to them, and what it feels like to receive information this way. P11 conveyed that dialysis patients are not informed appropriately:

> [We need] something more than just them giving you a pamphlet, a bunch of material to read. There should be more classrooms, more group discussions, with people that are going through similar situations. Instead of just one-on-one, with a doctor and a bunch of nurses at a table sitting there just telling you that you need to do this, you need to do that, you got to do this, you got to do that, you're beating down on a person that has no understanding of what's going on. (P11)

As P11 alluded to, other participants expressed frustration with how vital information was communicated concerning recommended health behavior. P16 expressed frustration with the information provided by the nutritionist. Despite the nutritionist being present at his dialysis treatments, the information provided did not address his information needs, which centered on how to lose weight, "[the nutritionist] mostly tries to tell us what not to eat, for our kidneys . . . every day she's there, but it's not about weight loss. It's more about learning how to eat [while receiving dialysis], what foods you are not supposed to have."

Many participants attended group sessions to learn more about transplants and dialysis, specifically the RISE program sponsored by the NKF. P13 stated:

> The RISE program is what saved me. Before that, they wasn't telling me anything about none of my lab work or nothing. They weren't telling me the results or none of that, they were just doing it, and I didn't know what to ask them and stuff, but when I came back from the first RISE [information session] I asked him [dialysis technician] myself, 'what's my blood level? What's my creatine at this time? Where you getting all this stuff from?' So they started printing out monthly lab work and gave it to me.

Several participants were quite complimentary of the RISE program:

> If people were on dialysis Monday, Wednesday, and Friday, they would schedule a two-week program that would be held on Tuesdays and Thursdays. We would go in, sit and talk to the people

> about what the kidney was all about . . . they had people come in to do presentations. They were educating us. Not just about a transplant but how to take care of yourself, the things that you were eligible for, how you could help yourself so that you would know what was going on with the body. They talked to you about nutrition, they talked to you about what you are eligible for with social security or SSI. And it was a very educational program because a lot of people, including myself, had no knowledge of exactly what end-stage renal [disease] was about, even though we were on dialysis. (P10)

Despite several participants stating how informative the RISE program was, participants expressed regret that the RISE program no longer exists, "From what I can understand, the Kidney Foundation no longer has the money to sponsor that program." (P10)

Shock upon hearing diagnosis and uncertain about future – I was kinda devastated. Several participants indicated that they were diagnosed with ESRD and told they would need to receive dialysis at the hospital during an emergency room visit. While these participants had heard of "kidney failure" and "dialysis," they were shocked upon learning of the diagnosis because they did not recall a blood test, urine test, or imaging test to assess their kidney function. Many did not recall being informed of the transplant treatment option. Others were unsure how to assess if a transplant waitlist was right for them. Being told that their kidneys had "failed" was overwhelming, in part because of *how* they were told, and they had trouble interpreting what this meant for them:

> It was a shock to me because I thought it was something else, but the way they actually described it to me, he [ER physician] said "you got stage four kidney failure," then they [ER physician and others who may have been residents] walked out the room. They didn't tell me what dialysis was or nothing. They just walked out of the room. (P14)

Another participant described what he felt when he was told during an emergency room visit that his kidneys had "failed." He recounted, "Well, initially, I was like . . . I just kind of said, 'This was my heritage.' That was my initial perception of it. Then, I had to kind of wrap my mind around, 'Is this thing gonna be fatal or not?'" (P10) A participant who received his diagnosis during an emergency room visit and subsequent hospital admission shared:

> I cried a little bit, and I called my mother I told her, and I tried to see if she knew anything about it. She really didn't know nothing about it, because ain't nobody in our family ever been on dialysis . . . I guess I cried 'cause I didn't understand what was going on, really. And I didn't know what dialysis was. I don't know [why the physician did not explain it to me]. I think he was making his rounds so he was kinda . . . trying to get everybody taken care of. But I feel that he could have gave me a little more information. (P14)

Another participant described the emotion he felt. Although he received the ESRD diagnosis during a physician office visit, the jolt was evident, "well, I was shocked, 'cause I didn't really notice anything wrong at that particular time. You just say, 'Hey, what me? How could that happen to me?'" (P03) Similarly, P08 described her experience, "I had no acceptance at the beginning, it was devastating to me you know. I was working, I was taking care of my children, and it was a critical moment for me to have to adjust my life."

Some participants also described the shock they felt when they first began receiving dialysis. One participant described her feelings when she first started dialysis, which happened to be in the same hospital where she had received her treatments for breast cancer:

> When I first went to dialysis it was kind of scary, the machines . . . hooking you up to the machine and stuff. And it just . . . I don't know. I never knew . . . as many times I had been to the hospital, I never knew dialysis was in there. I never thought about dialysis. I didn't know what dialysis was. (P17)

For one participant, simply walking into the dialysis center was overwhelming for her:

> I was kinda devastated because I didn't really know what dialysis entailed . . . when I walked into that place, I was in shock. I just stood in the middle of the clinic and just looked because I had never seen that many machines and that many people hooked up to machines. (P23)

Participants described that simply being aware of transplant information was not enough for them to make a final decision. The decision to be placed on a waitlist is significant requiring deliberation and consideration. One participant (P03) described his reaction to being told by clinicians that he should consider the waitlist, "I didn't tell them no. I just said, 'I don't think I'm ready yet.' They said, 'well ok, just keep up the good work and get yourself stabilized and we'll talk again.'" This deliberation was also associated with the decision to receive a kidney, even when a family member has agreed to donate. One participant (P14) described how his brother was willing to donate a kidney to him and his brother wanted to go through the necessary steps to be assessed, but P14 needed more time to consider the magnitude of this decision. He explained:

> I was kinda mad at first . . . because I wasn't actually ready for it, because they tell you, "you can get a kidney, a transplant, a organ from a family member." But a lot of people, they will have second thoughts about it, because your body can reject it . . . and they can't put it back in that person [donor]. So you just got an organ for nothing. And then like a situation might come up like they end up with stage four kidney failure . . . then they'd need a kidney. (P14)

Despite the crushing realization upon the ESRD diagnosis and that they would need to receive dialysis, some participants were interested in transplant. And after learning about the waitlists they managed their uncertainty by reflecting on their circumstances and expressed confidence in their ability to meet the stipulations to get on, and stay on, a waitlist. P03 described how his motivation and control over his dietary behavior ultimately determined his status on the waitlist, "it's all up to me. If you wanna do it, you do the right thing. If you don't, you won't do the right thing." P03 also described he was taken off of a waitlist previously due to his own dietary choices, "I took one drink out of that Pepsi and the next thing you know. I was hooked again."

Kidney function will be restored – It can come back. Some participants believe that their kidney function may be restored. They indicated that they understand that kidney function can return after starting dialysis, "they told me there was a 50% chance my kidneys can start back working." (P21) For some participants, the chance of their kidney function returning was sufficient to dissuade them from seeking a transplant. P21 also shared that he was still producing urine while on dialysis which indicated to him that his kidney function may return, "I really don't wanna take that chance of trying to get a kidney that might kill me when they're saying there's a good chance that it [kidney function] can come back." Even after speaking with a social worker, P21 expressed reluctance. The social worker asked her if she would accept a kidney if one was ready for her and P21 said, "I'm not sure . . . I don't know how to deal with that."

Survival chances better on dialysis – I see more people living than dying. Participants observed the difficulties of others in receiving a transplant or in persisting on a waitlist, so they simply believe that their chances of survival are better on dialysis. "I've heard people say they've been on dialysis for 18 years . . . They give me the courage to go forward. Because I see more people living than I see dying." (P23) This also illustrates how uncertainty at the layer of the self can be interconnected as the uncertainty is associated with information gathered from others who have been on dialysis.

Uncertainty at the layer of others

Mistrust due to racism – We don't trust the doctors and the nurses because of racism. Participants also reported that, as Black people, they did not trust institutions (e.g., hospitals, insurance companies) or individuals (e.g., doctors, nurses, social workers) who may have a role in their care. One participant elaborated on her frustration with how she was told about the transplant option, but she was not able to take advantage of it. This resulted in her questioning health care providers' motivations:

> They told you you're sick, and your kidneys no longer work. Okay," why can't I get some new kidneys then?" That was my first question. They said, "eventually, but you're gonna have to deal with these other things first." I believe they wanna guinea pig on you for a little while. Because if they really wanted to put a kidney in you, then they could probably put one in you. (P02)

Another participant (P03) described how financial incentives are a source of his mistrust:

> I thought they were putting people on dialysis on purpose. They tell us, "your kidneys are bad. We gonna put you on dialysis. Hemodialysis." Well I never thought that my kidney was bad. I mean, I'm still urinating and everything. I never thought my ass was bad. But then every day I see new faces in there, and there's so many people on [dialysis]. I don't know how to [explain it] . . . The money. The money is the root of all evil, man. And they get so much money off of each dialysis patient. It ain't even funny. They charge you for that little piece of cotton and the tape that they put on your arm. Everything. If I require a Band-Aid, they write it down. I had a list one time. I usually just throw it on the dresser, but I come home one day, and I look at it, and itemized all that and it's like, about, maybe, eight, 10,000 USD a month for dialysis? The insurance. That's what the insurance get. Yeah, that's a lot of money. Almost better than the casino.

One participant expressed how mistrust dissuades her and other Blacks from organ donation:

> We (Black people) figure that if I agree to donate my heart or my liver or whatever, then if something happened to us and we went in a hospital, they would just take it, whether we gave them permission to do it or not. A lot of people believe that. They would just take it [kidney] without our permission. Let us die and give it [our kidney] to somebody else. (P17)

One participant (P24) expressed that mistrust kept them awake while receiving dialysis, "I'm not comfortable going to sleep at dialysis. I'm not comfortable because I fear that they're not gonna do what they're supposed to do." Another participant (P17) described how mistrust is common for Black people, "we [Black people] don't trust the system. That's what it is. We don't trust the doctors and the nurses and these people who are gonna be doing the surgery on us to remove a kidney." This participant described how racism from their past is the cause of current mistrust, "[When I was growing up] we [could only go to] the Black dentist. We didn't get the same health care [as Whites] simply because of racism."

How participants perceive that clinical staff treats them is vital given the regular contact with staff and the considerable demands of the dialysis regimen. Participants expressed discouragement when they perceived that staff was unwilling to support them. For example, P21 recounted a circumstance in which she attempted to reschedule an appointment and went to the dialysis clinical staff for help, "they'll have the head nurse up there who don't want to listen to the social worker, she wanna keep walking away while the social worker is trying to tell her [that I need to reschedule]." This participant continued with how witnessing the dialysis staff not coordinating her care appropriately made her feel, "and so, I feel like since you can't hear the important thing that's going on with me and why I can't make it here, at least I'm trying to reschedule the appointment, then why am I even gonna waste my time?" (P21) In some cases, participants would not pursue assessments for the transplant list and would avoid specific dialysis centers, because of how they were treated by dialysis staff. For example, during an assessment for a waitlist P01 described how he volunteered that he had a history of drug use, but he maintained that he was completely drug free at the time of the assessment, "it was like I became a second-class citizen after that . . . I just told them I wasn't interested in a transplant."

Some participants reported avoiding specific dialysis centers or hospitals and not signing up for transplant waitlists because of how they were treated by staff, "no, I don't want to go to [names dialysis center]. I did not like their attitude. If they like you, okay. If they don't care for you then you waitin' . . . it's like they pick and choose who gets [a kidney]." (P24) Also, P13 recalled when he believed he was going into surgery to receive a kidney, the transplant surgeon stopped the transplant because of his hypertension. He shared that his primary care physician had already documented that he had hypertension and told him that he was approved for a transplant. Because of the surgeon's decision, he had to go back through the entire evaluation process in order to return to the transplant waitlist. Afterward, he decided to discuss this with a social worker, "the social worker said 'well you probably need to talk to the surgeon if you want to.' I said, 'No, not really . . . No, I don't think I want to see her.'"

Several other participants similarly expressed perceptions that they were not listened to by clinicians before their ESRD diagnosis and that lead to a delay in a diagnosis. For example, before ESRD diagnosis P11 expressed how he had reduced his caloric intake to 400 calories per day, yet he was not losing weight. His physician would not listen when he expressed that his diet was not the issue:

> To me, it came off like she thought I was lying but then when I went on dialysis and the weight came off, I told her, "look, I told you it was something else." And she said, "well, you know it's hard to diagnose." I said, "well it's easy to listen." (P11)

One participant detailed her attempts to get a kidney screen before having to receive dialysis, which she attributed to not being listened to:

> I didn't have any insurance so they sent me to a free clinic. The free clinic lady was supposed to write me out referrals but she didn't do it. And I kept calling her but they told me I couldn't come up there, "you just can't walk in here to see her." And I said, "well, I don't wanna lose my kidney. I wanna get to the referral, so I could see what's going on with my kidney." When she finally did that, it was 3 months later . . . and she sent me to a pulmonary doctor. So I'm [saying to myself], "why are you sending me to the lung doctor? I wanna get to the kidney doctor." She said, "This is my job and I know what I'm doing." That's what she said. So I get to the lung doctor, now my kidney is completely ate up. She said, "you have no business being here. You need to be in the kidney department." (P22)

Uncertainty at the contextual layer

Achieving BMI thresholds – They want me to lose around 50 pounds. Meeting the Body Mass Index (BMI) threshold was the most commonly cited clinical barrier to eligibility for transplant. Eight participants stated that they were told to lose a specific number of pounds to be eligible for transplant. P14, who indicated that he is "on hold" (i.e., on a waitlist but inactive), recounted the discussion with the transplant team, "the doctor looked at the paper and stuff, and he said that by me being in the lower percentile [blood type and other stipulations], I could (sic) have gotten a kidney by now, but they want me to lose around 50 pounds first." Another participant indicated that she identified her cousin as a potential live donor. She confirmed that her cousin was a match, but he was not eligible to donate his kidney because of BMI, "he was too big to be a donor." (P09)

In addition to citing BMI as a barrier, participants explained the multiple reasons why meeting the BMI requirement was difficult for them. Access to exercise equipment can be difficult for those on fixed or low incomes. P16 explained her reaction to the fitness program which was recommended during a recent hospital stay, "I'm on a fixed income. I [did not have] the 200 USD [plus] to pay for [a health club membership]." Furthermore, participants who had access to the recommended physical activity described feeling too tired after dialysis to engage in the physical activity recommended to reduce their BMI. P11 described how he felt after beginning dialysis, "I'm too tired to do anything . . . I couldn't bowl anymore, I couldn't play basketball, no contact sports, no football. I would go swimming but I kept getting pneumonia."

Challenges to the recommended dietary behavior were another barrier to meeting BMI thresholds. Dialysis requires dietary restrictions which some participants indicated were too difficult for them to maintain to meet weight loss goals, "Most of the diet food we can't have . . . anything dark green. Any type of dietary supplements. A lot of vegetables we can't have. [We can] basically have boiled chicken. That's it. Boiled chicken and rice, all day. Could you eat boiled chicken every [day]?" (P14) Some participants recounted that they were on a waitlist but they could not maintain the necessary dietary behavior to persist, "I stopped following what I'm supposed to do. I started back to drinking all of that dark cola I wasn't supposed to drink and foods I wasn't supposed to eat." (P03)

Age – after 60 you can't even get a transplant. Uncertainty regarding age thresholds for transplant eligibility influences the decision to pursue transplant. Some participants indicated a specific age requirement for a transplant, "I think after age 60 you can't even get a transplant." (P16) Other participants expressed that older age was disqualifying without indicating a specific age, "the older I get, the less of a chance I think I have [of receiving a transplant]." (P17) Upon probing about how they learned of these age qualifiers, patients confirmed that they did not learn about them from clinicians or dialysis staff. P12 explained her understanding of how age is a factor in eligibility, "I found out later [after being on dialysis for 3 years] that a person got one [transplant] that was 80 years old." Also, some older participants expressed that they had lived life and felt that it would be better if someone else received the kidney "at my age, it [transplant] really don't matter to me. I just keep doing dialysis." (P16). Another participant expressed her perspectives on transplant, "Cause my age, I'm 70. It makes a difference. And I'd rather see somebody younger get one." (P12)

Post-transplant care regimen – I don't wanna put myself through that. Participants expressed concern given their understanding of what would be required of them to maintain their kidney function after transplant. Many expressed worry concerning the required medication behavior, specifically the stipulation of taking the anti-rejection medication regularly. They were concerned because they felt that their current medication behavior was irregular, "I don't want [a transplant] because you're stuck to all these pills, every day, about 20 pills for the rest of your life. I'm bad with pills." (P03) Another participant stated, "all the pills you gotta take. I'm not good at taking pills. So if you don't take them pills, the kidney could stop. So, I don't wanna put myself through that." (P19) Participants recalled previous medical conditions with treatment regimens that included several medications, "I think I'll just go ahead on and do the dialysis . . . Cause I don't wanna go back to all that medicine." (P12) Another participant who had already received a kidney transplant indicated that the graft failed because she did not consistently follow the recommended medication behavior, "I stopped taking my medication . . . I was taking them, but I'd skip." (P07)

Another apprehension concerning the medication regimen is the ability to pay for necessary medications. Participants knew there would be changes to their existing medication regimen, and they expressed concerns with being able to afford them. Patients who need dialysis who do not have another form of insurance are eligible for Medicare; however, if they receive a transplant then their eligibility lapses three years after receiving the transplant (Centers for Medicare & Medicaid Services, 2020). Some participants were fully aware of this provision, "you must sustain yourself three years after transplantation. They automatically take you off if you're not 65. Let's say you're 50, and you get three years, and then you come off" (P02). Some also indicated reliance on disability benefits, and eligibility may be affected by receiving a transplant, "you only got like a year's time [of disability coverage]." (P01)

Multiple participants managed uncertainty by observing others' experiences of going back to dialysis after having a transplant. For some, this would be worse than never having a transplant, "I've seen people get on the waitlist, get that kidney, and be off dialysis, and it rejects, and they'd be put right back on dialysis, and have to go through that whole process again, and I don't wanna go through that, I'm not gonna go through that." (P23) One participant who had a transplant described his experience with having to go back to receive dialysis treatments, P13 who went through that process said:

> The second time, when I had the transplant, and then they said "hey you've got to go back to dialysis," man, that was, I don't get depressed, but I believe I was depressed then. Aww man, I was just sad, man. I mean, just dragging, dragging. Didn't wanna do nothing. (P13)

Several participants have already endured various health conditions, including surgeries, and the uncertainty of enduring another procedure influenced their decisions. One participant offered her experience with other medical procedures, "a surgery is not easy. You might come back out of it, and you might not." (P16) Another participant expressed the sentiment this way, "I was actually scared to have the surgery 'cause I done had so many surgeries in my life. It's just like, this is a big surgery." (P04) One participant expressed that they were not having any more surgeries, "they not cutting on me no more, period." (P19)

Certainty derived from perceptions of life after transplant

Several participants expressed certainty that receiving a transplant would improve their lives. These perceptions tended to reduce uncertainty. Disdain for receiving dialysis helped inform their perspectives on how their lives would improve. Faith resulted in optimism for a better future. Through spirituality, they derived meaning from their experiences for a better future. Some expressed faith that a transplant will help them "live life" again.

Several participants expressed certainty in their dislike of receiving dialysis and this influenced their perspectives on how receiving a transplant would greatly improve their lived experience, "the good part is that you don't have to take dialysis no more. Let me tell you something, I'm being disfigured getting stuck with a needle twice, three days a week. I'll take 100 pills to stay out of dialysis." (P09) Another participant expressed just wanting to enjoy simple pleasures like drinking water, "that's what getting me, the water part. I love water and you can't drink so much." (P15)

Optimism and spiritual faith provided a measure of certainty for some participants that their health will eventually improve. Their faith gave them motivation, "my experience, just have faith. You have to, I have to have a strong mind." (P06) Religious faith provided comfort, optimism, and certainty, "I have something to believe in. When you have something to believe in, it means you know there's something more . . . it's a sense of there's something out there that's bigger and better than you. And you try to achieve it and you strive to go get it." (P11) Spiritual faith elicits feelings that they will not face a challenge that they cannot meet, "He [God] is not going to let us be burdened with more than we can handle physically in our own bodies." (P20) One participant (P09) had to receive dialysis after receiving a kidney donated by his daughter. He shared that the graft failed because he did not take the antirejection medication as directed. He stopped taking his medications because "he felt fine" shortly after his transplant. He recounted, "I don't need this medication. I don't need doctor appointments. I'm feeling good. I was feeling brand new. I was back playing ball [sports], everything was going good." He asserted with certainty that having to receive dialysis again was a test to help him prepare mentally for his next transplant, "God is putting me through a test to say . . . 'this time I'm gonna make it hard for you to do everything necessary until you realize the importance of this'." Spirituality provided a solid source of certainty for participants.

Many participants expressed a certain desire to live life to the fullest again. P02 expressed the will to live several times as influencing his perspectives on receiving a transplant, "I like living and I like doing the things that help me do that . . . I don't wanna just die!" They were certain of being able to do the various activities that they cannot do while on dialysis, and some were certain that they could follow the recommended post-transplant regimen. For example, P09 did not understand why some individuals would refuse a transplant to avoid anti-rejection medication. He recounted his retort to that concern, "don't you wanna live a normal life . . . don't you wanna be able to sleep in . . . don't you wanna play with your grandkids." P10 was also perplexed as to why some did not want a transplant, "[getting a transplant enables you to] do things like a normal person, why wouldn't you want a kidney?" For some participants, the regular dialysis schedule made travel virtually impossible, "I wanna travel and everything, 'cause on my bucket list is to take a cruise, but so far I haven't found a cruise that can take me. One told me, "it's too expensive [to provide dialysis services] for just one person."

In addition to leisure travel, socialization was also a motivator. P22 also relayed a poignant account of traveling to Cleveland to see his brother before he died, then after he died how he could not spend as much time with his family as he would have preferred because he had to return to Detroit to receive dialysis:

> I couldn't go straight to him on that Sunday because that Monday I had to be on dialysis. So I had to wait until that Tuesday and get up early that morning and drive to Cleveland so I could see my brother before he passed away. When he died my family was getting ready for the funeral. I wanted to be there with the family and everything but I couldn't because Wednesday and Friday I gotta go to dialysis. So I had to go to dialysis Friday and then leave as soon as I got out [of dialysis] to go to Cleveland. What

good did it do me to go there when I still couldn't really be with the family. I gotta spend four hours out of my day just to go to dialysis.

The role of social support

The level and type of social support influenced participants' perspectives on transplant and waitlists. Unwillingness to seek or the inability to access social support (e.g., to ask family members to be a donor), and low social support impacted eligibility for some.

Barriers due to lack of social support – When i got sick, she left me

Lack of social support was a factor for some participants. Eligibility for waitlists includes a psychosocial assessment, which includes having someone who commits to supporting the patient in the period following the transplant. Multiple participants described their own situations in which access to support is difficult. For example, P06 described how her grandmother was a source of support when she was on a waitlist, but when her grandmother became ill, and her mother was not able to provide support, she was forced to ask different people to attend her assessment and evaluation meetings:

> I would just choose whoever I could to come to my meetings. But my social worker just kinda said, "You know what? I know that this support is not good for you. You're bringing multiple different people each time you come to your transplant evaluation. It's not gonna work." (P06)

P06 shared that she was removed from a waitlist due to lack of support, despite having individuals present at her assessments. Because she no longer had one consistent individual, her level of support was deemed insufficient. Other participants shared accounts of how they were removed from a waitlist due to insufficient support. One participant shared how his older brother consistently accompanied him at his regular assessments, but his brother's incarceration left him without a consistent source of support, "my older brother was my support team. My older brother encountered some legal issues and he was no longer able to be the support person." (P01) Another participant described how the mother of his children and his partner of 17 years was his support. She attended his regular assessments, but when his health declined, she ended their relationship, leaving him with no one to play the support role, "I was with my children's mom for 17 years but when I got sick, she left me." (P19) His relationship ending resulted in his removal from the waitlist. Participants expressed confusion as to what constitutes sufficient social support to persist on the waitlist. Some were aware of stipulations practiced by other transplant teams which differed from the stipulations they were subject to, "I don't really understand because I have a friend who was on dialysis with me as a child, she went to [the University of Michigan transplant center] . . . for her transplant and they don't require family consultations." (P06)

Participants indicated that having adequate social support was important in helping them follow the dialysis regimen, which includes regular attendance at dialysis treatments. Participants indicated that regular attendance was an important requirement to getting on a waitlist and persisting on it. Participants expressed that other demands, such as caregiving responsibilities, at times presents barriers to their ability to attend treatments. They also described how dialysis center staff were indifferent to their efforts to attend treatments amid competing demands. One participant offered a detailed account of her efforts to attend her dialysis treatments, but her caregiving demands at times presented barriers:

> The [dialysis] staff up there where I'm at, they expect you to be there every day. And I told them, by me going through what I'm going through . . . I was in the process of moving and I was going through stuff with my landlord and trying to take care of my kids. And my kids was having problems in school. I mean I understand that [I need to attend dialysis appointments], but it's kind of hard to not take care of your responsibilities, just so I can be up there [at the dialysis center]. And I do, I try to be there as much as I can, but I don't have no family that really can help me with the stuff I'm going through. (P21)

Participants who had experience on a waitlist also offered accounts of how insufficient social support presented barriers. One participant (P24) described how he was under a strict deadline to get to the hospital once he was notified that a kidney was available for transplant. He indicated that once his initial graft failed and he attempted to be placed back on a waitlist, he was denied because he could not travel quickly enough, "I had to get there in less than 45 minutes . . . I don't have a car and my son didn't have a car."

Unwillingness or inability to access social support – I don't want a kidney from my family

Participants described their experiences of having other family members who have had ESRD, so they did not want to receive a kidney from their family because family members may need both of their kidneys. P05 described how her family history of ESRD influences her decision not to want a live donor:

> My father was on dialysis, his mother was on dialysis, his brothers were on dialysis. It [ESRD] runs in my family. I don't want a kidney from my family member, the simple fact is I got seven kids. Okay, if I get one of my kid's kidneys, they might have kidney trouble in the [future] . . . So I wouldn't want it from none of my family members.

Another participant described the stiff reaction from family members when he sought a live donor from his family, "I went to a family reunion and I told everybody that I needed a transplant, and everybody got quiet." (P13) Another participant described concerns about organ donations from other Black people who did not have ESRD and who may be eligible to donate:

> They [other Black people] would tell you, "I may need my kidney later on. My kidney may go bad, I may need my kidney." Or they may say, "one of my children may need my kidney" . . . a lot of people don't even want their organs removed when they're dead. They say, "I wanna go to heaven with everything. I want my body intact". (P17)

Several participants described how they socializing and shared information bonded with others who were also receiving dialysis during the same time at the same center. These other patients who were receiving dialysis are information sources, and the stories they exchanged informed them of some of the risks and negative outcomes, "I heard bad stories about transplant, and I heard good stories. But the majority of the stories I heard have been bad . . . all the bad stories just got me kinda nervous." (P18) Some participants pointed out that they do not have access to the stories of positive transplant outcomes, because those people do not return to the dialysis center and the participants indicated that they never hear about what happens to them, unless they need to return to dialysis, "some people have them [transplant] and they keep going. When they have them, you don't hear from them no more, that's the thing though, you don't hear from them." (P16)

In addition to the information from others who were receiving dialysis at the same time, multiple participants told stories of people who received a kidney transplant and had either died or the graft failed and they needed to return to dialysis, "I had a girlfriend who had a sister on dialysis, and she was on dialysis for only a year and they called her for a transplant. She had the transplant, was in the hospital for a week, and the day she was supposed to go home, she died ... that was very devastating, that really scared me." (P22)

These stories included uncertainty about the health condition of the donor, and de facto the graft, "they explained to me, 'I might get an old lady's kidney ... and an old person's kidney might not last as long because they've lived and used it'." (P22) Another participant expressed fear that a donation may expose them to illness:

> "[I] heard different people talk and they say if somebody donated a kidney and they got AIDS, then if you get their kidney you gonna have it ... and then I heard that if they got hepatitis, and they give you their kidney you gonna get it, and I was like, 'oh no, I got enough going on.'" (P24)

Attending dialysis is a source of social support – I enjoy the people when i go to dialysis

Attending dialysis was a form of important socialization. As mentioned, the dialysis "family" is an important source of information, but the "family" also provides socialization. P12 stated, "I think I'll just go ahead on and do the dialysis ... 'cause that way you know you will be with people" She elaborated:

> I mean because I'm going to dialysis I get to see them, you know. We all get together, we talk, joke, have fun. They call me the Candy Lady 'cause I pass out the candy. I just enjoy 'em. I enjoy the people when I go to dialysis. You know 'cause in the morning everybody says, "Good morning. Hey. How you? What you doing?".

If she were to receive a transplant, then she would not be able to socialize with others who are also receiving dialysis, "I wouldn't see nobody." She elaborated on her family, and how little contact she has with them:

> I have four children, four sons. I don't even hear from them, they don't call. I was in the hospital, they didn't even come see me or call me. [I saw] the youngest about three, about four weeks ago ... [he] could have stayed where he was. Yeah, but that's alright though. I learned how to just forget 'em. I got, I got four boys. They got kids. I got 19 grand and 10 great-grands ... and I see the great grands. I seen them last year, Easter. I didn't see them this Easter but I was with them last Easter.

While receiving dialysis may be difficult, the prospect of losing the social connection is why some participants prefer dialysis. Another participant spoke to the social connections at the dialysis center among the patients, "everybody there is talking and discussing things with each other. It's like a big old family in the whole front area ... a lot of us talk right there in the front before we go in." (P11) Another participant shared her perspectives:

> We are all concerned about each other. When we don't see someone, we know something's wrong. That mean you sick, or you've passed away. One of the two. Basically everybody in my particular clinic, when they get sick they're going to Providence Hospital. When I don't see them for a day or two, I'll go to [the hospital]. I ask before I go. I'll call and ask. If they're in the hospital, I'll go and see them. (P24)

Motivation derived from social support – I wanna live for them

Social support provided motivation for some participants to pursue transplant. Participants indicated that their family, peers who also receive dialysis, and dialysis staff are all motivators.

Biological family provides participants a certain motivation to pursue a transplant. P03 explained that his motivation stems from being the primary caregiver for his grandchildren, "I wanna live for them. I do not want to leave my wife in a situation where she's alone taking care of the kids, that's kinda bad. I don't want to leave my wife alone like that." Similarly, P04 cited wanting to live for her son and being able to see him grow up, "my son is the reason why I do everything, if it wasn't for my son, I would have gave up." She shared that her son wants to go to Disney World for his 12th grade trip, "so I wanna be able to go with him ... but dialysis has you tied down." P19 expressed wanting to see his grandkids grow up, but he offered a sobering possibility, "you can't do that when you're dead."

Participants also described how family members provided direct motivation and a measure of certainty to continue to do what was required of them to be approved to be put on a transplant waitlist. P21 describes how his brother keeps him motivated, "my brother is my biggest support system ... when it gets rough he talks to me, he encourages me to keep going." P15 shared that he needs to lose weight to be placed on a waitlist, and his daughter is encouraging him, "me and my daughter just joined the gym together."

Multiple participants had family members who expressed interest in donating their kidney. Some found creative ways to ensure that they were tested to confirm a match. For example, P09 explained his confusion when he was notified to come to an office to start the transplant process because he had a live donor match. But he was unaware who he had been matched with. Upon arriving at the office for the transplant consultations, he found his daughter waiting there and said, "I was like, 'why, why would you?' She said, 'Daddy, I love you and you wasn't doing good, and I don't wanna lose you, and we are a perfect match'." Similarly, P14 was uncertain about his brother donating his kidney, and afraid that he would lose the kidney his brother donated, or he was uncertain if his brother would need both of his kidneys, but P14 expressed that his brother "was insistent."

Participants also spoke of friends who motivated them and provided them certainty to pursue the transplant waitlist. For example, P05 detailed how one of her friends motivated her, "[my friend] told me a long time ago, 'don't ever think that it won't work, 'cause if you think it don't work, then it won't work. You gotta keep yourself positive that it will work.'" P11 spoke about how friends who are also on dialysis served as motivation which resulted in reassurance and certainty:

> it's helpful when you've got one person who's struggling in the same fight you are, and he says, "here man, let me show you how to help, how do you do this." And then you help the next person and then everybody's helping. It becomes . . . easier.

Several participants also described the impact of the death of friends they had made during dialysis. These experiences made them more aware that getting a transplant could be lifesaving, "there's so many of us leaving [dying] at dialysis since I've been on dialysis, it's about 30 people that left, that didn't get to [receive a kidney donation]." (P05). Participants expressed deep sorrow from seeing so many people who they used to receive dialysis with die. These deaths struck a particular loss for participants, in part because they become quite close to their peers, and participants were adamant that they did not want that to happen to them. Losing so many people that they are close enough to call "family" is upsetting and further motivated participants, "it's kind of scary, actually, because you'll be thinking if you're gonna be next? I know that's how I feel." (P21). Also, P22 describes her reaction to discovering that a man who also received dialysis in the chair next to her had died, she said "I cried. Each time I lose somebody I cry, and I just hope that it doesn't happen to me."

In contrast to participants who related how their experiences with dialysis staff had discouraged them from pursuing the waitlist, dialysis staff motivated some participants to get on a waitlist. P01, who had been deterred from a waitlist by his interactions with certain clinical staff after disclosing his history of drug use, described how a social worker on the transplant team encouraged him to get back on a waitlist, "she [social worker] helped me with getting past revealing my drug history." Nurses also play an integral role in encouraging patients. For example, P05 described how he had trouble with limiting fluid intake, but the nurses where he received dialysis would encourage him by saying "don't do that this weekend, watch your weight. You know you got them grandkids to live for."

Discussion

This research represents an important contribution to further understanding disparities in progress to kidney transplant for Black patients. This is the only investigation that focuses solely on the perception, understanding, and belief of Black ESRD patients who are on dialysis and who are not active on a transplant waitlist. Findings contribute to the literature by illuminating transplant perceptions and should be used to enhance current approaches of communicating treatment options and targeting health information interventions.

Participants expressed considerable uncertainty when contemplating their current health circumstances, yet they also expressed certainty about their future should they be fortunate to receive a transplant. Uncertainty derived from the layer of the self (e.g., perceptions based on their understanding of age eligibility/restrictions, ability to follow the post-transplant care regimen) and others (e.g., clinical staff informing them of BMI thresholds) and social and/or familial relationships (e.g., dialysis provides socialization/support, reluctance to ask family members to be donors). Interestingly, *unwillingness* to seek social support (seeking a live donor) and *low* social support influenced their perceptions.

Uncertainty at the layer of the self-stemmed from participants lacking information about treatment options. Participants expressed that they did not know that the transplant treatment option may be an alternative to dialysis. Participants expressed several areas in which they simply lacked information on transplant eligibility (e.g., age thresholds) and did not know that the transplant process may be initiated by the patient. Clearly, access to reliable information needs to be enhanced. Given the intense emotions upon diagnosis, particularly in the hospital setting, the timing of when to communicate health information concerning treatment options should be considered. Attending dialysis provided participants with a vital source of information. This distinction was clear, participants who were receiving dialysis had access to information, specifically the dialysis treatment option, and access to this information reduced uncertainty. This is consistent with prior studies which describe the importance of peer support, particularly in the dialysis center (Kazley et al., 2012). Simply receiving dialysis provides a source of information. Attendance at dialysis treatments also provides vital social support. Patients exchanged information at the dialysis center, both before and during dialysis; however, clinic staff did not necessarily share information concerning other treatment options, which is consistent with literature concerning information sharing in dialysis centers (Veinot et al., 2010).

Uncertainty at the layer of others was most apparent in participants' expression of racism which resulted in mistrust. Consistent with this study, previous studies have also shown that patients from racial minority groups mistrust physicians at rates higher than individuals from majority groups, due to perceived racial bias and cultural discordance (Peek et al., 2013). Previous health communication interventions have been effective in reducing mistrust between groups (Matsaganis et al., 2014). These interventions utilize peer health advocates ("peer mentors") to bridge information gaps much like the peer mentors referenced in this study. There is a difference, however, in that peer health advocates are trained on outreach methods and how to provide pertinent health information so that they are not only trusted as a peer, but they are formally trained which may enhance their ability to provide accurate information. Utilizing these existing resources in the dialysis centers could enhance the efficacy of an intervention designed to provide treatment option information, especially after initial diagnosis. Peer mentors, situated in dialysis centers, who provide health information may also discuss with both patients and caregivers' issues and concerns in attempts to address uncertainty.

Communicating health information concerning treatment options and assessments for transplant waitlists should include social support assessments. These assessments should be attentive to types of social support. Comprehensive assessments will include determining to what degree receiving dialysis may play in a patient's emotional and social life. Social workers are particularly well-positioned to perform these assessments, given their proximity to dialysis patients and their caregivers (Senteio & Callahan, 2020). For some patients, receiving dialysis may provide essential socialization. Regular visits to the dialysis center represent a crucial source of social support. Further, the literature is consistent in describing the importance of social support as patients from racial minority groups attempt to follow care recommendations (Senteio & Veinot, 2014), and associations have been described between social support and health behaviors (e.g., dialysis patients' adherence to diet restrictions) (Sousa et al., 2019). Patient education should also include the likelihood of kidney function recovery given that such a small proportion of patients who are on dialysis experience the return of their kidney function. In large study populations, rates of recovery are between 1– 2%, and almost one-third of patients who experience recovery have a primary diagnosis of acute kidney injury as the reason for renal failure (Mohan et al., 2013).

Last, participants were quite complimentary of the RISE program, the Rehabilitation, Information, Support and Empowerment program which has been used by affiliates of the NKF. The patient education program was established in 1999 to "assist patients return to meaningful activity" (National Kidney Foundation, 1999, 2002). This program should be consulted to inform patient education and support for this population.

Limitations

There are two limitations to the study. First, we only investigated patient perceptions. We did not include dialysis staff who have experience treating this population. Future work should include investigating perspectives of individuals in clinical roles which play a vital role in providing dialysis services and referral for transplant evaluation. (e.g., nephrologists, primary care physicians, nurses, health educators, nutritionists, and nephrology social workers). Second, we did not explicitly ask about patient satisfaction surveys. Literature shows associations between dialysis patient satisfaction and quality of care at the facility level, with significant differences observed by specific providers (Kshirsagar et al., 2019). Therefore, focused efforts should be taken to collect patient satisfaction information from this population to inform interventions addressing dissatisfaction. Future research should focus on refining validated patient satisfaction instruments for dialysis patients from racial minority populations to understand the specific barriers to information and quality care they may face. Special attention should be given to mistrust and its effect on health behaviors.

Dialysis centers should develop and implement regular patient satisfaction surveys to understand the concerns and when patients may request or need additional information. Little is known of dialysis patients' satisfaction rates and experiences of care for those that do not respond to surveys, and for those that do respond White patients report higher satisfaction than Black patients (Richardson et al., 2015). No participant indicated that they had ever responded to a satisfaction survey or had another formalized way to express dissatisfaction to dialysis staff. Since staff perceptions have such a profound influence on barriers to pursue transplantation, providing a conduit for patients to express concerns warrants immediate attention.

Acknowledgments

The authors want to thank the NKF of Michigan whose help was paramount in contacting and recruiting participants for the study. The authors would also like to thank the participants of the study who shared deeply personal and moving stories.

Disclosure of potential conflict of interest

The authors declared no potential conflicts of interest with respect to the research, authorship, and/or publication of this article.

ORCID

Charles R. Senteio http://orcid.org/0000-0002-0254-3127
Matthew K. Ackerman http://orcid.org/0000-0002-0506-9037

References

Albrecht, T. L., & Adelman, M. B. (1984). Social support and life stress: New directions for communication research. *Human Communication Research*, *11*(1), 3–32. https://doi.org/10.1111/j.1468-2958.1984.tb00036.x

Axelrod, D. A., Schnitzler, M. A., Xiao, H., Irish, W., Tuttle-Newhall, E., Chang, S.-H., Kasiske, B. L., Alhamad, T., & Lentine, K. L. (2018). An economic assessment of contemporary kidney transplant practice. *American Journal of Transplantation*, *18*(5), 1168–1176. https://doi.org/10.1111/ajt.14702

Bonner, A., & Lloyd, A. (2012). Exploring the information practices of people with end-stage kidney disease. *Journal of Renal Care*, *38*(3), 124–130. https://doi.org/10.1111/j.1755-6686.2012.00258.x

Brashers, D. E. (2001). Communication and uncertainty management. *Journal of Communication*, *51*(3), 477–497. https://doi.org/10.1111/j.1460-2466.2001.tb02892.x

Brashers, D. E. (2007). A theory of communication and uncertainty management. In B. B. Whaley & W. Samter (Eds.), *Explaining communication: Contemporary theories and exemplars* (pp. 223–242). Lawrence Erlbaum Associates.

Brashers, D. E., Goldsmith, D. J., & Hsieh, E. (2002). Information seeking and avoiding in health contexts. *Human Communication Research*, *28*(2), 258–271. https://doi.org/10.1111/j.1468-2958.2002.tb00807.x

Centers for Disease Control and Prevention. (2019). *Chronic kidney disease in the United States, 2019*. https://www.cdc.gov/kidneydisease/pdf/2019_National-Chronic-Kidney-Disease-Fact-Sheet.pdf

Centers for Medicare & Medicaid Services. (2020). *End-stage renal disease (ESRD)*. Retrieved August 2, 2020, from https://www.cms.gov/Medicare/Coordination-of-Benefits-and-Recovery/Coordination-of-Benefits-and-Recovery-Overview/End-Stage-Renal-Disease-ESRD/ESRD

Corbin, J., & Strauss, A. (2007). *Basics of qualitative research: Techniques and procedures for developing grounded theory* (3rd ed.). SAGE Publications.

Costello, K. L., & Murillo, A. P. (2014). "I want your kidney!" Information seeking, sharing, and disclosure when soliciting a kidney donor online. *Patient Education and Counseling*, *94*(3), 423–426. https://doi.org/10.1016/j.pec.2013.11.009

Creswell, J. W. (2006). *Qualitative inquiry and research design: Choosing among five approaches* (2nd ed.). SAGE Publications.

Crews, D. C., Bello, A. K., & Saadi, G. (2019). Burden, access, and disparities in kidney disease. *Kidney International*, *95*(2), 242–248. https://doi.org/10.1016/j.kint.2018.11.007

Glaser, B. G. (1965). The constant comparative method of qualitative analysis. *Social Problems*, *12*(4), 436–445. https://doi.org/10.2307/798843

Glaser, B. G. (1978). *Theoretical sensitivity: Advances in the methodology of grounded theory*. Sociology Press.

Grams, M. E., Massie, A. B., Schold, J. D., Chen, B. P., & Segev, D. L. (2013). Trends in the inactive kidney transplant waitlist and implications for candidate survival. *American Journal of Transplantation*, *13*(4), 1012–1018. https://doi.org/10.1111/ajt.12143

Jagdale, A., Cooper, D. K. C., Iwase, H., & Gaston, R. S. (2019). Chronic dialysis in patients with end-stage renal disease: Relevance to kidney xenotransplantation. *Xenotransplantation*, *26*(2), e12471. https://doi.org/10.1111/xen.12471

Kazley, A. S., Simpson, K. N., Chavin, K. D., & Baliga, P. (2012). Barriers facing patients referred for kidney transplant cause loss to follow-up. *Kidney International*, *82*(9), 1018–1023. https://doi.org/10.1038/ki.2012.255

Kilambi, V., Bui, K., Hazen, G. B., Friedewald, J. J., Ladner, D. P., Kaplan, B., & Mehrotra, S. (2019). Evaluation of accepting kidneys of varying quality for transplantation or expedited placement with decision trees. *Transplantation*, *103*(5), 980–989. https://doi.org/10.1097/TP.0000000000002585

Kshirsagar, A. V., Tabriz, A. A., Bang, H., & Lee, S.-Y. D. (2019). Patient satisfaction is associated with dialysis facility quality and star ratings. *American Journal of Medical Quality*, *34*(3), 243–250. https://doi.org/10.1177/1062860618796310

Lipford, K. J., McPherson, L., Hamoda, R., Browne, T., Gander, J. C., Pastan, S. O., & Patzer, R. E. (2018). Dialysis facility staff perceptions of racial, gender, and age disparities in access to renal transplantation. *BMC Nephrology*, *19*(1), 5. https://doi.org/10.1186/s12882-017-0800-6

Matsaganis, M. D., Golden, A. G., & Scott, M. E (2014). Communication infrastructure theory and reproductive health disparities: Enhancing storytelling network integration by developing interstitial actors. *International Journal of Communication*, *8*, 1495–1516. https://ijoc.org/index.php/ijoc/article/view/2566/1145

Miles, M. B., Huberman, A. M., & Saldaña, J. (2014). *Qualitative data analysis: A methods sourcebook*. Sage.

Mohan, S., Huff, E., Wish, J., Lilly, M., Chen, S.-C., & McClellan, W. M. (2013). Recovery of renal function among ESRD patients in the US medicare program. *PLoS ONE*, *8*(12), e83447–e83447. https://doi.org/10.1371/journal.pone.0083447

Morgan, S. E. (2006). Many facets of reluctance: African Americans and the decision (not) to donate organs. *Journal of the National Medical Association*, *98*(5), 695–703. https://www.ncbi.nlm.nih.gov/pmc/articles/PMC2569263/

National Kidney Foundation. (1999, June 25). *National Kidney Foundation offers new series on rehabilitation*. Retrieved August 3, 2020, from https://www.kidney.org/news/newsroom/newsreleases/0128

National Kidney Foundation. (2002, June 11). *NKF seeks Wayne Nix Award nominee*. Retrieved August 3, 2020, from https://www.kidney.org/news/newsroom/newsreleases/0035

Patzer, R. E., McPherson, L., Redmond, N., DuBay, D., Zayas, C., Hartmann, E., Mulloy, L., Perryman, J., Pastan, S., & Arriola, K. J. (2019). A culturally sensitive web-based intervention to improve living donor kidney transplant among African Americans. *Kidney International Reports*, *4*(9), 1285–1295. https://doi.org/10.1016/j.ekir.2019.05.771

Peek, M. E., Gorawara-Bhat, R., Quinn, M. T., Odoms-Young, A., Wilson, S. C., & Chin, M. H. (2013). Patient trust in physicians and shared decision-making among African Americans with diabetes. *Health Communication*, *28*(6), 616–623. https://doi.org/10.1080/10410236.2012.710873

Purnell, T. S., Luo, X., Cooper, L. A., Massie, A. B., Kucirka, L. M., Henderson, M. L., Gordon, E. J., Crews, D. C., Boulware, L. E., & Segev, D. L. (2018). Association of race and ethnicity with live donor kidney transplantation in the United States from 1995 to 2014. *JAMA*, *319*(1), 49–61. https://doi.org/10.1001/jama.2017.19152

Richardson, M. M., Paine, S. S., Grobert, M. E., Stidley, C. A., Gabbay, E., Harford, A. M., Zager, P. G., Miskulin, D. C., & Meyer, K. B. (2015). Satisfaction with care of patients on hemodialysis. *Clinical Journal of the American Society of Nephrology*, *10*(8), 1428–1434. https://doi.org/10.2215/CJN.11241114

Robinson, J. D., & Tian, Y. (2009). Cancer patients and the provision of informational social support. *Health Communication*, *24*(5), 381–390. https://doi.org/10.1080/10410230903023261

Saldaña, J. (2009). *The coding manual for qualitative researchers*. SAGE Publications.

Scott, A. M., Martin, S. C., Stone, A. M., & Brashers, D. E. (2011). Managing multiple goals in supportive interactions: Using a normative theoretical approach to explain social support as uncertainty management for organ transplant patients. *Health Communication*, *26*(5), 393–403. https://doi.org/10.1080/10410236.2011.552479

Senteio, C. R., & Callahan, M. B. (2020). Supporting quality care for ESRD patients: The social worker can help address barriers to advance care planning. *BMC Nephrology*, *21*(1), 55. https://doi.org/10.1186/s12882-020-01720-0

Senteio, C. R., & Veinot, T. C. E. (2014). Trying to make things right: Adherence work in high-poverty, African American neighborhoods. *Qualitative Health Research*, *24*(12), 1745–1756. https://doi.org/10.1177/1049732314549027

Sousa, H., Ribeiro, O., Paúl, C., Costa, E., Miranda, V., Ribeiro, F., & Figueiredo, D. (2019). Social support and treatment adherence in patients with end-stage renal disease: A systematic review. *Seminars in Dialysis*, *32*(6), 562–574. https://doi.org/10.1111/sdi.12831

Talamantes, E., Norris, K. C., Mangione, C. M., Moreno, G., Waterman, A. D., Peipert, J. D., Bunnapradist, S., & Huang, E. (2017). Linguistic isolation and access to the active kidney transplant waiting list in the United States. *Clinical Journal of the American Society of Nephrology*, *12*(3), 483–492. https://doi.org/10.2215/CJN.07150716

Tong, A., Hanson, C. S., Chapman, J. R., Halleck, F., Budde, K., Josephson, M. A., & Craig, J. C. (2015). 'Suspended in a paradox'–patient attitudes to wait-listing for kidney transplantation: Systematic review and thematic synthesis of qualitative studies. *Transplant International*, *28*(7), 771–787. https://doi.org/10.1111/tri.12575

Traino, H. M., Nonterah, C. W., Cyrus, J. W., Gillespie, A., Urbanski, M., & Adair-Kriz, M. (2015). Disparities in the completion of steps to kidney transplantation: Protocol for a systematic review. *BMJ Open*, *5*(9). https://doi.org/10.1136/bmjopen-2015-008677

United States Renal Data System. (2019). *US renal data system 2019 annual data report: Epidemiology of kidney disease in the United States*. National Institutes of Health. https://www.usrds.org/annual-data-report/

Veinot, T. C. E. (2010). '"We" have a lot of information to share with each other'. Understanding the value of peer-based health information exchange. *Information Research*, *15*(4). http://informationr.net/ir/15-4/paper452.html

Veinot, T. C. E., Meadowbrooke, C. C., Newman, M. W., Zheng, K., & Perry, E. E. (2010). Routines that ease the pain: The information world of a dialysis clinic. *Proceedings of the American Society for Information Science and Technology*, *47*(1), 1–4. https://doi.org/10.1002/meet.14504701254

Yuan, C. M., Bohen, E. M., & Abbott, K. C. (2012). Initiating and completing the kidney transplant evaluation process: The red queen's race. *Clinical Journal of the American Society of Nephrology*, *7*(10), 1551. https://doi.org/10.2215/CJN.08680812

Zheng, K., Newman, M. W., Veinot, T. C., Hanratty, M., Kim, H., Meadowbrooke, C., & Perry, E. E (2010). Using online peer-mentoring to empower young adults with end-stage renal disease: A feasibility study. *AMIA Annual Symposium Proceedings*, *2010*, 942–946. http://www.ncbi.nlm.nih.gov/pmc/articles/PMC3041447/

In Our Sacred Voice – An Exploration of Tribal and Community Leader Perceptions as Health Communicators of Disease Prevention among American Indians in the Plains

Crystal Y. Lumpkins, Ryan Goeckner, Jason Hale, Charley Lewis, Jordyn Gunville, River Gunville, Chris M. Daley, and Sean M. Daley

ABSTRACT

American Indians (AI) are disproportionately and significantly impacted by disease morbidity, mortalityand poor behavioral health outcomes. Health promotion and health communication programs exist to address these health disparities and health conditions; however, few programs fully integrate holistic approaches when targeting AI populations. The objective of this study was to explore how tribal and community leaders throughout the Central Plains (Kansas, Iowa, Missouri, and South Dakota) viewed themselves as health communicators and health promoters within their communities. Members of the Center for American Indian Community Health (CAICH) conducted 39 in-depth interviews with members of federally recognized tribes living in reservation communities as well as urban tribal communities across the region. Results from the sample show that these individuals do not necessarily see themselves as the "authority" health communicator or health promoter within their tribe or community. They did perceive themselves and others as gatekeepers of pertinent health information. Social and cultural authority within culturally centered messaging and collective delivery of this type of health information from trusted sources within tribes and communities is perceived to bolster health communication programs and positively impact health outcomes among AI populations.

Introduction

Health communication and health promotion programs exist to address health disparities and health conditions among American Indian peoples and communities; however, more is needed to fully integrate Native community members and leaders into the health promotion and health communication process. The integration of American Indian cultural, social, and spiritual values and norms, as well as oral traditions have shown impactful on American Indian health and wellness (Heaton et al., 2018; F. S. Hodge et al., 2002). Historically, and counter to the positive outcomes on these traditions, many cultural, social, and spiritual aspects of American Indian life have been impaired by Western cultures and the accompanying ethnocentrism, ethnocide, and genocide, resulting in many instances of historical trauma (Brave Heart, 1998; Duran & Duran, 1995; Evans-Campbell, 2008). These factors have perpetuated a cascade of negative health outcomes and other health issues among American Indians (Heckert & Eisenhauer, 2014, 2014; Morgan & Freeman, 2009; Szlemko et al., 2006, 2006).

Due to colonization, Westernization, and the paternal nature of the Euro-American biomedical model, health communication and health promotion about health disparities and disease prevention shared with American Indian peoples and communities may actually dissuade Native individuals from seeking better health because of cross-cultural miscommunication (Kagawa Singer, 2012; Kagawa-Singer & Kassim-Lakha, 2003). Disease prevention information provided to Native peoples and communities through culturally responsive and inclusive health communication strategies is plausible to increase awareness and impact attitudes toward positive health behavior (Geana et al., 2012; Gearhart & Trumbly-Lamsam, 2017; Kalbfleisch, 2009; Rentner et al., 2012). Health communication and health promotion shared by medical personnel or researchers can also have a deleterious impact and contribute to health information inequalities and inequities (Kreps & Sparks, 2008). These forms of strategic communication with minimal inclusion of lived experiences of historical trauma, mistrust and other adverse events among Indigenous populations may hinder disease prevention. Further, exclusion of Indigenous health beliefs and behaviors in health communication and health promotion also minimizes message effectiveness (Hinnant et al., 2019). The present study aims were to explore perceptions that tribal leaders and elders in the Central Plains have about their role as promoters and communicators of disease prevention among Native peoples and communities. Our inquiry to explore credible and reliable sources within a communicative infrastructure (Dutta, 2018) among this sample was guided through an historical trauma and critical cultural communication lens. To our knowledge, this is one of the first community-based studies to explore perceptions that Native leaders have about being health communicators in their communities.

Health disparities among American Indians

According to the 2010 U.S. Census, 0.9% of the population, or about 2.9 million people, identify as solely American Indian or Alaska Native, while 1.7%, or about 5.2 million people claim to be either solely American Indian, Alaska Native or American Indian or Alaska Native in combination with one or more races (Norris et al., 2012). Currently, American Indian populations are disproportionately and significantly impacted by disease morbidity, mortality (Espey et al., 2014; Heron, 2013; Jacobs-Wingo et al., 2016; National Center for Health Statistics [NCHS], 2019) and poor behavioral health outcomes. These outcomes reflect a dire picture of overall health where American Indian populations have an almost 5-year shorter life span than all other racial/ethnic groups (Indian Health Service [IHS], 2015). Based on the U.S. Department of Health and Human Services data from 2017, American Indians have the highest infant mortality at 9.2 per 1,000 live births as compared to 4.7 for non-Hispanic Whites and 5.8 for all races (Office of Minority Health [OMH], 2020). A 2019 National Vital Statistics Report shows the five leading causes of death among American Indian populations are heart disease (18.1%), cancer (17.1%), accidents (11.6%), diabetes (5.8%), and chronic diseases of the liver (5.5%) (Centers for Disease Control [CDC], 2020). In the Midwest, health disparities among American Indian populations also reflect a deficit in oral health care and access to dental services (NCHS, 2019).

Health disparities among American Indian populations can, in part, be described by a variety of phenomena, barriers, and lived experiences. Within these populations historical trauma (Sotero, 2006) informs experiences with medical authority, medical conditions, distribution of power, and existing public narratives that impact health (Mohatt et al., 2014). These experiences then are probable to shape identified perceptions, attitudes, and beliefs toward health and wellness narratives and information (Larkey & Hecht, 2010). Reaching these populations with relevant communication and language that is culturally inclusive (Kreuter et al., 2003; Kreuter & McClure, 2004; Thomas et al., 2004), culture centered (Larkey & Hecht, 2010) and reflective of a diverse and vast American Indian population may assist in the mitigation of disease.

Historical trauma and medical mistrust

Historical trauma is multigenerational trauma experienced by a specific cultural, racial, or ethnic group. It is related to inhumane acts that have oppressed a particular group of people and have included slavery, the Holocaust, forced migration, and the violent colonization of Native Americans (Administration for Children and Families [ACF], 2020). Lakota clinician and researcher Maria Yellow Horse Brave Heart describes historical trauma as the "cumulative emotional and psychological wounding over the lifespan and across generations, emanating from massive group trauma experience," (Brave Heart, 2003, p. 7). The traumas American Indian populations face include both the lived experiences of individuals, as well as the secondary responses by subsequent generations, allowing the traumas to persist past the generation of people on which it was initially inflicted (Brave Heart, 1998; Danieli, 1998; Figley, 1995; Motta et al., 1994). American Indian experiences tied to colonization, and the accompanying ethnocide and genocide, as well as the continued colonization and persecution of Native peoples are examples of these traumas (Brave Heart & DeBruyn, 1998; Denham, 2008; Evans-Campbell, 2008; Morgan & Freeman, 2009; Szlemko et al., 2006). Historical trauma has contributed to high rates of alcohol and drug abuse, family violence, suicide, homicide, and other violence and mental health issues American Indian peoples face today (Kunitz, 2006; Poupart, 2003). The negative effects of unresolved historical trauma among American Indian individuals and communities may also damage individual and/or community cultural identity (Sotero, 2006).

American Indian mistrust of the Euro-American biomedical establishment also presents barriers to positive health outcomes, as well as influences encounter with medical establishments and personnel. Mistrust of the scientific community is a significant reason for the lack of Native participation in medical activities (Baker, 1999; Beal, 2011; Cook & de Mange, 1995; Corbie-Smith, Flagg et al., 2002; Corbie-Smith, Thomas et al., 2002; Corbie-Smith et al., 2019; Pacheco et al., 2013; Wasserman et al., 2019). The mistrust of medical research and medical practice contribute, in part, to perceived overt racial/ethnic discrimination in healthcare settings (Colclough & Brown, 2014) and mistrust of researchers. Documented examples of unethical medical research (F. Hodge et al., 2000) and activity are grounded into incidences where, in one case, blood samples were taken from members of the Havasupai Nation by geneticists (Mello & Wolf, 2010; Santos, 2008). Racial/ethnic minorities have also participated in studies where researchers failed to obtain informed consent, modified protocols without consulting participants, withheld information, and failed to follow up, resulting in a lack of trust. Other studies have directly examined attitudes of racial/ethnic minorities, fear, and mistrust of medical research and identified them as deterrents to research participation (Moreno-John et al., 2004; Pacheco et al., 2013). Knowledge of these factors and, also historical, cultural, and medical abuses may provide a guide to overcoming gaps in health communication barriers. There also is an opportunity to explore how trusted communication of tribal leaders and elders serves as building blocks for effective disease prevention health promotion programming.

Tribal leaders and elders as health communicators and health promoters of culture-centered communication among American Indians

Health communication and health disease prevention promotion programs exist to address health disparities and health conditions. However, few programs fully integrate holistic approaches when targeting American Indian populations (Walters et al., 2020). Culturally tailored communication, focused on individual characteristics (Kreuter et al., 2003) (e.g., readiness to screen for colorectal cancer) and culturally targeted health communication (e.g., American Indians who are 45 and older who have never screened for colorectal cancer), that emphasize group characteristics have shown impactful among racial/ethnic minority populations. Tailoring has been beneficial when employed to create awareness, increase knowledge, health literacy (Kreps & Neuhauser, 2015; Parker & Kreps, 2005), and intent to influence individual health behavior and foster positive health outcome (Kreuter & Wray, 2003; Rimer & Kreuter, 2006). Trusted individuals, the senders and source of information, and culture-specific communication tools resonate among racial/ethnic minorities, American Indians (LeMaster & Connell, 1994), Native Hawaiians, (Ka'opua et al., 2011), Latinos (Baezconde-Garbanati et al., 2014; Briant et al., 2018; Huerta & Macario, 1999), Asians (Nguyen & Bowman, 2007; Todd & Hoffman-Goetz, 2011; Wang et al., 2006), African Americans (Allicock et al., 2011; Campbell et al., 2007; Lumpkins et al., 2013; McNeill et al., 2018) and optimize effective health communication (Giri et al., 2020). Culturally tailored and targeted information promulgated and co-created from within the culture is inclusive of the population with health risk and maximizes the potential of relevance among recipients who receive culturally tailored or targeted information (Hicks et al., 2012; Lumpkins et al., 2016) through a culturally grounded process (Walters et al., 2020). Tailored and targeted communication at any part of the communication process (sender, message, receiver) may address and include information that is relevant at the individual level and to segments of the population. These strategies fall within the cultural-sensitivity approach according to Dutta (Dutta & Basu, 2008; Dutta-Bergman, 2005) and are used to bolster health communication strategies by including individual and group characteristics that will increase the cultural appropriateness of health communication. However, cultural sensitive health communication that includes tailored and targeted information that draws on the characteristics of a culture as the primary focus of the approach is a starting point. A culture-centered approach, according to Dutta, addresses hegemonic influences – incorporating culture within the process for not only how culture shapes health communication but also how the inclusion of structural and societal factors (e.g., economic, social, and political influences) may address communication inequities and subsequently health disparities that are an indirect result of these inequities. Greater, the communicative discursive spaces and meaning making of communication infrastructure between senders and receivers (actors) are centered to address power and dominant communicative structures that have contributed to the exclusion of marginalized voices (Dutta, 2018; Dutta & Basu, 2008). This approach builds on both tailored and targeted communication strategies and is inclusive of culture, society, shared power, dominance, and authority.

Social capital and cultural networks of health communication

Examples of viable communicative infrastructure components and thus representations of how healthy communication may be optimally exchanged and shared within any given community or culture are found in affinity or trusted organizations. Among African Americans, faith-based and community-based organizations (Butler-Ajibade et al., 2012) including faith leaders or pastors of these organizations perceive themselves to be strong channels of health communication and health promotion (Bopp et al., 2013; Lumpkins et al., 2013). There also is evidence to support that faith-based organizations are efficacious in health promotion of cancer prevention, heart disease, and nutrition (Campbell et al., 2007; DeHaven et al., 2004; Peterson et al., 2002). These and other similar affinity and trusted organizations as communicative infrastructures have been theorized as meta-channels to optimize health and wellness (Stephens et al., 2004). Further, these trusted and affinity channels as culturally appropriate and relevant factors (e.g., source, message, communication channel, receiver) (McGuire, 1981) are woven into health communication programming to appeal to the target audience. Among American Indian populations, the necessary communication components include: a trusted source, message, communication channel, and receiver. These are viable modes of health communication and represent communicative infrastructures for relatable, credible, and reliable health information. Culture defined here moves beyond mere cultural group factors inclusive of racial/ethnic identification and social economic status but is the "processes of language acquisition and socialization; shared by all members of the cultural group; an adaptation to specific environmental and technical conditions; and therefore is a dynamic and ever-changing process" (Kagawa Singer, 2012, p. 357). The shared health communication of tribal leaders and elders within American Indian communities are networks of cultural exchanges, ideas, and information. Health information shared via a trusted cultural network (i.e., American Indian tribal leaders and elders) builds on social capital concepts of normative and trust factors and are conceptualized as facilitators of action and cooperation for mutual benefit processes and also a facilitator of interpersonal cooperation (Putnam et al., 1993, p. 35). Stephens and colleagues further theorized that social capital concepts of norms and obligations, trust and social (cultural) networks and voluntary associations are proposed to serve primarily two functions in health communication: instrumental (material support) and affinity (social support) (Stephens et al., 2004). Culturally relevant information disseminated through trusted channel(s) and cultural networks of communication (tribal leaders and elders), connected to the tribe, traditions, and the infrastructure/group dynamics fulfill these functions and thus the viability of impactful health communication. These entities of trust and culture become networks or meta channels of health communication.

Cultural authority

Cultural authority, one that "defines reality and judgements of meaning and value will prevail as valid and true," and is a construction of reality. Cultural authority among American Indian tribal leaders and elders is embedded into the meaning making of communication about health and everyday lived experiences. Social authority, the type of authority that belongs to social actors and "involves the control of action through the giving of commands," (Starr, 1982, p. 13) is integral to lived experiences and also dialogs about health but, rests within the action of actors who are often outside of the culture. These actors have adopted a dominant approach and thus non-culture centric approach or view. Cultural authority juxtaposed to social authority, captures more appropriately naturally occurring cultural exchanges of health information among Native elders and leaders within their communities. While these programs have aided in mitigating some health disparities and reducing health information inequities among Indigenous populations, little is known about how American Indian tribal leader and elders perceive themselves as health communicators among their own people and how these narratives may inform culture-centric health communication and health promotion among American Indian populations.

Critical communication components in health programming (e.g., health literacy, health information seeking, social marketing) and identification of public health factors including environmental, social, epidemiological (downstream and upstream) are included however these programs are not fully integrated into holistic and culture-centric approaches targeting American Indian populations. Culturally appropriate health communication aimed to address diverse audiences strengthens the health communication process by infusing cultural beliefs and lived experiences to impact health behavior change and outcome. The primary goal is to create communication that is inclusive *of* and relevant *to* Native people. The primary purpose *then* of this study, was to explore how tribal leaders and elders perceived themselves as trusted entities of health communication and health promotion of disease prevention within their own communities. We also wanted to see how these perceptions informed a communicative infrastructure that addresses health communication inequities within these communities.

Given culturally tailored and targeted health communication approaches have shown as impactful among racial/ethnic minority populations (Kreuter & McClure, 2004; Rimer & Kreuter, 2006) and reflect a cultural-sensitive approach, it is a starting point (Dutta, 2018; Dutta & Basu, 2008). The centrality of opinions and perceptions among community American Indian tribal leader and elder perceptions as health communicators and promoters of disease prevention in culture-centered health communication was explored. We asked the following research question: *How do American Indian tribal community leaders/elders in urban and tribal communities from the Central Plains perceive themselves as health communicators and or health promoters of disease prevention?*

Materials and methods

Using a community-based participatory research (CBPR) approach, that involved community members from project conception to analysis, the research team set out to understand how tribal leaders perceive themselves as health communicators in their communities.

CBPR approaches continue to be more effective in American Indian communities than others, in part because the development of culturally appropriate programs is nearly impossible without the full participation of community members (Holkup et al., 2004; Whitewater et al., 2016). The team that conducted this research is composed of Native and non-Native members and represented what was at the time of this project, the Center for American Indian Community Health (CAICH) and the Center for American Indian Studies (CAIS).[1] CAICH and CAIS were the two founding centers of the not-for-profit American Indian Health Research and Education Alliance (AIHREA). AIHREA is a national organization dedicated to addressing health and educational disparities among Native peoples and in their communities. AIHREA's network of connections spans the United States and includes reservation, rural, and urban Indian communities, American Indian focused organizations, and academic institutions.

Semi-structured interview guides – Symbolic interactionism and CCA

Tailored and targeted health communication and health promotion to underserved populations involves understanding *how* audience or community members perceive, understand, and act on information. From within the community, those who recognize and understand the culture, may increase effectiveness. Tribal leaders and elders are from within the community and can provide a non-threatening viewpoint. In-depth interviews included a grounded theoretical process whereby the individuals' experiences helped guide researchers in understanding how tribal and elder communication can impact health communication and health promotion of disease prevention. Health behavior theory, historical trauma, and the concepts of culture, critical cultural communication, and social capital were also applied. Grounded theory draws from symbolic interactionism, a perspective that uses lived experiences and perceptions of the population as a lens to query or investigate a phenomenon (Denzin, 1992). Constructs from the health belief model (Janz & Becker, 1984; Rosenstock, 1966) and components from the Culture-Centered Approach (CCA) framework (Dutta, 2018) were included to account for American Indian Culture, individual perceptions, and beliefs about their own barriers to health, health promotion, and health communication. As a meta-theory, the CCA served as a guide to investigate tribal and community members' insights and views via these in-depth interviews. Through the CCA, investigators were able to analyze knowledge of health communication and promotion of disease prevention among tribal and community leaders and how this knowledge contributes to the communication infrastructure within their communities. Social capital concepts allowed for an exploration of perceptions and beliefs about community investment in health promotion efforts and what the tribal leader or elder thought about the tribal community and environment for health promotion and health communication of disease prevention.

A semi-structured interview guide was developed by the research team through an iterative process that ultimately resulted in the coverage of a variety of topic areas including perceptions of the health of the participant's community; health promotion messaging in the community; role and participation in health promotion; beliefs about health promotion;

messaging; attitudes related to the importance of cultural communication in American Indian communities; and demographics. Following KUMC Institutional Review Board approval (#00141131), a series of semi-structured, ethnographic interviews (N = 39), lasting between 30 and 100 minutes, were conducted in English and recorded by team members. Study staff also approached tribal council for study approval however it was determined that individuals participating in the project were representing themselves and their own views as health communicators and not as an official voice for their respective tribes.

Participants were self-identified American Indian individuals and leaders in their communities representing four tribal nations and two urban communities from the Central Plains (see Table 1) and were recruited via word-of-mouth through the AIHREA Community Advisory Board, our broader network of community partners, personal connections, and recruitment at AIHREA powows and other community events. Our definition of tribal leaders was understood broadly to include any community member that might be viewed as an authority figure by members of their own community on health and their community generally. Thus, participants included formally elected officials in Tribal government, community health workers, educators, youth program organizers, cultural revitalization directors, spiritual leaders, and elders. This flexibility captured a more comprehensive representation of leadership in American Indian communities and allowed for representation in urban communities as well. Participants also provided informed consent prior to their interview and received a $100 gift card for participation. Interviews were subsequently transcribed verbatim.

Transcriptions were analyzed using a grounded theory approach (Strauss & Corbin, 1990) an analysis method developed by researchers at CAICH (Daley et al., 2010) that included a team of four coders, representing both emic (within) and etic (outside) perspectives. The inclusion of emic and etic coders takes into consideration the differing experiences, backgrounds, and cultural contexts of our team members. Etic coders on our research team were researchers who have worked with American Indian populations and projects and emic researchers were from our American Indian staff and communities. Prior to formal analysis, these coders met, along with other members of the research team, to develop a codebook for analysis based upon preliminary review of the transcripts. This inductive codebook covered topic areas that included health, types of health communication programming, access to healthcare, modes of communication, and ideas about health promoters or communicators. Using this codebook, coders analyzed each stratum separately before comparing across strata, allowing thematic statements to emerge from the text. Each coder developed their own set of "pre-themes" and met, along with other members of the research team, to discuss their findings and develop the final set of themes. Disagreements among coders were resolved through consensus, taking into consideration both emic and etic perspectives of the data. The inclusion of the researcher perspective from outside the culture and American Indian within the culture was integral to capturing formative data. This data analysis process was followed to increase reliability and replicability for future studies and to limit bias. Although emic coders were paid staff from CAICH, these were trained coders who had participated in coding for several other AI studies. Further, the process will lay a foundation for how these tribal and elder leader perceptions may inform measurement of indigenous capacity and its role in cultural communication within these populations (Oetzel et al., 2011).

Table 1. In-depth interview demographics.

Central Plains Tribe (N = 39)	Gender	Age Group	Self-Identified Role*
Kansas, Iowa, Missouri and South Dakota Tribes and Communities	Female 51% Male 48%	25–34/ 3% 35–44/ 18% 45–54/ 28% 55+/ 38%	Tribal Government 20% Youth Outreach 5% Education 28% Healthcare/Social Services 28% Cultural Promotion 10% Religion/Spiritual/Traditional Teaching Leader 15% Other 2%

*Some Missing Data (Participants did not provide data and/or gave multiple answers in category).

Results

Most participants in the sample were women (51%) who were 45 years old or older (66%) (Table 1). Nearly 60% of participants were from reservation communities as opposed to non-reservation and urban communities (41%) in the Central Plains (Kansas, Missouri, Iowa, and South Dakota).

Overall, six themes emerged from the interviews and reached saturation across all demographic variables (see Table 2). No unique themes within demographic categories reached saturation.

Participants Infrequently Recognized Themselves as Health Communicators and Promoters. Despite being identified by the research team and their fellow community members as eligible participants, interviewees often did not think of themselves as health communicators and promoters within their communities. Participants had a variety of backgrounds including community health workers, educators, and tribal officials serving in administrative and political positions. Notably, spirituality was a sub-theme and thus component that some participants saw as central to health and wellness communication and as a characteristic that leaders in Native communities should possess.

"Culturally I think that . . . spiritually we need to connect to the environment. We need to connect to the, you know, things that we do with the trees and the plants and make sure that everything that we're eating is safe, good soil health. I'm doing some training on that too."

"You have to have folks who are known in the community to be a spiritual leader," another participant explained, "it can't be someone who is a spiritual leader once in a while."

Other participants mentioned specific spiritual leaders within the tribe and the critical role that this individual had in disseminating health messages within the tribe.

"You know, a lot of us believe in traditional ways. And I think there should be some kind of support from the tribe for our medicine men. To go around and have ceremonies for

Table 2. Focus group themes.

1. *Participants infrequently recognized themselves as health promoters*
2. *Health promoters should be viewed as people who "practice what they preach"*
3. *Programs focusing on youth could affect entire households*
4. *Transportation to and from healthcare providers is the most significant barrier to receiving healthcare and health information*
5. The majority of health programs focus on diabetes or obesity while *mental health programming is still needed*
6. *Some degree of cultural tailoring is important for health communication programs in American Indian communities*

the families that want it from the medicine man, you know. I think it would be great to do something like that for us. Especially us elderly who believe our way, you know? Our way brought us, thousands of years up to this point and I don't see nothing wrong with it."

Spiritual positions (e.g., medicine man) that tribal members recognized as possessing significant authority within respective communities were compartmentalized as those who had cultural authority in the areas of health and wellness. Participants self-identified (see Table 1) as community health worker, educator, tribal official but did not self-identify as a spiritual authority although these narratives were woven into their conversation about communicating disease prevention.

The other most frequently identified communicator and promoter of health in these communities were the Indian Health Service and contract health providers. Participants also identified representatives from nonprofit organizations, urban Indian centers, as well as community elders as potentially effective health communicators and promoters. Most importantly, it was agreed that any health promoter must have broad notoriety in their communities and that health efforts should begin with tribal leadership.

"These initiatives should start with the tribal chairman and the [tribal] council members who are aware of the avenues that we need to take to improve our health."

"My community expands in such a way that most of my interactions are coming with tribal leaders across our region so I talk about health disparities and health issues as a part of my job all the time. . . .so it's an ongoing discussion, fundamentally, I think we've been missing the conversations with the right people."

The recognition of *other* leaders in the community as having the authority to speak about health and act as a health communicator or promoter points to participants' perceptions about their authority and others. The participants' collective identification of individuals with specific medical positions, roles, and affiliations were perceived to be those who would and could successfully fulfill and execute the role of a health communicator or health promoter. The defined and specific role of a health communicator and/or health promoter personally was perceived to be outside the scope of who they were, and the authority held within the community.

Health Communicators/Promoters Should be Viewed as People Who "Practice What They Preach." A central concern for many participants was the perceptions of health communicators and promoters in their communities. While they agreed that certain community members, by virtue of their position in the community, would make better health communicators and promoters than others, it was clear that these individuals must also participate in the practices that they themselves are promoting to be taken seriously. While reflecting on how they saw themselves as a community health communicator and/or promoter, participants expressed the importance of being a representation of what you teach and preach.

"I think you need to live that lifestyle if that's what you believe in [and] promote."

Another explained that health promoters needed to lead by example and that this should factor into who qualifies for this role.

"I think that I need to try and practice what I preach, live that lifestyle and live that way. You know people like to criticize you if you're saying you shouldn't drink, you shouldn't smoke and then you turn around and do it yourself. I think you need to live that lifestyle if that's what you believe in what you promote . . . .so that's what I try to do."

A second participant echoed these sentiments.

"I think everybody's got a role in that (health promotion). Um, but again, it's kind of, you kind of have to lead by example. Everybody's got a role, but do they take that role? Do they know, are we – what are they doing for themselves? Ultimately, it's gotta be, you have to find those people that um, aren't doing it for themselves . . . because they want to, not because they're pushed, and try and get all of them involved and come with a plan."

A participant from another tribe reflected on the need and importance of being more involved in these health communication roles.

"I think like if our tribal leaders started being more active in the community and regaining the trust and the sense of community perhaps we could become you know, healthier as a unit and maybe if they took the lead or if they wanted to be invited maybe in some of our group chats, that you know like the cancer survivors have, then maybe they (community) would buy into it."

Participants' reflections here also echo the theme of *who* and *what* constitutes an authority figure as a health promotor and health communicator but also the importance of this individual's role. Here, the qualification and thus authenticity of living a life that represents the role of a health communicator or promoter is paramount. The leadership position role, and duties that these individuals have are often unspoken, nonverbal and are also important in the verbal process of health promotion and health communication.

Programs Focusing on Youth Could Affect Entire Households. Highlighting the importance of youth in many American Indian communities, interview participants suggested that mobilizing the power of youth in their communities to promote healthy living could be an effective strategy.

"Involve the youth and then the parents will come along, and then maybe even have some activities for the whole family."

Another participant spoke of the busyness of life and how this should be minimized to increase involvement among youth.

"We see some participation with the younger people, but the problem we have today is everybody is so busy with school activities and activities outside the Native community, that we don't have the participation with the younger people that we need and um that's one of the issues that we are trying to improve with."

A third participant spoke of the need for youth involvement and their impact however the challenges of getting youth involved.

"We are doing everything we can to get younger folks involved, get on the board of directors, you know anything we can do to get them involved. And it's difficult. It's really difficult to get younger people involved in leadership training."

Participants' identification of youth within their community signals a need to fill a gap in the health promotion and health communication process. Youth were identified as a missing link in communicating health to the parent and an ally in communicating health. Compared to the specific leaders within the community who were identified as having medical and cultural authority to serve as health promoters and communicators at the community level, youth were perceived as viable channels of communication at the local and familial levels. The inclusion of youth was also seen as a beneficial option to diversify health communicators and broaden the distribution of health information.

Transportation to and from Healthcare Providers is the Most Significant Barrier to Receiving Healthcare and Health Information. While an overall lack of healthcare providers continues to be a concern, access to reliable transportation to these services was a key barrier identified by participants. Interviewees living in both reservation and urban communities expressed concern about accessibility to healthcare and health education programming. Particularly for elderly community members, securing transportation, including funds to cover fuel costs, limits the reach of healthcare and health education programming in many American Indian communities.

"We have to drive about 47 miles to commute to get our medicine," one community member noted.

Another urban community member explained that the scarcity of Indian Health Service clinics required her to drive more than a hundred miles to receive care, illustrating that access to care is not solely an issue for reservation communities, but urban communities as well.

"Since we're urban we don't have any Indian Health clinics which would be nice. We do have AIHREA where we have check-ups at the powwow where you can get your blood checked, your weight, your breathing ... Then we have (a) mental health counselor, but we only have one in XX area. And then of course our nearest Indian Health service is in XX which is like 130 away."

Another participant suggested that the need was so severe that it necessitated outside assistance for basic transportation needs. "Some kind of program to help us with fuel ... and car repairs or anything like that to get us to where we have to go to see the doctor."

The prevalence of transportation barriers and limited number of health care providers among participants represents the overwhelming need for assistance but also speaks to missing communication components that contribute to a void in societal structures that reinforce inequity. Advocacy through health communication and health promotion points to identifying barriers and opportunities to positively change and impact health outcome on societal and systemic levels. The community's involvement and experiences help to inform the communication infrastructure and mitigate communication gaps and inequities between actors such as community members, community leaders, and policy makers.

The Majority of Health Programs Focus on Diabetes or Obesity While Mental Health Programming is Still Needed. Overall, participants explained that the health programming in their communities tend to focus on the prevalence of diabetes and obesity.

"We do have programs that bring about awareness and give you knowledge about what your diet should be and how you should eat, how you should exercise," one female participant explained when discussing the programs available in her community.

Another participant recalled a similar emphasis on this type of health programming. "Maybe in the last ten years there's been more of an initiative to do preventive type [programs] like with the diabetes program and weight programs."

However, participants noted that mental health programming and services were the areas most in need of attention in their communities. Recalling an earlier discussion about accessibility issues, one female community member explained the dire need for mental health services.

"We need the suicide prevention program; we need a facility here."

Another suggested programming specifically to deal with the impact of losing someone from mental health. "The trauma that a person goes through [when someone they know passes away]."

A female participant from one of the reservations spoke about the need also for programs that were culturally responsive. "I know a lot of clients or the patients you know just from personal knowledge, from them, just talking to them, they don't like some of the places that they get referred out to. Maybe that culturally relevant mental health aspect would be something that they would be more open to cause you know, there is a lot of stigma with mental health."

Similar to participants' identification of characteristics and the *type* of health communication leader; structural and societal factors are potential barriers to health promotion and communication among American Indians. The topic of mental health is seen as a top health priority among these participants. Cultural tailoring and targeting efforts from dominant communication efforts have brought diabetes and obesity to the forefront; participants' reflections point to the prevalence of mental health issues within the community and personally speak to their perceptions of the urgency when compared to other health topics deemed priority. This underscores the evolving landscape of communication and dosage of information that individuals, communities, and other entities deem culturally relevant, appropriate, or critical at different time points.

Some Degree of Cultural Tailoring is Important for Health Communication Programs in American Indian Communities. When asked about the content of programming designed to be used in American Indian communities, interview participants strongly encouraged future programs to be culturally tailored at least to some degree. They explained that it is particularly important for these programs to draw on and organize themselves around cultural values, languages, and spiritual traditions from the Native communities in which they will be implemented.

"When you're dealing with Native people, you have to respect ... these values ... and I think that you should probably know some of the language," one woman from a reservation explained.

One man expressed similar ideas. "Whoever does go and spread the [health] message, they definitely need to be culturally aware of the way that Native American people are."

To account for the rich diversity of tribal nations represented in many urban communities, urban community members suggested that health (communication/promotion) programming should not be as tribally specific in their communities.

"I think just a little, just enough to make it feel like it's for them without getting bogged down in too much detail because the variation is just too wide in [this] community."

This final theme that captures participants' opinions about cultural tailoring and how they believe that it should work also points to appropriate dosage of health information detail but also points to the limitations of cultural tailoring. Participant experiences with cultural tailoring here show that they are *familiar* with the process and that it involves specific steps. Cultural inclusion by way of engaging community members in the communication process and including characteristics of the culture is expected and should be expanded. Participant expressions represent a continuum of health communication and health promotion that is reflective of what is needed beyond cultural tailoring to appropriately reach American Indian communities from one tribe or many through a culturally centered process.

Discussion

To our knowledge this is one of the first research projects that explores how American Indian tribal leaders and elders perceive themselves as health communicators and/or health promoters in their tribal communities. These exploratory interviews with tribal leaders and elders from Native communities in the Central Plains yield important lived experiences that highlight and suggest new strategies for employing American Indian populations in the health communication process of disease prevention. While participants infrequently identified themselves as "authorities" of health promotion and communication, they did see themselves as gatekeepers in at least some capacities and knowledgeable about *who* or *what* community agencies and entities were important and trusted to disseminate pertinent health information. This recalls differential notions of perceived authority of medical practitioners delineated by sociologist Starr (1982). He argues that medical authority can be broken down into different types, social and cultural, based on the context of their authorization. Specifically, Starr suggests that social authority is established through organizational certification or executive means. Individuals and entities in these positions (the Indian Health Service and elected tribal officials, for instance) were those who participants identified as potential communicators of health information and health promoters, generally. Starr further characterizes those possessing cultural authority as being granted through community consent because of shared cultural values and practices (Pescosolido & Martin, 2004; Pippin, 1996; Starr, 1982). Individuals and institutions with this kind of authority were often mentioned by participants when discussing who "practices what they preach." The relationship between these two types of authoritative figures and institutions suggests that effective health promotion and communication programming in American Indian communities must mobilize both types of authority to be successful.

Emphasizing the importance of longstanding relationships with Native communities coupled with a working knowledge of perceptions of authority figures within the communities in question, stresses the importance of CBPR approaches in health communication, promotion, and culture-centered research with Native communities. These findings suggest that health communication and health promotions programming among American Indians would be most effective when it is sanctioned and disseminated by community partners possessing social authority, while also prioritizing individuals with cultural authority (e.g., medicine man, tribal council member) as examples of fellow community members who "practice what they preach." Further, these findings reflect the need for culture centeredness in the health communication processes and inclusion of indigenous knowledge (Belone et al., 2016). The role of spirituality also was a sub-theme and part of participant expressions of what characteristics health communicators in Native communities possessed. Those within the Native community that held cultural authority to disseminate health information were characterized as not only spiritual but as individuals who practiced what they preached. Participants saw others in the community as spiritual leaders but self-identified themselves as community members who fulfilled traditional roles within their respective communities. Study staff identified participants as leaders; however, participants most likely did not see themselves as the "authority" on health communication because of perceptions about possessing authority (social or cultural). The perceptions might also point to Native culture that de-emphasizes centralized leadership, power, and authority (Bryant, 1998) and emphasizes collectivism.

Health communication messaging disseminated through shared processes and trusted-network sources is plausible and feasible to overcome mistrust of the medical establishment, address levels of historical trauma and other health-related issues among American Indian community members. Culturally appropriate channels of health communication are positioned as critical purveyors of health information that impact community health and health behavior (Gearhart & Trumbly-Lamsam, 2017). Modern medicine limits medical encounters (Pippin, 1996) while American Indian populations emphasize and describe medical problems "related to their own bodies and lives without the medical references or language to assist in facilitating the interaction," (Kalbfleisch, 2009). Employing American Indian messengers in the capacity described above is important in establishing trust and increasing the veracity of the message. The identification of specific types of health topics to prioritize (mental health), engagement of under-utilized voices (youth) and barriers (transportation) also signaled critical components in the role of health communication of disease prevention. The inclusion or absence of these factors among American Indians may bolster or dilute important health communication.

The CCA in particular served as a central part of the framework to guide our understanding of how these tribal and elder leaders saw themselves as health communicators within their communities, As a meta-theoretical framework, in-depth interviews with participants allowed an exploration of the existing communication infrastructure within these communities and opportunities to address dominant communication structures that may compete, dilute, or even block authentic indigenous knowledge and voices. These findings are central to cultural grounding within American Indian experience and important for cultural validation of (indigenous) community capacity for American Indian communication (Oetzel et al., 2011)

Linkage or adoption of other health communication strategies conducted among other racial/ethnic groups also provide a guide to centralize culture in interventions and programming. Community Health Workers (CHWs), also referred to as promotora/os among Latinx and immigrant populations have shown essential in addressing disease prevention programs and health outcome. Within other cultural groups, trusted community members and leaders also are positioned to promote and communicate disease prevention and impact health outcome (Han et al., 2017; Santos et al., 2017). While racial/ethnic groups in the U.S. share similar cultural values, the process for defining culture in the experiences of the population and determination for health information shared within a community's trusted cultural network will differ. Strategic positioning of culturally responsive health communication and health promotion among American Indian populations is dependent on intended and intentional senders, messages, and recipients rather than predetermined components minimally informed by culture. Culturally grounded interventions that centralize community engagement and also indigenous knowledge may lead to culturally valid communication programs and (messages) products (Walters et al., 2020)

Some of the limitations of the study were that CAICH interviewers, the majority of who were from tribal communities and part of the research team, were familiar and knew some of the interviewees through previous research and community activities. This could have primed interviewees and or limited transparency however, following a CBPR process the goal is to work intimately with the community and incorporate community members into every phase of the research process (Israel et al., 2001). The sampling also was purposive and may not have included additional individuals who were considered leaders in the community such as representatives from the Indian Health Service and other agency interviewees named in data collection. Interviews also significantly varied in length where some were completed in 30 minutes while others were more than 90 minutes. The consensus of some of the data may have been overrepresented in certain parts of the Central Plains areas, however, data saturation was achieved.

Implications of this research can help shape and bolster health communication and health promotion program planning processes of development, execution, and evaluation on multiple levels, particularly when including tribal leader and elder perspectives. This is an opportunity for health communication and promotion professionals and researchers to more fully integrate American Indian tradition and trust of tribal elders and leaders into the health communication strategies that inform practice and program intervention research among this population at individual, organizational, community, and societal levels (Dickerson et al., 2020; Hicks et al., 2012; Walters et al., 2020). Health communication programs and evidence-based research that are inclusive of culture in addition to trusted sources of health communication and information is an avenue to achieve culturally appropriate approaches and communication that resonate with American Indians about disease prevention.

There are 574 federally recognized American Indian and Alaska Native tribes (Saenz, 2020); this culture-centered approach is comprehensive and responsive to include tribe-specific targeting (American Indians nationally) or tailoring (tribe-specific) health communication where culture, values and language of elders and tribal leaders are infused into health communication messages and programming. Efforts with the Centers for Disease Prevention & Control (CDC) are examples of national initiatives to incorporate culture into health promotion among American Indians. The CDC's National Center for Chronic Disease Prevention and Health Promotion (NCCDPHP) was tasked to include Indigenous experience and knowledge into its process to build culturally responsive interventions (Lawrence & James, 2019). Those sessions included listening to tribal health leaders and visiting tribal organizations and other tribal areas. The Good Health and Wellness in Indian Country (GHWIC) program is centered on the knowledge of the community to help guide healthy living and chronic disease prevention (Williams et al., 2019). Inclusion of tribal leader and elder perspectives and lived experiences into health communication initiatives and programs has potential to increase cultural relevance in regional and local disease prevention strategies/programs targeting American Indian populations. Nationally, The National Congress for American Indians also (National Congress of American Indians, 2020) recognizes the importance of effective communication among tribes and created its own communication resource to facilitate effective health communication among tribes across the country. Tribal Communication officers representing tribes throughout the nation were interviewed about messaging, outreach, engaging with media to identify ways to effectively communicate and advocate for Native people. Communication goals and efforts are to further the success of tribal nations through these tactics and create opportunities for policy change through health and media advocacy.

The present study was a beginning to explore how regional tribal leaders and elders in the Central Plains perceived themselves as health promoters and health communicators in their communities. Additional research that explores perceptions among tribal and community members may provide additional insight and a comparison to how community members think of health communication via these trusted leaders. Formative research then can serve to test the effectiveness of cultural-centered tribal and elder health communication compared to other tailored and targeted or culture-sensitive health communication. Strategies inclusive of these elements are well positioned to capture and reflect American Indian cultures and help reduce disease burden among American Indian populations.

Note

1. The research teams and centers have combined and transitioned to a new university and is now known as the Institute for Indigenous Studies at Lehigh University in Bethlehem, PA.

Acknowledgments

The authors would also like to thank the tribal communities for their contributions to this study.

Disclosure statement

No potential conflict of interest was reported by the author(s).

Funding

This study was supported by a CTSA grant from NCATS awarded to the University of Kansas for Frontiers: University of Kansas Clinical Translation Science Institute [#UL1TR002366].

ORCID

Crystal Y. Lumpkins http://orcid.org/0000-0003-0963-0706

References

Administration for Children and Families. (2020). *Trauma: What is historical trauma?* www.acf.hhs.gov/trauma-toolkit/trauma-concept

Allicock, M., Campbell, M. K., & Walsh, J. (2011). Tailoring health interventions: An approach for working with African American churches to reduce cancer health disparities. In A. Lemelle., W. Reed., & S. Taylor (Eds.), *Handbook of African American health* (pp. 235–251). Springer. https://doi.org/10.1007/978-1-4419-9616-9_16

Baezconde-Garbanati, L. A., Chatterjee, J. S., Frank, L. B., Murphy, S. T., Moran, M. B., Werth, L. N., Zhao, N., Amezola de Herrera, P., Mayer, D., Kagan, J., & O'Brien, D. (2014). Tamale lesson: A case study of a narrative health communication intervention. *Journal of Communication in Healthcare*, *7*(2), 82–92. https://doi.org/10.1179/1753807614Y.0000000055

Baker, R. (1999). Minority distrust of medicine: A historical perspective. *Mount Sinai Journal of Medicine*, *66*(4), 212–222. PMID: 10477472.

Beal, A. C. (2011). High-quality health care: The essential route to eliminating disparities and achieving health equity. *Health Affairs (Millwood)*, *30*(10), 1868–1871. https://doi.org/10.1377/hlthaff.2011.0976

Belone, L., Tosa, J., Shendo, K., Toya, A., Straits, K., Tafoya, G., Rae, R., Noyes, E., Bird, D., & Wallerstein, N. (2016). Community-based participatory research for cocreating interventions with Native communities: A partnership between the University of New Mexico and the Pueblo of Jemez. In N. Zane, G. Bernal, & F. T. L. Leong (Eds.), *Evidence-based psychological practice with ethnic minorities: Culturally informed research and clinical strategies* (pp. 199–220). American Psychological Association. https://doi.org/10.1037/14940-010

Bopp, M., Baruth, M., Peterson, J. A., & Webb, B. L. (2013). Leading their flocks to health? Clergy health and the role of clergy in faith-based health promotion interventions. *Family & Community Health*, *36*(3), 182–192. https://doi.org/10.1097/FCH.0b013e31828e671c

Brave Heart, M. L., & DeBruyn, L. M. (1998). The American Indian holocaust: Healing historical unresolved grief. *American Indian and Alaska Native Mental Health Research*, *8*(2), 56–78. PMID: 9842066.

Brave Heart, M. L. (1998). The return to the sacred path: Healing the historical trauma and historical unresolved grief response among the Lakota through a psychoeducational group intervention. *Smith College Studies in Social Work*, *68*(3), 287–305. https://doi.org/10.1080/00377319517532

Brave Heart, M. L. (2003). The historical trauma response among Natives and its relationship with substance abuse: A Lakota illustration. *Journal of Psychoactive Drugs*, *35*(1), 7–13. https://doi.org/10.1080/02791072.2003.10399988

Briant, K. J., Sanchez, J. I., Ibarra, G., Escareño, M., Gonzalez, N. E., Jimenez Gonzalez, V., Marchello, N., Louie, S., & Thompson, B. (2018). Using a culturally tailored intervention to increase colorectal cancer knowledge and screening among Hispanics in a rural community. *Cancer Epidemiology, Biomarkers & Prevention: A Publication of the American Association for Cancer Research, Cosponsored by the American Society of Preventive Oncology*, *27*(11), 1283–1288. https://doi.org/10.1158/1055-9965.EPI-17-1092

Bryant, M. T. (1998). Cross-cultural understandings of leadership: Themes from Native American interviews. *Educational Management & Administration*, *26*(1), 7–20. https://doi.org/10.1177/0263211x98261002

Butler-Ajibade, P., Booth, W., & Burwell, C. (2012). Partnering with the Black church: Recipe for promoting heart health in the stroke belt. *Association of Black Nursing Faculty (ABNF), Inc. Journal*, *23*(2), 34–37. https://ezproxy.jocolibrary.org/login?url=https://search.ebscohost.com/login.aspx?direct=true&db=c9h&AN=75297974&site=ehost-live&scope=site

Campbell, M. K., Hudson, M. A., Resnicow, K., Blakeney, N., Paxton, A., & Baskin, M. (2007). Church-based health promotion interventions: Evidence and lessons learned. *Annual Review of Public Health*, *28*, 213–234. https://doi.org/10.1146/annurev.publhealth.28.021406.144016

Centers for Disease Control. (2020). *Underlying Cause of Death 1999–2019*. CDC Wonder. http://wonder.cdc.gov/ucd-icd10.html

Colclough, Y. Y., & Brown, G. M. (2014). End-of-life treatment decision making: American Indians' perspective. *American Journal of Hospice and Palliative Medicine*, *31*(5), 503–512. https://doi.org/10.1177/1049909113489592

Cook, L. S., & de Mange, B. P. (1995). Gaining access to Native American cultures by Non-Native American nursing researchers. *Nursing Forum*, *30*(1), 5–10. https://doi.org/10.1111/j.1744-6198.1995.tb01277.x

Corbie-Smith, G., Flagg, E. W., Doyle, J. P., & O'Brien, M. A. (2002). Influence of usual source of care on differences by race/ethnicity in receipt of preventive services. *Journal of General Internal Medicine*, *17*(6), 458–464. https://doi.org/10.1046/j.1525-1497.2002.10733.x

Corbie-Smith, G., Hoover, S. M., & Dave, G. (2019). Connecting dots to bridge the health disparities gap: Implementation of a scalable electronic medical record-integrated community referral intervention at the clinic visit. *American Journal of Public Health*, *109*(4), 531–533. https://doi.org/10.2105/AJPH.2019.304993

Corbie-Smith, G., Thomas, S. B., & St George, D. M. (2002). Distrust, race, and research. *Archives of Internal Medicine*, *162*(21), 2458–2463. https://doi.org/10.1001/archinte.162.21.2458

Daley, C. M., James, A. S., Ulrey, E., Joseph, S., Talawyma, A., Choi, W. S., Greiner, K. A., & Coe, M. K. (2010). Using focus groups in community-based participatory research: Challenges and resolutions. *Qualitative Health Research*, *20*(5), 697–706. https://doi.org/10.1177/1049732310361468

Danieli, Y. (1998). *International handbook of multigenerational legacies of trauma*. Plenum Press.

DeHaven, M. J., Hunter, I. B., Wilder, L., Walton, J. W., & Berry, J. (2004). Health programs in faith-based organizations: Are they effective? *American Journal of Public Health*, *94*(6), 1030–1036. https://doi.org/10.2105/ajph.94.6.1030

Denham, A. R. (2008). Rethinking historical trauma: Narratives of resilience. *Transcultural Psychiatry*, *45*(3), 391–414. https://doi.org/10.1177/1363461508094673

Denzin, N. K. (1992). *Symbolic interactionism and cultural studies: The politics of interpretation*. Blackwell. https://search.library.wisc.edu/catalog/999706178102121

Dickerson, D., Baldwin, J. A., Belcourt, A., Belone, L., Gittelsohn, J., Keawe'aimoku Kaholokula, J., Lowe, J., Patten, C. A., & Wallerstein, N. (2020). Encompassing cultural contexts within scientific research methodologies in the development of health promotion interventions. *Prevention Science*, *21*(1), 33–42. https://doi.org/10.1007/s11121-018-0926-1

Duran, E., & Duran, B. (1995). *Native American postcolonial psychology*. State University of New York (SUNY) Press.

Dutta-Bergman, M. J. (2005). Theory and practice in health communication campaigns: A critical interrogation. *Health Communication*, *18*(2), 103–122. https://doi.org/10.1207/s15327027hc1802_1

Dutta, M. J., & Basu, A. (2008). Meanings of health: Interrogating structure and culture. *Health Communication*, *23*(6), 560–572. https://doi.org/10.1080/10410230802465266

Dutta, M. J. (2018). Culture-centered approach in addressing health disparities: Communication infrastructures for subaltern voices. *Communication Methods and Measures*, *12*(4), 239–259. https://doi.org/10.1080/19312458.2018.1453057

Espey, D. K., Jim, M. A., Cobb, N., Bartholomew, M., Becker, T., Haverkamp, D., & Plescia, M. (2014). Leading causes of death and all-cause mortality in American Indians and Alaska Natives. *American Journal of Public Health*, *104*(S3), S303–S311. https://doi.org/10.2105/AJPH.2013.301798

Evans-Campbell, T. (2008). Historical trauma in American Indian/Native Alaska communities: A multilevel framework for exploring impacts on individuals, families, and communities. *Journal of Interpersonal Violence*, *23*(3), 316–338. https://doi.org/10.1177/0886260507312290

Figley, C. R. (Ed.). (1995). *Compassion fatigue: Coping with secondary traumatic stress disorder in those who treat the traumatized*. Brunner/Mazel.

Geana, M. V., Greiner, K. A., Cully, A., Talawyma, M., & Daley, C. M. (2012). Improving health promotion to American Indians in the Midwest United States: Preferred sources of health information and its use for the medical encounter. *Journal of Community Health*, *37*(6), 1253–1263. https://doi.org/10.1007/s10900-012-9564-x

Gearhart, S., & Trumbly-Lamsam, T. (2017). The scoop on health: How Native American newspapers frame and report health news. *Health Communication*, *32*(6), 695–702. https://doi.org/10.1080/10410236.2016.1168001

Giri, V. N., Selvan, P., Mohanty, S., Lum, R., Serrao, S., & Leader, A. E. (2020). Exploring Asian Indian views about cancer and participation in cancer research: An evaluation of a culturally tailored educational intervention. *Journal of Community Genetics*, *11*(2), 193–203. https://doi.org/10.1007/s12687-019-00436-5

Han, H. R., Song, Y., Kim, M., Hedlin, H. K., Kim, K., Ben Lee, H., & Roter, D. (2017). Breast and cervical cancer screening literacy among Korean American women: A community health worker-led intervention. *American Journal of Public Health*, *107*(1), 159–165. https://doi.org/10.2105/ajph.2016.303522

Heaton, B., Gebel, C., Crawford, A., Barker, J. C., Henshaw, M., Garcia, R. I., Riedy, C., & Wimsatt, M. A. (2018). Using storytelling to address oral health knowledge in American Indian and Alaska Native communities. *Preventing Chronic Disease*, *15*, E63. https://doi.org/10.5888/pcd15.170305

Heckert, W., & Eisenhauer, C. (2014). A case report of historical trauma among American Indians on a rural Northern Plains reservation. *Journal of Forensic Nursing*, *10*(2), 106–109. https://doi.org/10.1097/jfn.0000000000000028

Heron, M. (2013). Deaths: Leading causes for 2010. *National Vital Statistics Reports*, *62*(6), 1–97.

Hicks, S., Duran, B., Wallerstein, N., Avila, M., Belone, L., Lucero, J., Magarati, M., Mainer, E., Martin, D., Muhammad, M., Oetzel, J., Pearson, C., Sahota, P., Simonds, V., Sussman, A., Tafoya, G., & Hat, E. W. (2012). Evaluating community-based participatory research to improve community-partnered science and community health. *Progress in Community Health Partnerships: Research, Education, and Action*, *6*(3), 289–299. https://doi.org/10.1353/cpr.2012.0049

Hinnant, A., Subramanian, R., Ashley, R. R., Perreault, M., Young, R., & Thomas, R. J. (2019). How journalists characterize health inequalities and redefine solutions for Native American audiences. *Health Communication*, *34*(4), 383–391. https://doi.org/10.1080/10410236.2017.1405482

Hodge, F. S., Pasqua, A., Marquez, C. A., & Geishirt-Cantrell, B. (2002). Utilizing traditional storytelling to promote wellness in American Indian communities. *Journal of Transcultural Nursing: Official Journal of the Transcultural Nursing Society*, *13*(1), 6–11. https://doi.org/10.1177/104365960201300102

Hodge, F., Weinmann, S., & Roubideaux, Y. (2000). Recruitment of American Indians and Alaska Natives into clinical trials. *Annals of Epidemiology*, *10*(8 Suppl), S41–S48. https://doi.org/10.1016/s1047-2797(00)00196-4

Holkup, P. A., Tripp-Reimer, T., Salois, E. M., & Weinert, C. (2004). Community-based participatory research: An approach to intervention research with a Native American community. *Advances in Nursing Science*, *27*(3), 162–175. https://doi.org/10.1097/00012272-200407000-00002

Huerta, E. E., & Macario, E. (1999). Communicating health risk to ethnic groups: Reaching Hispanics as a case study. *Journal of the National Cancer Institute (JNCI) Monographs*, *1999*(25), 23–26. https://doi.org/10.1093/oxfordjournals.jncimonographs.a024202

Indian Health Service. (2015). *Disparities*. https://www.ihs.gov/newsroom/factsheets/disparities/

Israel, B. A., Schulz, A. J., Parker, E. A., & Becker, A. B. (2001). Community-based participatory research: Policy recommendations for promoting a partnership approach in health research. *Education for Health (Abingdon)*, *14*(2), 182–197. https://doi.org/10.1080/13576280110051055

Jacobs-Wingo, J. L., Espey, D. K., Groom, A. V., Phillips, L. E., Haverkamp, D. S., & Stanley, S. L. (2016). Causes and disparities in death rates among urban American Indian and Alaska Native populations, 1999–2009. *American Journal of Public Health*, *106*(5), 906–914. https://doi.org/10.2105/ajph.2015.303033

Janz, N. K., & Becker, M. H. (1984). The health belief model: A decade later. *Health Education Quarterly*, *11*(1), 1–47. https://doi.org/10.1177/109019818401100101

Ka'opua, L. S. I., Park, S. H., Ward, M. E., & Braun, K. L. (2011). Testing the feasibility of a culturally tailored breast cancer screening intervention with Native Hawaiian women in rural churches. *Health & Social Work*, *36*(1), 55–65. https://doi.org/10.1093/hsw/36.1.55

Kagawa Singer, M. (2012). Applying the concept of culture to reduce health disparities through health behavior research. *Preventive Medicine*, *55*(5), 356–361. https://doi.org/10.1016/j.ypmed.2012.02.011

Kagawa-Singer, M., & Kassim-Lakha, S. (2003). A strategy to reduce cross-cultural miscommunication and increase the likelihood of improving health outcomes. *Academic Medicine*, *78*(6), 577–587. https://doi.org/10.1097/00001888-200306000-00006

Kalbfleisch, P. J. (2009). Effective health communication in Native populations in North America. *Journal of Language and Social Psychology*, *28* (2), 158–173. https://doi.org/10.1177/0261927X08330607

Kreps, G. L., & Neuhauser, L. (2015). Designing health information programs to promote the health and well-being of vulnerable populations: The benefits of evidence-based strategic health communication. In C. Arnott Smith & A. Keselman (Eds.), *Meeting health information needs outside of healthcare* (pp. 3–17). Chandos Publishing. https://doi.org/10.1016/B978-0-08-100248-3.00001-9

Kreps, G. L., & Sparks, L. (2008). Meeting the health literacy needs of immigrant populations. *Patient Education and Counseling*, *71*(3), 328–332. https://doi.org/10.1016/j.pec.2008.03.001

Kreuter, M. W., Lukwago, S. N., Bucholtz, D. C., Clark, E. M., & Sanders-Thompson, V. (2003). Achieving cultural appropriateness in health promotion programs: Targeted and tailored approaches. *Health Education & Behavior*, *30*(2), 133–146. https://doi.org/10.1177/1090198102251021

Kreuter, M. W., & McClure, S. (2004). The role of culture in health communication. *Annual Review of Public Health*, *25*, 439–455. https://doi.org/10.1146/annurev.publhealth.25.101802

Kreuter, M. W., & Wray, R. J. (2003). Tailored and targeted health communication: Strategies for enhancing information relevance. *American Journal of Health Behavior*, *27*(Suppl 3), S227–S232. https://doi.org/10.5993/ajhb.27.1.s3.6

Kunitz, S. J. (2006). Life-course observations of alcohol use among Navajo Indians: Natural history or careers? *Medical Anthropology Quarterly*, *20* (3), 279–296. https://doi.org/10.1525/maq.2006.20.3.279

Larkey, L. K., & Hecht, M. (2010). A model of effects of narrative as culture-centric health promotion. *Journal of Health Communication*, *15*(2), 114–135. https://doi.org/10.1080/10810730903528017

Lawrence, T. J., & James, R. D. (2019). Good health and wellness: Measuring impact through an indigenous lens. *Preventing Chronic Disease*, *16*, E108. https://doi.org/10.5888/pcd16.180655

LeMaster, P. L., & Connell, C. M. (1994). Health education interventions among Native Americans: A review and analysis. *Health Education Quarterly*, *21*(4), 521–538. https://doi.org/10.1177/109019819402100413

Lumpkins, C. Y., Greiner, K. A., Daley, C., Mabachi, N. M., & Neuhaus, K. (2013). Promoting healthy behavior from the pulpit: Clergy share their perspectives on effective health communication in the African American church. *Journal of Religion and Health*, *52*(4), 1093–1107. https://doi.org/10.1007/s10943-011-9533-1

Lumpkins, C. Y., Vanchy, P., Baker, T. A., Daley, C., Ndikum-Moffer, F., & Greiner, K. A. (2016). Marketing a healthy mind, body, and soul: An analysis of how African American men view the church as a social marketer and health promoter of colorectal cancer risk and prevention. *Health Education & Behavior*, *43*(4), 452–460. https://doi.org/10.1177/1090198115604615

McGuire, W. J. (1981). Behavioral medicine, public health, and communication theories. *Health Education*, *12*(3), 8–13. https://doi.org/10.1080/00970050.1981.10618148

McNeill, L. H., Reitzel, L. R., Escoto, K. H., Roberson, C. L., Nguyen, N., Vidrine, J. I., Strong, L. L., & Wetter, D. W. (2018). Engaging Black churches to address cancer health disparities: Project CHURCH. *Frontiers in Public Health*, *6*(191). https://doi.org/10.3389/fpubh.2018.00191

Mello, M. M., & Wolf, L. E. (2010). The Havasupai Indian tribe case: Lessons for research involving stored biologic samples. *New England Journal of Medicine*, *363*(3), 204–207. https://doi.org/10.1056/NEJMp1005203

Mohatt, N. V., Thompson, A. B., Thai, N. D., & Tebes, J. K. (2014). Historical trauma as public narrative: A conceptual review of how history impacts present-day health. *Social Science & Medicine*, *106*, 128–136. https://doi.org/10.1016/j.socscimed.2014.01.043

Moreno-John, G., Gachie, A., Fleming, C. M., Nápoles-springer, A., Mutran, E., Manson, S. M., & Pérez-stable, E. J. (2004). Ethnic minority older adults participating in clinical research. *Journal of Aging and Health*, *16*(5_suppl), 93S–123S. https://doi.org/10.1177/0898264304268151

Morgan, R., & Freeman, L. (2009). The healing of our people: Substance abuse and historical trauma. *Substance Use & Misuse*, *44*(1), 84–98. https://doi.org/10.1080/10826080802525678

Motta, R. W., Suozzi, J. M., & Joseph, J. M. (1994). Assessment of secondary traumatization with an emotional Stroop task. *Perceptual and Motor Skills*, *78*(3 Pt 2), 1274. https://doi.org/10.2466/pms.1994.78.3c.1274

National Center for Health Statistics. (2019). *National Center for Health Statistics*. https://www.cdc.gov/nchs/hus/contents2018.htm#Table_006

National Congress of American Indians. (2020). http://www.ncai.org/

Nguyen, G. T., & Bowman, M. A. (2007). Culture, language, and health literacy: Communicating about health with Asians and Pacific Islanders. *Family Medicine*, *39*(3), 208–210. PMID: 17323213.

Norris, T., Vines, P., & Hoefel, E. M. (2012). *The American Indian and Alaska Native population: 2010 census briefs*. https://www.census.gov/prod/cen2010/briefs/c2010br-10.pdf

Oetzel, J., Wallerstein, N., Solimon, A., Garcia, B., Siemon, M., Adeky, S., Apachito, G., Caston, E., Finster, C., Belone, L., & Tafoya, G. (2011). Creating an instrument to measure people's perception of community capacity in American Indian communities. *Health Education & Behavior*, *38*(3), 301–310. https://doi.org/10.1177/1090198110379571

Office of Minority Health. (2020). *Infant mortality and American Indians/Alaska Natives*. U.S. Department of Health and Human Services, Office of Minority Health. https://minorityhealth.hhs.gov/omh/browse.aspx?lvl=4&lvlid=38

Pacheco, C. M., Daley, S. M., Brown, T., Filippi, M., Greiner, K. A., & Daley, C. M. (2013). Moving forward: Breaking the cycle of mistrust between American Indians and researchers. *American Journal of Public Health*, *103*(12), 2152–2159. https://doi.org/10.2105/AJPH.2013.301480

Parker, R., & Kreps, G. L. (2005). Library outreach: Overcoming health literacy challenges. *Journal of the Medical Library Association: JMLA*, *93*(4Suppl), S81–S85. https://pubmed.ncbi.nlm.nih.gov/16239962

Pescosolido, B. A., & Martin, J. K. (2004). Cultural authority and the sovereignty of American medicine: The role of networks, class, and community. *Journal of Health Politics, Policy and Law*, *29*(4), 735–756. https://doi.org/10.1215/03616878-29-4-5-735

Peterson, J., Atwood, J. R., & Yates, B. (2002). Key elements for church-based health promotion programs: Outcome-based literature review. *Public Health Nursing*, *19*(6), 401–411. https://doi.org/10.1046/j.1525-1446.2002.19602.x

Pippin, R. B. (1996). Medical practice and social authority. *The Journal of Medicine and Philosophy*, *21*(4), 417–437. https://doi.org/10.1093/jmp/21.4.417

Poupart, L. M. (2003). The familiar face of genocide: Internalized oppression among American Indians. *Hypatia*, *18*(2), 86–100. https://doi.org/10.1111/j.1527-2001.2003.tb00803.x

Putnam, R. D., Leonardi, R., & Nanetti, R. (1993). *Making democracy work: Civic traditions in modern Italy*. Princeton University Press.

Rentner, T. L., Dixon, L. D., & Lengel, L. (2012). Critiquing fetal alcohol syndrome health communication campaigns targeted to American Indians. *Journal of Health Communication*, *17*(1), 6–21. https://doi.org/10.1080/10810730.2011.585692

Rimer, B. K., & Kreuter, M. W. (2006). Advancing tailored health communication: A persuasion and message effects perspective. *Journal of Communication*, *56*(s1), S184–S201. https://doi.org/10.1111/j.1460-2466.2006.00289.x

Rosenstock, I. M. (1966). Why people use health services. *Milbank Memorial Fund Quarterly*, *44*(3), 94–127. https://doi.org/10.1111/j.1468-0009.2005.00425.x

Saenz, M. (2020). *Federal state and recognized tribes*. National Conference of State Legislatures. https://www.ncsl.org/research/state-tribal-institute/list-of-federal-and-state-recognized-tribes.aspx#federal

Sancar, F., Abbasi, J., & Bucher, K. (2018). Mortality among American Indians and Alaska Natives. *Journal of the American Medical Association*, *319*(2), 112. https://doi.org/10.1001/jama.2017.20760

Santos, L. (2008). Genetic research in native communities. *Progress in Community Health Partnerships: Research, Education, and Action*, *2*(4), 321–327. https://doi.org/10.1353/cpr.0.0046

Santos, S. L. Z., Tagai, E. K., Scheirer, M. A., Bowie, J., Haider, M., Slade, J., Wang, M. Q., & Holt, C. L. (2017). Adoption, reach, and implementation of a cancer education intervention in African American churches. *Implementation Science: IS*, *12*(1), 36. https://doi.org/10.1186/s13012-017-0566-z

Sotero, M. (2006). A conceptual model of historical trauma: Implications for public health practice and research. *Journal of Health Disparities Research and Practice*, *1*(1), 93–108. https://ssrn.com/abstract=1350062

Starr, P. (1982). *The social transformation of American medicine*. Basic Books.

Stephens, K. K., Rimal, R. N., & Flora, J. A. (2004). Expanding the reach of health campaigns: Community organizations as meta-channels for the dissemination of health information. *Journal of Health Communication*, *9*(Suppl. 1), 97–111. https://doi.org/10.1080/10810730490271557

Strauss, A., & Corbin, J. (1990). *Basics of qualitative research: Grounded theory procedures and techniques*. Sage Publications.

Szlemko, W. J., Wood, J. W., & Thurman, P. J. (2006). Native Americans and alcohol: Past, present, and future. *Journal of General Psychology*, *133*(4), 435–451. https://doi.org/10.3200/genp.133.4.435-451

Thomas, S. B., Fine, M. J., & Ibrahim, S. A. (2004). Health disparities: The importance of culture and health communication. *American Journal of Public Health*, *94*(12), 2050. https://doi.org/10.2105/AJPH.94.12.2050

Todd, L., & Hoffman-Goetz, L. (2011). Predicting health literacy among English-as-a-second-language older Chinese immigrant women to Canada: Comprehension of colon cancer prevention information. *Journal of Cancer Education*, *26*(2), 326–332. https://doi.org/10.1007/s13187-010-0162-2

Walters, K. L., Johnson-Jennings, M., Stroud, S., Rasmus, S., Charles, B., John, S., Allen, J., Kaholokula, J. K., Look, M. A., de Silva, M., Lowe, J., Baldwin, J. A., Lawrence, G., Brooks, J., Noonan, C. W., Belcourt, A., Quintana, E., Semmens, E. O., & Boulafentis, J. (2020). Growing from our roots: Strategies for developing culturally grounded health promotion interventions in American Indian, Alaska Native, and Native Hawaiian communities. *Prevention Science*, *21*(1), 54–64. https://doi.org/10.1007/s11121-018-0952-z

Wang, J. H., Liang, W., Schwartz, M. D., Lee, M. M., Kreling, B., & Mandelblatt, J. S. (2006). Development and evaluation of a culturally tailored educational video: Changing breast cancer-related behaviors in Chinese women. *Health Education & Behavior*, *35*(6), 806–820. https://doi.org/10.1177/1090198106296768

Wasserman, J., Palmer, R. C., Gomez, M. M., Berzon, R., Ibrahim, S. A., & Ayanian, J. Z. (2019). Advancing health services research to eliminate health care disparities. *American Journal of Public Health*, *109*(S1), S64–S69. https://doi.org/10.2105/AJPH.2018.304922

Whitewater, S., Reinschmidt, K. M., Kahn, C., Attakai, A., & Teufel-Shone, N. I. (2016). Flexible roles for American Indian elders in community-based participatory research. *Preventing Chronic Disease*, *13*, E72. https://doi.org/10.5888/pcd13.150575

Williams, S. L., Kaigler, A., Armistad, A., Espey, D. K., & Struminger, B. B. (2019). Creating a public health community of practice to support American Indian and Alaska Native communities in addressing chronic disease. *Preventing Chronic Disease*, *16*, E109. https://doi.org/10.5888/pcd16.190193

A Comparative Analysis of Health News in Indigenous and Mainstream Media

Victoria L. LaPoe, Candi S. Carter Olson, Cristina L. Azocar, Benjamin R. LaPoe, Bharbi Hazarika, and Parul Jain

ABSTRACT

It is important to evaluate the media's health coverage of Indigenous communities both because these communities have been hit very hard by health inequities, and because misinformation can negatively affect the future health of Indian Country. This study takes the unique angle of examining both Indigenous and non-Indigenous ("mainstream") news publications to evaluate information gaps in health, health policy, and health efficacy coverage. The Indigenous media examined, which covered 14 times more health stories than mainstream media, highlighted health issues in Indian Country through the lens of resilience by using framing to emphasize unequal power, while at the same time providing depth and specificity. Instead of putting Indigenous health stories into historical and cultural context, mainstream media focused on the lack of resources and the chronic struggle of Indigenous communities. Mainstream media often only covered the topic once per outlet; however, those outlets with connections to Indigenous communities did provide more balanced coverage. Instead of promoting change, most mainstream media stories blamed Indigenous people for their situation and offered a doom trajectory for tribes hit hardest by health disparities. This study reveals how embedded framing and mediatization direct non-Native readers' attention away from the systemic deprivation of support to U.S. Indigenous tribes that was guaranteed to them by the U.S. government in tribal agreements. The implications for journalism and policy are discussed.

The first outbreak of the novel coronavirus – a.k.a., COVID-19, SARS-CoV-2, corona, coronavirus, or, in the Navajo language, Dikos Ntsaaígíí-Náhást'éíts'áadah – was reported on December 31, 2019 in Wuhan, Hubei Province, China and by March 11, 2020 the World Health Organization (WHO, 2020a) officially declared a pandemic. The U.S. documented its first-known case of the virus on January 21, 2020 (AJMC Staff, 2020). By the spring of 2020, hospitals and intensive care units were at risk of becoming overrun with patients. By November 25, 2020, the U.S. accounted for 21% of the global number of cases and 18% of the deaths (AJMC Staff, 2020). Communities of color were hit the hardest. The Navajo Nation, one of the largest tribes in the U.S., led national headlines in late spring 2020 as infection rates spread quickly across tribal lands and elders fought for funding and support from the federal government, as part of their trust relationships. By the middle of May 2020, the Navajo Nation had the highest per-capita COVID-19 infection rate in the U.S., about 1,100 per 100,000 individuals (COVID-19 in Indian Country: Indian Country's COVID-19 syllabus, 2020). In contrast, the country as a whole saw around 400 cases per 100,000 individuals (COVID-19 in Indian Country, 2020).

The spike in cases in Indigenous communities revealed health inequities for Indigenous people in the U.S. Those inequities include a lower life expectancy of at least 5.5 years, and a disease burden which is disproportionate to the greater population and which is rooted in both economic and social adversity (Indian Health Service, 2019). Indigenous communities face multiple health inequities such as low levels of insurance rates, lack of access to reliable healthcare, health issues including high rates of chronic diseases (James et al., 2009). While Indian Health Service does provide some relief to these communities, the low levels of funding make it difficult to provide timely and adequate services at a larger scale (James et al., 2009). Lack of access to healthcare information compounds the situation. But access to news media reporting on healthcare has been shown to influence healthcare decision-making (Schwitzer, 2004) and so may provide information to Indigenous people on how to access services and about health-related information in general. In addition, policy leaders use news media to guide legislation about healthcare programs that affect Native American tribes (Bakir, 2006; Herbst, 1998).

It is important to evaluate the health coverage of Indigenous communities by both Indigenous and non-Indigenous news sources because media coverage has the potential to influence policy decisions (Gollust et al., 2019; Kim et al., 2010). National media coverage of the COVID-19 impact in Indian Country, in general, and the Navajo Nation, in particular, began soon after outbreaks were reported in Indigenous communities across the U.S. The Navajo Nation, which has more than 350,000 residents, didn't start seeing COVID-19 cases until early March 2020 (COVID-19 across the Navajo Nation, 2020). As of June 20, 2020, however, the Nation had a total of 6,990 cases, including 354 deaths, and 3,603 people recovered (COVID-19 across, 2020). Throughout the outbreak, news coverage both inside and outside of Indian Country became an important way for tribal leaders across the U.S. to get their voices heard in Washington, D.C., where policy makers held power over millions of dollars in relief funds.

The pandemic provided an opportunity to compare the framing of stories about Indian Country in Indigenous-produced and focused media sources to mainstream news sources. For the purposes of this article, mainstream news sources are defined as those produced for a broad audience without a particular interest in or tie to Indigenous communities. Indigenous media are defined as, "those media or forms of media where expression is created, owned, controlled, and managed by Indigenous Peoples to produce and exchange culturally appropriate information in the languages that they speak and understand" (Sunuwar, 2019, para. 1). This study is one of the first to compare the health and medical coverage of both Indigenous and mainstream news stories. The article begins by outlining literature on race framing of healthcare coverage and how race framing has negatively impacted racial and ethnic minorities' health.

Literature review

Although there are some studies that examine Australian and Canadian Indigenous health disparities (e.g., Cooper et al., 2021; Kerry, 2014), current studies, which are focused specifically on news coverage of health disparities in U.S. Indigenous communities, are mainly absent from academic databases, and even fewer compare sources within this media. This leads to an incomplete picture of what happens in Indian Country as a result of health inequities.

Mediatization theory

Our current study relies on mediatization theory and framing to understand how U.S. mainstream media and Indigenous U.S. media coverage of the COVID-19 pandemic affected government and individuals' reactions to, and preparations for, the healthcare crisis. Mediatization theory suggests that media has become so ingrained in our culture and society that it cannot be analyzed as a separate entity (Ampuja et al., 2014; Hjarvard, 2008).

Mediatization theory sheds light on the ways that publics ingest mediated messages without understanding that their opinions and subsequent actions toward a group of people are actually being guided by messages that have been cultivated by mass media sources. According to Hjarvard (2008), "the media are at once part of the fabric of society and culture and an independent institution that stands between other cultural and social institutions and coordinates their mutual interaction" (p. 105). As such, the media acted as information intermediaries between tribal leaders and U.S. policy makers when it came to formulating informed, Indigenous-community-focused responses to the pandemic in tribal communities. Mediatization theory relies on two foundational media theories: framing and agenda setting. Agenda setting is the act of directing audience attention to certain topics – what to think about, but not *how* to think about it; framing is the act of delivering messages to audiences that influence individual thoughts and actions (Entman, 1993; McCombs & Shaw, 1972). These theories are particularly important for understanding how media influences public perception and policy makers' actions on social issues, particularly those pertaining to minority populations, including Black, Latinx, and Indigenous people (Kim et al., 2010).

Racialized frames

Scholars have published a range of studies addressing racializing framing and health news coverage, many of which consider obesity and eating disorders. These scholars found that frames consistently place blame on minority racial and ethnic groups for their situations, while not considering the broader social constructs that lead to inequality and health disparities and that framing can influence audience perceptions and policy outcomes (Amzel & Ghosh, 2007; Kim et al., 2010; Saguy & Gruys, 2010). Thematic frames, which focus on broader social issues, lead to public opinion that holds government responsible, but news coverage about racial issues blames the victim, which decreases White support for governmental programs designed to reduce racial disparities (Kim et al., 2010).

According to research, health news coverage on Indigenous populations is not a priority for many mainstream journalists (Gearhart et al., 2017). The limited coverage tends to focus on episodic framing (news coverage of one specific event), rather than thematic framing. This event coverage places blame on the subject and does not address environmental causes; it also varies in its inclusion of information that might help mobilize action to remedy the health disparity or crisis situation (Gearhart & Trumbly-Lamsam, 2017; Hoffman-Goetz et al., 2003; Starr & Oxlad, 2020).

To compound this issue of limited health news coverage by mainstream media, the subject of Indigenous communities generally is often not included at all. Research on media coverage of Indigenous communities in Australia found that Indigenous communities were often ignored; instead, reporters used policy makers to talk *about* Indigenous people rather than speaking to Indigenous sources (McCallum et al., 2012).

In the U.S., the absence of Indigenous voices in news coverage has led to inappropriate policy decisions for Indian Country. In contrast to mainstream media coverage, Indigenous media provided different framing of the COVID-19 crisis (Arviso et al., 2020) by explaining the difficulty and nuances of data collection. Most importantly, they published feature articles about the deaths of the many people who were loved and lost by their relatives (Arviso et al., 2020).

Indigenous media perspectives

Indigenous-produced media offers a counterpoint to most mainstream media, which continues to include stereotypical portrayals of Indigenous people that perpetuate inaccurate understandings of these communities (Jarding, 2004; National Congress of American Indians, 2020a). Indigenous media messages empower their communities by directly communicating Native American communities' concerns and perspectives (Sunuwar, 2019). Indigenous media provide more information, more detail, and more alternative viewpoints then mainstream news (Jarding, 2004). However, most Americans do not regularly consume Indigenous media. Consumers must intentionally seek out Indigenous media sources, or counter-mainstream narratives about Indigenous people, to find this perspective (Gregory et al., 2011; Jarding, 2004; Lam et al., 2017; McCallum et al., 2012).

Our study examines both Indigenous and mainstream publications to evaluate information gaps in health, health policy, and health efficacy coverage. With the prominence of social media like #NativeTwitter, tribal citizens are drawing attention to Indigenous communities in mainstream media coverage. By comparing and contrasting the health coverage and the potential impacts on policy makers on a range of issues, from COVID-19 test availability in Indian Country to the release of federal funds from COVID-19 relief on highly impacted Nations, this study seeks to understand the ways media impacted the social and cultural views of the pandemic's impact on Indian Country. This article seeks to answer the following research questions:

> RQ1a: In what ways did mainstream media cover health in Indian Country as the COVID-19 pandemic became public?
>
> RQ1b: Was there a difference in news coverage among Indigenous supported mainstream media, such as those with Indigenous reporters on staff?

RQ2: How did Indigenous media cover COVID-19?

> RQ3: How did COVID-19 coverage illustrate healthcare equality in Indigenous communities?

Method

We conducted a qualitative textual analysis of Indigenous and mainstream digital news sources from February 26, 2020, when the pandemic became a widespread news story in the U.S., until June 24, 2020, when businesses across the nation began to consistently reopen. We collected content noting the news source, headline, themes, and whether the author was identified as Indigenous, or if an author was a part of a diversity-focused news beat. Stories were found via online search-engine by searching "Native," "news." Health content considered for this study includes any digital COVID-19 "news" with a specific focus on health; we did not want to hinder our data collection and so cast a wide net. If a website contained content as a news source, we included it. Therefore, the articles came from radio, business, television, newspaper, and digital entities at the tribal, local, regional, national, and international levels.

Textual analysis assists in describing and interpreting messages such as news (Morris, 2004). Utilizing textual analysis means that our qualitative research will be primarily descriptive but represented by the themes we uncovered. To interpret our data's messages, we conducted our analysis by reading through texts and sorting each news story based on recurrent themes as well as noting author diversity. We selected a term or phrase from the news story that we determined to be the main point. Some stories had more than one main point, so they were categorized with more than one term or phrase. This method was born out of the NAJA Bingo Card – a rubric that was created from what U.S. Indigenous journalists repeatedly saw as stereotypical coverage (Native American Journalists Association, 2020a, 2020b). This bingo card includes often-covered topics in Indian Country, but if a reporter *bingos* on it, they should reconsider their work because their writing reinforces stereotypes. For our research, we looked for these single word "themes" throughout the coverage. To calculate a reliability for themes, we drew on O'Connor and Joffe (2020) guidelines and utilized Holsti's calculation (M. Allen, 2017). We selected less than 10% of the sample, which included 30 total themes. We then calculated how many themes we both agreed on and divided by the total number of possible themes. This gave us an acceptable Holsti agreement of .90 (M. Allen, 2017). We were confident as we moved toward our analysis, once we saw the same themes consistently repeating amongst the two groups of news sources (Denzin & Lincoln, 1998).

We collected a total number of 326 news stories for analysis. As Table 1 shows, we were aware we may not get a large number of stories about Indigenous communities within a single news outlet. For example, 122 mainstream news outlets produced close to the same amount of news coverage during this time period as nine Indigenous media outlets.

Indigenous media produced 14 times the amount of health news coverage per outlet, clearly showing its importance to the outlets' communities. Knowing most mainstream media tend to sparsely report on Indigenous communities (LaPoe & LaPoe, 2017), we conducted a substantial search that included business news such as gaming and legal sources. For context, as the National Congress of American Indians (NCAI) notes, these sites are relevant because "tribal governments use gaming revenues to fund social service programs, including scholarships, health-care clinics, substance abuse programs, education, law enforcement, and tribal courts" (National Congress of American Indians, 2020a, para. 2).

Diverse reporters

Indigenous reporters have consistently represented less than 0.5% of the staff in mainstream media newsrooms and most of these do not have diversity-focused beats or tribal affairs desks (Azocar et al., 2021; Native American Journalists Association, 2019a). We felt that this underwhelming number was important when considering health reporting in Indian Country. To accurately report on Indian Country, media outlets must understand Indigenous communities and cultural norms, such as how funding pandemic healthcare responses from community-run businesses are connected to community healthcare.

Findings

Mediatization theory acknowledges that media are naturally part of our culture – not separate entities reporting on stories to an audience. News coverage becomes part of the dominant ideology's knowledge about other communities (Hjarvard, 2008). Therefore, we analyzed the coverage of Indigenous and mainstream media to examine thematic differences that

Table 1. Indigenous and Non-Indigenous News Sources Included in Study-.

Mainstream Media News Outlet	Number of Articles Published
12News.com (Phoenix)	1
ABC News	2
ABC 7 Eyewitness News Southern California	1
Aberdeen News	1
Al Jazeera	1
Associated Press	2
Arizona Republic	1
Auburn Reporter	1
AZ Central	1
Axios	1
Bizjournals.com	1
Borderreport.com	1
BridgeMI.com	1
CBS News	1
CNN	2
Cardplayer.com	1
Casino.org	1
Claimsjournal.com	1
Chicago Sun Times	1
Courthousenews.com	2
Crain's Detroit Business	1
Cronkite News	6
Cruxnow.com	1
CTMirror.org	1
Desert Sun	1
Detroit Free Press	1
Duluth News Tribune	1
EcoWatch	1
Fox News Channel	1
Fresno Bee	1
Gambling News	1
Green Bay Gazette	2
Harvard Gazette	1
Health Affairs	1
Heraldonline.com	1
HeraldNet Everett, Washington	1
High Country News (Mainstream media with Indigenous Affairs Desk)	4
History News Network	5
Inside Edition	6
Journaltimes.com	1
Kaiser Health News	2
KDRV.com	2
KEPR-TV News & KOMO	2
KGW	1
Kitsap Sun	2
KOB 4	2
KOTA-TV	3
KPBS	5
KPIX5	2
KQED	1
KRQE	5
KREM	2
KTAR.com	1
KTVZ	2
KVAL-KOIN	1
Law.com	1
Madison.com	1
Marketplace	1
Marketwatch	1
MedPage Today	1
Miami Herald	1
Michigan Radio/NPR	1
Mille Lacs Messenger	1
Milwaukee Journal Sentinel	1
MLive (Michigan)	1
Mohave Daily News	1
NBC-LA	1
NBC News	1
NPR	1
New Mexico In-depth	1
News Break	1
"Newscast" (Internewscast.com)	1
Newsweek	1
News World Casino	1
Online Poker Report	1
PBS Newshour	1
Phoenix News Times	1
Pine River Times	2
Politico	2
Portland Monthly	1
PlayUSA	2
Pro Publica	2
Q13Fox.com	1
Quarles.com	1
Reuters	1
Salt Lake Tribune/republished Indian Country Today	1
San Francisco Chronicle	1
SBsun.com	1
Schwab.com/newsroom	2
Seattle Times	1
Sioux Falls Argus Leader	1
Slate	1
South Dakota News Watch	1
South Florida Sun-Sentinel	1
Spectrum News California	1
Spectrum News Charlotte	1
Star Tribune	1
The Albuquerque Journal	1
The Bellingham Herald (Washington/reposting Seattle Times)	1
The Guardian	1
The Hill	1
The Lewiston Tribune	1
The Los Angeles Times	1
The Mercury News (CA)/AP	1
The Morning Call	1
The New York Times	1
The Philadelphia Inquirer	1
The Ponca City News	1
The Washington Post	1
The San Diego Tribune	2
The Santa Fe New Mexican	1
Time	2
Times Union	1
US News	1
Underscore.news	1
Vox	1
Voice of American News	1
WAFB	1
WITL 100.7 radio	1
WLBT	1
WPR	1
YahooSports	1
Yogonet Gaming News	1
Total	*169*
Indigenous Media News Outlets	Number of Articles Published
Osage News	2
Indianz.com	4
Indian Country Today	103
Native News	1
Cherokee Phoenix	3
Navajo Times	41
Indigenous New England	1
Navajo-Hopi Observer	1
Native Business Magazine	1
Total	*157*

served as frames within coverage. Indigenous media were more connected to these stories and therefore, had more diversity within their coverage. Indigenous media applied five themes versus mainstream media's three themes. Most mainstream themes were negative with the leading frames being the following: Indigenous communities' *chronic disproportionate struggle*; Indigenous communities *lacking resources* needed to survive through and combat COVID-19; and coverage that reinforced *stereotypes* by lacking specifics or reiterating negative generalized stories about Indigenous people. In contrast, Indigenous media's health news coverage frames included: *clarity and depth* through investigative reporting on topics like what it means to follow health orders in some parts of Indian Country or the specific numbers of Indigenous people statistically impacted by the pandemic in a certain location; *honoring culture and tradition*, whereby reporters didn't assume that the progression of the virus, or deaths from the virus, were experienced in the same way in every community; *community focused solution reporting* that highlighted citizens working together for positive collective health outcomes; *unpacking government relationships to community health* and what that means at the tribal, state, and federal level to Indigenous areas; and *specificity on community health impact* that detailed ways the pandemic impacted access to resources like water, food, and supplies.

Despite these differences, we found that when mainstream media appeared to support Indigenous reporters, allowing them space to tell specific stories, coverage was often more inclusive. There were times, however, when this seemed to not happen. Overall, our research findings are descriptive and capture the frames that emerged in the mainstream and Indigenous media.

Mainstream media frames

Chronic disproportionate struggle and lacking resources

Mainstream media coverage reported on specific medical issues and tracked COVID-19 deaths in Indian Country. Specifically, the coverage noted *chronic disproportionate struggle* and emphasized historical health epidemics and historical trauma. Statistics on diabetes, heart disease, and obesity were often present. This coverage also included what was *lacking* in Indigenous communities, such as deficiency in federal aid and scarcity of resources some may take for granted, such as water, electricity, transportation, internet, money, and housing. These articles often cited health statistics without adding historical context, including information about the federal government's refusal to honor treaties and fund health services.

The following example from *Albuquerque Journal* highlights where this economical and historical context is not included: "Researchers, advocates and lawmakers point to poor access to a health care system that has been chronically underfunded, high rates of chronic illnesses and environmental factors of heavy metals exposure and poor air and water quality" (Kaplan & Davis, 2020, para. 11). While the health disparity information may have been factual, it did not include the historical context needed to understand why this occurred in some parts of Indian Country.

Dissecting a COVID-19 story that appeared in *The Washington Post*'s health section on April 4, 2020 also highlighted the frames of *lacking resources* and *chronic disproportionate struggle* (Hedgpeth et al., 2020a). The article began with a headline framing a doom-filled situation: "Indian Country, whose residents suffer disproportionately from disease, is bracing for coronavirus." The subheading under the title reinforced this theme: "Conditions in Indian Country are ripe for a rapid spread of the coronavirus. Rates of infection among Navajos is a major concern." The reporters working on this piece included an Indigenous reporter. To the report's credit, sources such as Cherokee Nation's chief, John Hoskin and the Navajo Nation's president, Jonathan Nez were included, as well as research from a journal focused on American Indians. Despite these efforts, the tone within the story still highlighted despair. " . . . The beds aren't needed yet, but on a reservation where residents suffer high rates of diseases that exist throughout Indian Country, the Lummi Tribal Health Clinic is taking every precaution to prepare for the deadly coronavirus" (Hedgpeth et al., 2020a, para. 1). The article also illustrated the negative health conditions associated with Indigenous communities:

> And they suffer disproportionately from hypertension, asthma, cancer, heart and cardiovascular disease — maladies that put them at a higher risk of fatal complications from the coronavirus. American Indians are 600 times more likely to die of tuberculosis and nearly 200 times more likely to die of diabetes than other groups. More than a quarter under age 65 lack health insurance (Hedgpeth et al., 2020a, para. 8).

The history of the why these conditions exist is missing, which might include information on the chronically underfunded Indian Health Service as well as specificity about the tribe or tribes being reported on. This information matters to the community and matters to health providers to understand and decontextualize negative narratives. Health disparities in Indian Country have long-term causes including genocide, relocation and termination policies, and the federal government ignoring its trust responsibilities.

This negative, non-contextual health narrative cited a credible journal, but failed to include easily accessible information that could enlighten the reader's understanding of present challenges. By adding historical context to their story, such as the following detail from a report about the 1918 Spanish Flu outbreak, these *Washington Post* reporters would have presented more balanced and nuanced coverage:

> . . . Although local authorities across the country closed public schools during the worst of the outbreak to stem the spread of the virus — much like schools and universities have closed today due to COVID-19 — the Indian Office decided that indigenous children had 'as good a chance to escape the disease in a boarding school as they [had] in their reservation homes' and thus refused to close these residential schools. Federal officials justified this decision on the grounds that boarding schools had better medical facilities than reservations, which, they argued, meant that children had 'a better chance for recovery at school than at home.' Yet, financial incentives lay at the heart of this decision since Congress funded boarding schools on the basis of average annual attendance (Adams, 2020, para. 5).

The Washington Post's reporting is problematic because it paints a broad stroke of history and appears to blame the victims. Adams (2020) analysis shows financial greed is a past historical factor influencing relations between Indigenous communities and the federal government; how this plays out today should also be investigated and included when referencing previous pandemics.

The *Washington Post* article continued with a common stereotype that Indigenous people are stuck in the 19th century: "Conditions a century ago were similar to what exist today in Indian Country: multigenerational families living in close quarters, struggling with poverty, poor nutrition and underfunded health-care programs" (Hedgpeth et al., 2020a, para. 11). Two days later, *The Philadelphia Inquirer* ran the same story. However, a quote in the headline included the same catastrophic history trajectory as the article. The *Inquirer*'s headline read: "'We could get wiped out': Native Americans have the highest rates of diseases that make COVID-19 more lethal" (Hedgpeth et al., 2020b, para. 1). Re-running a national news organization's story highlights the life cycle of reporting and how news produced by a national news organization might be reprinted in local news outlets, with the most dramatic negative portion of the story in a headline to gain readership.

For *The Washington Post*, it appeared that the packaging of this report may have become problematic through the publishing cycle. For example, the article lacked the breadth and depth that could be included through additional sourcing that would provide a clear picture of COVID-19 throughout Indigenous communities. The *Washington Post* newsroom has had questionable coverage of Indian Country in the past, including concerning methodologies and reporting on mascots, which the American Psychological Association has noted are harmful to Indigenous and non-Indigenous people (American Psychological Association, 2011; Native American Journalists Association, 2019b).

Stereotypes

As seen in the example above, many aspects of mainstream reporting, from the headlines to the stories themselves, included stereotypes of Indigenous peoples. *The New York Times* often resorted to highlighting these negative themes, which strategically may have been used to entice readers. Examples included: "On Tribal Lands, a Time to Make Art for Solace and Survival" (Brown, 2020, para. 1); "Opinion: The Top U.S. Hot Spots Are All Indian Lands" (Kristof, 2020, para. 1); "Tribal Nations Face the Most Severe Crisis in Decades as the Coronavirus Closes Casinos" (Romero & Healy, 2020, para. 1); and "Native American Tribes Sue Treasury Over Stimulus Aid as They Feud Over Funding" (Walker & Cochrane, 2020, para. 1). While there may be truth within each of these stories, and there appeared to be reporters who had experience in covering Indian Country, the packaging of the story mattered. *Specificity* is essential – and ethically needed – to avoid resorting to stereotypes. Collectively, these headlines focused on art, casinos, feuds, and problem locations. There are multiple issues with these headlines, which is not surprising as *The New York Times* has also been criticized for the way they cover Indian Country (Native American Journalists Association, 2019c). Tribes and their experiences vary dramatically, and so details matter in headlines, especially because many readers do not read beyond the headline (American Press Institute, 2014). For example, the fourth headline about aid (Walker & Cochrane, 2020) lacks specificity about whether the aid is for federal or state tribes, or both. If both, that number includes more than 600 tribes. It would be very rare to lump 600+ cities into one news story when covering a health issue and policy as large as the COVID-19 pandemic.

Research notes that stereotypes do not lead to better understanding, even if people have used them subconsciously to try to understand people dissimilar from themselves (Lippmann, 1922). Education, experience, and exposure helps alleviate the psychological barriers this schema-making creates (LaPoe et al., 2018; Lippmann, 1922). Regurgitating stories, which falsely presents a monolithic situation for millions of people within underserved populations, is harmful to the understanding of health and policies needed to make change. Few mainstream reporters provided coverage that added nuance to this perspective. Even when there was an Indigenous reporter presented in the bylines, it appeared that perhaps the news holes, corporate biases, or editing process led to the suppression of specificity in coverage.

Indigenous-supported media frames

Within our data set, 6% of the authors were Indigenous and 2% of those were from the only established tribal affairs desk at a mainstream news organization, *High Country News*. When journalists were provided reporting space on Indigenous communities, coverage from Indigenous reporters (and/or by reporters who have connections to Indigenous communities) included appropriate story context. Not all reporters on *High Country News*' tribal affairs desk are Indigenous, nor historically have all reporters been Indigenous at Indigenous media outlets, such as *Navajo Times*. However, all journalists should be connected with the communities they cover to provide balanced and ethical coverage on Indian Country.

Clarity and depth

Indigenous reporters covering COVID-19 added clarity when reporting on health guidelines. A story by two diversity-focused reporters, including an Indigenous journalist from a national mainstream news outlet, explained the implications of handwashing when some Indigenous families must drive miles to get water. *NBC News*' Chiara Sottile (Karuk) wrote a piece with Erik Ortiz (2020), a reporter focused on racial injustice and social inequality, which explored what washing your hands for 20 seconds meant in the Navajo Nation, and the history behind why this is so complicated for some residents: "The coronavirus is exposing underlying fractures in the infrastructure of Indian Country, including health care and basic needs, like water, that have long been underfunded and, some say, ignored by the federal government" (Sottile & Ortiz, 2020, para. 7). Another Indigenous reporter, Rebeca Nagle (2020) (Cherokee Nation), provided context in another international mainstream outlet, *The Guardian*, about the implications of lumping Indigenous people in the *other* category when reporting COVID-19 statistics:

> In states that do categorize Native Americans in the demographic results, early data indicates dramatically disproportionate rates of

> infection and death. Last week, the Arizona department of health services reported that Native Americans make up 16% of the state's Covid-19 related deaths, despite representing only 6% of the state's population. In New Mexico, Native Americans make up less than 10% of the population, but over one-third of coronavirus cases. This week, the health authority for the Navajo Nation, which includes areas of Arizona, Utah and New Mexico, reported 1,197 positive coronavirus cases and 44 deaths. If it were a state, it would rank third in the country for confirmed cases per 100,000 population, behind only New York and New Jersey (though the nation is also testing at a far higher rate than most states) (paras. 4–5).

Kalen Goodluck, who is Diné (Navajo), Mandan, Hidatsa, and Tsimshian tribes and is a tribal member of the Three Affiliated Tribes of the Fort Berthold Indian Reservation in North Dakota (Goodluck, 2020a), added tribal specificity to her article in *High Country News*:

> Tribes across the Southwest have been badly hit by the world's newest coronavirus, the virus that causes COVID-19. One pueblo, however, has seen fewer confirmed cases than neighboring communities, including other pueblos. Acoma Pueblo, a small tribal community with just over 4,800 citizens, lies 65 miles west of Albuquerque near El Malpais National Monument. Acoma Gov. Brian Vallo credits the pueblo's stringent response to the pandemic . . .
>
> . . . *High Country News* spoke with Vallo about the economic impacts of closing businesses like the Sky City Casino, which funds Acoma Pueblo's government services and programs, his frustration that Indian Country was a stimulus package afterthought, and the difficulty of informing spiritual leaders about the risks of public gatherings. This interview has been edited and condensed for length and clarity (Goodluck, 2020b, paras. 1–2).

While Goodluck's "question and answer" written interview was edited, it still provided close to 20 paragraphs of detail about one specific tribe.

Honoring culture and tradition

COVID-19 provided an interesting challenge to Indigenous media in places like the Navajo Nation. As LaPoe and LaPoe (2017) find, prior to COVID-19 death was not, historically, covered in the *Navajo Times*: "The CEO and Publisher of the *Navajo Times*, Tom Arviso, said his staff is continually cognizant that its reporting tends to incorporate the traditional Navajo beliefs. Navajo beliefs impact how the paper covers death, funerals, and domestic violence" (p. 86). Within the scope of our study, when addressing death, Indigenous media primarily reported the numbers of cases and deaths; however, we found that the national outlet *Indian Country Today*'s Vincent Shilling (Akwesasne Mohawk) covered it differently; he spoke with an Indigenous funeral director about their financial experience providing traditional burials during the pandemic:

> The difficulty for Gill in the midst of the COVID-19 pandemic is that there are no extra transportation costs for any deaths in North Dakota, South Dakota, Wisconsin, or Minnesota. All of this considered Gill personally to come to the family's home to make all the funeral arrangements. Today, we spoke with Gill about the difficulties in maintaining safe practices while maintaining the traditions of the families involved (It's hard, 2020, para. 3).

Gill also discussed the logistics of travel and preparing for a funeral, which included jurisdictions:

> It's hard when a death occurs because you have to, first of all, do the removal of the decedent, wherever they may be at a morgue. A lot of the tribes have morgues for pathologists, they'll go to like Sioux Falls. There's a federal pathologist way down to Ramsey, Minnesota and St. Paul. They take bodies from way over in the different tribes because the tribes aren't states they're their own sovereign nation. So federal takes over. (It's hard, 2020, para. 11).

Like much that has to do with Indigenous communities, understanding tradition as well as jurisdiction was essential to covering this topic from an Indigenous perspective, which was clear in how Schilling transcribed his interview on this culturally sensitive topic.

Community focused solution reporting

The majority of Indigenous news outlets in our data set reported death statistics. However, the largest proportion of Indigenous media's health reporting framed the reporting as *solutions*, specifically addressing resources focused on the betterment of the collective community. Following this category, Indigenous media framed what was *lacking*, but focused on the lack of well-being rather than on cultural deficiency. A lack of federal funding and tribal/state/federal tensions around money were the main focus.

The *Cherokee Phoenix*, the first Indigenous (U.S.) newspaper, established in 1828, focused on perseverance as a solution and the importance of covering the needed expansion of medical and mental health care:

> During these unprecedented times, many medical facilities have had to furlough and terminate employees, OKCIC Chief Human Resource Officer Monica Krienke said. "We have been fortunate. Not only have we been able to keep our whole workforce, but also continue to hire in areas that support our patients" (Oklahoma City Indian clinic continues to hire during COVID-19, 2020, para. 3).

In this paragraph, health solutions and growth are the focus – a solution to a need because of the pressure of the pandemic.

Meanwhile, *Indian Country Today*'s Joaqlin Estus (Tlingit) (2020) provided readers a solution to healthcare issues via telehealth for those who live in rural Alaska with difficult terrain and few doctors:

> . . . "We'd like to think that the things we do in an exam are so important. But in a relatively stable patient who we've known for many years that really doesn't add much, like, you know, very little." He said he gets most of the information he needs from talking with the patient, and less than 10 percent of it from "me actually putting my stethoscope to their lungs, listening to their heart, and pressing my finger into their ankles to see if they have any edema" (paras. 16–17).

With the healthcare challenges COVID-19 presented across the country, Estus provided a shift in health narrative and focused on how technology provided a solution to readers' medical needs.

Connectedness of community was also a prominent theme in Indigenous media coverage, which noted that solutions would not necessarily come from a single person, but from a community of medical experts:

> Yazzie has eight colleagues, all of whom are capable of adapting to any and every position at the clinic in Naatsis'áán, with a population of less than 500 people. But each of the women has her own place at Navajo Mountain Community Health Center, one

of nine clinics under the Utah Navajo Health System (K. Allen, 2020, para. 8).

This collective connectedness also appeared in *Navajo Times*. Krista Allen (Diné) (Kristof, 2020) reported on cultural upbringing that focused on endurance, therefore shifting the narrative from victims to survivors:

> When there's stuff that is hard for us to do, we just all come in a group and ask one another, "Who knows how to do this?" she said. "Most of us were raised here in Navajo Mountain. We all work together and fix it ourselves. Especially when we have an emergency patient and we can't lift that patient; we all work together to lift them up. And if we have a domestic violence, like if we can't hold down a patient, we still have strength to work together. But we stabilize the patient pretty well" (K. Allen, 2020, para. 5).

Community relationships also moved beyond just citizens working together. Government and government relationships are also important to community health in Indian Country.

Government relationships to community health

The relationship between a tribe, the state, and the federal government was also apparent in Indigenous media coverage. The states could not dictate tribes' mandatory shutdowns in their Nations. The federal government's lack of responsiveness reinforced the importance of reporters knowing history. *Indianz.com*'s Acee Agoyo (Ohkay Owingeh) (Agoyo, 2020) wrote:

> With coronavirus cases continuing to rise at disproportionate rates in Indian Country, advocates are calling on Congress to live up to its trust and treaty obligations by providing adequate funding for health care in tribal and urban communities.
>
> The Indian Health Service needs at least 9.1 USD billion to meet the needs of the first Americans, key lawmakers are being told at a hearing on Thursday afternoon, among the first in the COVID-19 era. The agency's budget currently falls far short of that amount.
>
> The COVID-19 pandemic has further exposed the vast deficiencies in health care funding, access, quality, and availability that exists across the Indian health system, Stacy Bohlen, Chief Executive Officer of the National Indian Health Board, says in written testimony (para. 1–3).

The article included a tweet from Indian Health Services and showed pictures of its director visiting a drive-up testing site on the Navajo Nation, and a tweet that provided information about where and when readers could watch the Interior-Environment Subcommittee hearing chair discuss the *disproportionate suffering* of Indigenous people from COVID-19 via YouTube (Agoyo, 2020, para. 8).

The inclusion of Indigenous knowledge was clear in how Indigenous media addressed relationships with funding, and how they highlighted sovereignty. *High Country News*' Indigenous Affairs reporter and NAJA board member Graham Brewer (2020) summed up this perspective best in a tweet on June 26th: "I don't know who needs to hear this, but when Indian Health Services doesn't have the money or resources it needs, it isn't 'underfunded,' it's because the US is not honoring treaty rights – in other words: breaking the law." By reporting in Indigenous news sources and on social media, Indigenous reporters emphasized history and unfulfilled promises to Inddiigenous communities; the same communities which mainstream media often cast as not their primary audience and instead the problematic "other."

Specificity on community health impact

In mainstream media coverage of the ways COVID-19 was impacting various communities in the U.S., articles emphasized the unequal healthcare available to Indigenous people. However, most mainstream media did not provide sufficiently descriptive language or specific detail, which served to perpetuate stereotypes and harm (LaPoe & LaPoe, 2017). For example, Lisa Deaderick's (2020) *San Diego Union-Tribune* article "History of Inequality making COVID-19 worse for Native Americans" reported:

> Indigenous communities have already experienced generations of disparities in areas such as poverty, education and access to health care, so something like the COVID-19 pandemic magnifies the ways in which our systems have failed to serve everyone appropriately. These failures have made the virus especially dangerous (para. 1).

While the reporter should be applauded for providing a lengthy question and answer e-mail interview with an Indigenous official, it would have also been helpful to unpack specific community issues in detail; this specificity in reporting would assist in moving the narrative forward.

In comparison, Arlyssa Becenti's (2020) *Navajo Times* article was specific about inequalities and reported on the absence of running water in the community of Wide Ruins. "Getting water to communities is a priority for fighting the pandemic – and with 600 USD million in federal funds now in the bank earmarked for COVID-19 mitigation, Wide Ruins may finally get its wish" (para. 3). With the U.S. allocating some COVID-19 relief funds to Indigenous communities, understanding that these funds may be used for very basic pre-pandemic needs is an essential part of this Indian Country story.

A mainstream media outlet, *NBCNews*, which has recently grown its Indigenous reporter cohort, illustrated the difference a journalist's knowledge about Indian Country makes when reporting on health inequity. NBC has also consistently funded relationships and programs with diverse journalism organizations such as Native American Journalists Association (2020c). This Indigenous relationship, awareness, and presence in the newsroom appears to impact the stories that are published. *NBCNews* reporter Erik Ortiz (Native American Journalists Association, 2020b) interviewed Navajo Nation citizen Cynthia Wilson in the story "As the coronavirus pandemic strains supplies, Native Americans fight food insecurity." The story reported how many of the food sources relied on limited supplies in Wilson's community, which also lacked running water:

> Prior to the coronavirus pandemic "people were dependent on the grocery store," Wilson said. "Now, they're in shock or worried about how they're going to keep their pantries filled when they can't go to the stores like they used to. It's a wake-up call that we need to go back to growing our own foods and tending to our own livestock" (para. 3).

Ortiz's reporting was community specific. This and his other stories reveal reporting that avoids the broad, monolithic, historical, negative narrative devoid of context. Ortiz shows a national mainstream audience what inequality in health care means to one Nation.

Discussion

State of health inequalities

The pandemic exposed Indigenous people's health inequalities to the world. A 2018 United Nations publication on the impact of structural racism and inequality on Indigenous healthcare internationally observed, "It is a noted irony that Indigenous people living in the richest countries of [the] U.S. and Canada are among their poorest citizens. In terms of addressing Indigenous people's health situation, there are structural issues that require consideration" (The Department of Economic and Social Affairs of the United Nations, 2018, p. 110). In July 2020, both the World Health Organization and Pan American Health Organization (PAHO) released alerts broadcasting a need for increased attention to the health care needs of Indigenous communities in the Americas writ whole. Both of these alerts uncovered the systemic inequalities that placed Indigenous communities at increased risk for large-scale COVID-19 outbreaks. These include remote locations with low access to basic sanitation and health services and the Indigenous community's higher rate of co-morbidities, such as Tuberculosis, that have the potential for increasing death rates (Pan American Health Organization & World Health Organization, 2020; World Health Organization, 2020b). Racial and ethnic discrimination are apparent in health policies that do not "reflect the social and cultural practices and beliefs of Indigenous peoples" (Hongbo, 2018, p. v. The PAHO argued that it is important to address ethnicity within the context of COVID-19 because "structural racism and historical domination against these populations, which continues today, makes them more vulnerable than the general population to the effects of the pandemic" (del Pino & Camacho, 2020, p. 4).

Theoretical research implications

The research presented in this article emphasizes the importance of the news media acknowledging systemic inequalities and addressing different cultural and ethnic contexts when reporting about the pandemic and Indigenous communities. The current analysis found most mainstream media, without a connection to Indian Country, focused on lack of resources and the chronic struggle of Indigenous communities instead of putting Indigenous health stories into context. Instead of promoting change, stories merely relied on stereotypical tropes, blamed Indigenous people for health inequities, and offered a doom trajectory for tribes hit hardest by health issues, especially COVID-19. Schemas, stereotypes, priming, and cognitive dissonance all contributed to producing episodic framing of the pandemic in mainstream media. In comparison, Indigenous media coverage included community solutions to COVID-19 and a focus on resilience versus crisis. They committed to community coverage and produced almost 14 times more coverage per outlet than mainstream media.

Framing theory emphasizes that media have two options when discussing a story: they can use episodic framing, which focuses on "case studies and discrete events"; or they can use thematic framing, which focuses on "trends over time, and highlighting contexts and environments" (Benjamin, 2007, para. 1). As shown in the current analysis, a majority of the mainstream media, without connections to Indian Country, relied on episodic framing when reporting about Indigenous people during the pandemic, while Indigenous media used both episodic and thematic framing by telling individual stories and placing those stories within the broader cultural and historical context of health issues within Nations. Episodic framing ignores one of the most important roles of journalism – to explain *why*; episodic framing attributes responsibility to the characters in a story, thus Indigenous people are blamed for lacking the resources needed to overcome the health disparities they face (London, 1993, para. 9). Findings indicate that this episodic framing is actually playing into deficit framing, meaning that Indigenous people are framed as having a surfeit of personal responsibility, or other qualities, that would enable them to handle the pandemic in the first place. A broad-based literature review of studies on the evolution of deficit framing in the media found that this kind of *blame the victim* framing ignores the systematic disenfranchisement of subaltern groups and has broad impacts on policy (Baumgartner & McAdon, 2017; Iyengar, 1996; Johnston et al., 2015; Rose & Baumgartner, 2013; Spence, 2010).

By using episodic framing in reporting about the pandemic outbreak on the Navajo Nation, mainstream media overall often played into the current conversations that ignore systemic disenfranchisement of Indigenous people and instead frame tribes as lax in taking care of their people and services, thus needing the U.S. government to *save* the tribes with undeserved funding. This caused delays in the distribution of governmental aid to the tribes and skewed outsider views of what was actually happening across the tribal lands.

This study reveals how embedded framing has mediatized society to direct mainstream readers' attention away from the systemic deprivation of support that is guaranteed to Native Nations in tribal agreements (Pevar, 2004). As Suzan Shown Harjo, curator of a 2015 Smithsonian National Museum of the American Indian display of treaties, said, "The people who are citizens of the U.S., these are your treaties. They aren't just the Indians' treaties. No one gave us anything. No one was dragging any land behind them when they came here. This was our land" (Wang, 2015, para. 16).

The continuous disregard by the federal government for Indigenous communities was once again made apparent when the lack of internet access in those communities affected their ability to get COVID-19 information. The National Congress of American Indians (2020b) called on the FCC to give tribes the same access as cable companies, by extending the application for the Tribal Priority Window to apply for broadband licenses. NCAI noted that this extension was critical to track and share health data during the pandemic (2020b). The FCC, NCAI stated, argued that to extend the window for more than 30 days would hurt those who already applied for licenses; NCAI disagreed and asks for the same treatment that cable companies received because of COVID-19 – an extension of 180 days.

Meanwhile, other Indigenous organizations hosted live online events to address overall coverage of COVID-19 in Indian Country, including what was missing in the news. On

July 23, 2020, during NAJA's webinar, Jourdan Bennett-Begaye (Dine'), Washington, D.C. bureau chief for *Indian Country Today*, said that media sources completely ignored the impact of the 1918 flu pandemic on Indigenous people, and "there's nothing left of our people" in those stories. Essentially, she said, Indigenous people "did not exist during the 1918 pandemic" (NAJA, 2020d).

Professional implications

The challenge to reporters is to record the true story of Indigenous people. A shift in overall mainstream news framing of Indian Country and the pandemic could move conversations forward about policies at the national level. This may relieve some of the pressures tribes are seeing placed on their resources, particularly if their income sources are significantly reduced when tribal businesses are forced to close. Findings also showed Indigenous media was just beginning to comprehend this pandemic in its early stages; that comprehension included trying to build statistics that encompassed Indian Country while also telling stories of individuals and specific Nations' responses to COVID-19. All of the reporters and editors on NAJA's July 2020 "Covering COVID-19 in Indian Country: Navajo Nation" panel mentioned how it was essential for Indigenous journalists to report on as many Indigenous communities as possible, versus crafting monolithic coverage. Donovan Quintero, photojournalist for *Navajo Times*, said his work was guided by the principle, "The more we know about who we are, the more empowered we become." Reporter Bennett-Begaye said that gathering the statistics dominated her life early in the pandemic because she had to make a lot of individual phone calls and build a lot of relationships because Indian Country's data was spread out across the various nations. Soon, though, it became important to her and her staff to tell individual stories, particularly of people who died, because each person was part of the community.

Our findings suggest that non-Indigenous journalists need to do their homework to avoid falling into centuries-old patterns of stereotyping, simplifying, and denigrating Indigenous communities as "others." Mainstream media need to take the simple steps of continuing to educate themselves, using the experience of Indigenous journalists, and exposing themselves to Indigenous media. Then, instead of producing stories that may generate unequal health policies for Indigenous communities, they may promote positive change. In contrast, the Indigenous media studied in this sample highlighted the health issues in Indian Country through the lens of resilience. This thematic framing helps emphasize unequal power, while at the same time providing understanding of the issues.

Conclusion

Only when mainstream news sources produce stories about Indigenous health issues that are free of the stereotypes that have inculcated enduring schemas about Indigenous people will they begin to have a positive policy impact on Indigenous communities. Non-Indigenous journalists have easy access to resources and should incorporate them into their daily practices.

A good first step is to reference the NAJA Bingo Card as a quick self-check. NAJA offers free seminars and holds an annual conference open to all. It also has a number of reporting guides on special topics. Many publications that serve Indian Country are available at no charge online, including *Navajo Times*, *Cherokee Phoenix*, and *Indian Country Today*. Journalists just need to make sure that they are using independent sources, as some publications are products of tribal governments. There are also articles written by Indigenous journalists and academics about the best way to cover Indian Country (e.g., Azocar, 2019).

Covering health in Indian country

This analysis also reinforces that 1) newsrooms need reporters connected to Indigenous communities so that there is diverse coverage; 2) news organizations must allow these reporters space to tell specific stories with breadth and depth; and 3) news managers must understand that when packaging stories about diverse communities, that each part of a news story – from headlines to hashtags to pictures – plays a role in ethical reporting. Guidelines for news reporting on Indian Country may be found at NAJAnewsroom.com.

ORCID

Candi S. Carter Olson http://orcid.org/0000-0001-5696-4907
Cristina L. Azocar http://orcid.org/0000-0001-5659-9858
Benjamin R. LaPoe http://orcid.org/0000-0002-9410-7946

References

Adams, M. M. (2020, April 16). #COVIDintheSouth: Social distancing in the age of assimilation. *UNC: Center for the Study of the American South*. https://south.unc.edu/2020/04/16/covidinthesouth-social-distancing-in-the-age-of-assimilation/

Agoyo, A. (2020, June 11). COVID-19 exposes inadequate funding levels at Indian Health Service. *Indianz.com*. https://www.indianz.com/News/2020/06/11/covid19-exposes-inadequate-funding-level.asp

AJMC Staff. (2020, November 25). A timeline of COVID-19 developments in 2020. *The American Journal of Managed Care*. https://www.ajmc.com/view/a-timeline-of-covid19-developments-in-2020

Allen, K. (2020, May 28). With bleach and a prayer: In a tiny town, a clinic run by women holds the front line. *Navajo Times*. https://navajotimes.com/ae/community/in-a-tiny-town-a-clinic-run-by-women-holds-the-front-line/

Allen, M. (2017). Intercoder reliability techniques: Holsti method. In M. Allen (Ed.), *The Sage encyclopedia of communication research methods* (pp. 1–4). SAGE Publications, Inc. https://doi.org/10.4135/9781483381411.n258

American Press Institute. (2014, March 17). *The Personal News Cycle: How Americans Choose to Get Their News*. https://www.americanpressinstitute.org/publications/reports/survey-research/personal-news-cycle/

American Psychological Association. (2011). *Summary of the APA Resolution Recommending Retirement of American Indian Mascots*. https://www.apa.org/pi/oema/resources/indian-mascots

Ampuja, M., Koivisto, J., & Väliverronen, E. (2014). Strong and weak forms of mediatization theory. A critical review. *Nordicom Review*, *35* (2014), 111–123. https://doi.org/10.2478/nor-2014-0107

Amzel, A., & Ghosh, C. (2007). National newspaper coverage of minority health disparities. *Journal of the National Medical Association*, *99*(10), 1120–1125. https://www.ncbi.nlm.nih.gov/pmc/articles/PMC2574402/

Arviso, T., Quintero, D., Smith, N., & Bennett-Begaye, J. (2020, July 23). Covering COVID-19 in Indian Country: Navajo Nation. *Native*

American Journalists Association, *99*(10), 1120–1125. https://najanewsroom.com/2020/07/10/naja-to-host-first-covering-covid-19-in-indian-country-virtual-roundtable-july-23-2020/

Azocar, C. (2019). *The diversity style guide*. Wiley Blackwell.

Azocar, C., LaPoe, V., Carter Olson, C., LaPoe, B., & Hazarika, B. (2021). Indigenous communities and COVID 19: Reporting on resources and resilience. *Howard Journal of Communications*, *32*, 1–17. https://doi.org/10.1080/10646175.2021.1892552

Bakir, V. (2006). Policy agenda setting and risk communication. *Press Politics*, *11*(3), 67–88. https://doi.org/10.1177/1081180X06289213

Baumgartner, F. R., & McAdon, S. (2017, May 11). There's been a big change in how the news media covers sexual assault. *The Washington Post*. https://www.washingtonpost.com/news/monkey-cage/wp/2017/05/11/theres-been-a-big-change-in-how-the-news-media-cover-sexual-assault/

Becenti, A. (May 14, 2020). Pipe dreams: Could coronavirus finally bring water to rez? *Navajo Times*. https://navajotimes.com/reznews/pipe-dreams-could-coronavirus-finally-bring-water-to-rez/

Benjamin, D. (2007, December). *Episodic vs. Thematic Stories*. https://www.frameworksinstitute.org/article/episodic-vs-thematic-stories/

Brewer, G. [@grahambrewer]. (2020, June 26). *I don't know who needs to hear this, but when Indian Health Services doesn't have the money or resources* [Tweet] Twitter. https://twitter.com/grahambrewer/status/1276380429281525761

Brown, P. L. (2020, June 5). On tribal lands, a time to make art for solace and survival. *The New York Times*. https://www.nytimes.com/2020/06/05/arts/design/native-americans-art-coronavirus.html

Cooper, R., Pollock, N. J., Affleck, Z., Bain, L., Hansen, N. L., Robertson, K., & Chatwood, S. (2021). Patient healthcare experiences in the Northwest Territories, Canada: An analysis of news media articles. *International Journal of Circumpolar Health*, *80*(1), 1–9. https://doi.org/10.1080/22423982.2021.1886798

COVID-19 across the Navajo Nation. (2020, April. 6). *Navajo Times*. https://navajotimes.com/coronavirus-updates/covid-19-across-the-navajo-nation/

COVID-19 in Indian Country: Indian Country's COVID-19 syllabus. (2020, March 17). *Indian Country Today*. https://indiancountrytoday.com/news/indian-country-s-covid-19-syllabus-EiN-p5Q-XkW-smnaebJV6Q

Deaderick, L. (2020, May 10). History of inequality making COVID-19 worse for Native Americans. *San Diego Union Tribune*. https://www.sandiegouniontribune.com/columnists/story/2020-05-10/history-of-inequality-making-covid-19-worse-for-native-americans

del Pino, S., & Camacho, A. (2020). *Considerations on indigenous peoples, Afro-descendants, and other ethnic groups during the COVID-19 pandemic*. Pan American Health Organization. Retrieved March 17, 2021, from https://iris.paho.org/handle/10665.2/52251

Denzin, N. K., & Lincoln, Y. S. (1998). *The landscape of qualitative research: Theories and issues*. SAGE Publications, Inc.

Entman, R. M. (1993). Framing: Toward clarification of a fractured paradigm. *Journal of Communication*, *43*(4), 51–58. https://doi.org/10.1111/j.1460-2466.1993.tb01304.x

Estus, J. (2020, May 9). Pandemic broadens use of telemedicine in Indian Country and beyond. *Indian Country Today*. https://indiancountrytoday.com/news/pandemic-broadens-use-of-telemedicine-in-indian-country-and-beyond-BJbQHsMWp0i-LpADXGuRiQ

Gearhart, S., & Trumbly-Lamsam, T. (2017). The scoop on health: How native American newspapers frame and report health news. *Health Communication*, *32*(6), 695–702. https://doi.org/10.1080/10410236.2016.1168001

Gearhart, S., Trumbly-Lamsam, T., & Adegbola, O. (2017). Why isn't health a priority? A survey of journalists serving Native American news media. *Journalism Practice*, *12*(9), 1183–1200. https://doi.org/10.1080/17512786.2017.1363658

Gollust, S. E., Fowler, E. F., & Niederdeppe, J. (2019). Television news coverage of public health issues and implications for public health policy and practice. *Annual Review of Public Health*, *40*, 167–185. https://www.annualreviews.org/doi/abs/10.1146/annurev-publhealth-040218-044017

Goodluck, K. (2020a). *Bio*. https://www.kalengoodluck.com/about.

Goodluck, K. (2020b, May 11). It's hurting in the short term. It's hurting now! *High Country News*. https://www.hcn.org/articles/indigenous-affairs-interview-its-hurting-in-the-short-term-its-hurting-now

Gregory, A., Borell, B., McCreanor, T., Barnes, A. M., Nairn, R., Rankine, J., & Kaiwai, H. (2011). Reading news about Māori: Responses from non-Māori media audiences. *AlterNative: An International Journal of Indigenous Peoples*, *7*(1), 51–64. https://doi.org/10.1177/117718011100700105

Hedgpeth, D., Fears, D., & Scruggs, G. (2020a, April 4). Indian Country, where residents suffer disproportionately from disease, is bracing for coronavirus. *The Washington Post*. https://www.washingtonpost.com/climate-environment/2020/04/04/native-americancoronavirus/

Hedgpeth, D., Fears, D., & Scruggs, G. (2020b, April 6). 'We could get wiped out': Native Americans have the highest rates of diseases that make COVID-19 more lethal. *Philadelphia Inquirer*. https://www.inquirer.com/health/coronavirus/coronavirus-native-americans-indians-20200406.html

Herbst, S. (1998). *Reading public opinion: How political actors view the democratic process*. Westview Press.

Hjarvard, S. (2008). The mediatization of society: A theory of the media as agents of social and cultural change. *Nordicom Review*, *29*(2), 105–134. https://doi.org/10.1515/nor-2017-0181

Hoffman-Goetz, L., Shannon, C., & Clarke, J. N. (2003). Chronic disease coverage in Canadian aboriginal newspapers. *Journal of Health Communication*, *8*(5), 475–488. https://doi.org/10.1080/10810730390233299

Hongbo, W. (2018). *Foreword to the state of the world's Indigenous People*. Department of Economic and Social Affairs of the United Nations. https://www.un.org/development/desa/indigenouspeoples/wp-content/uploads/sites/19/2018/03/The-State-of-The-Worlds-Indigenous-Peoples-WEB.pdf

Indian Health Service. (2019). *Disparities: Fact sheet*. https://www.ihs.gov/newsroom/factsheets/disparities

'It's hard when a death occurs' during COVID-19. (2020, June 18). *Indian Country Today*. https://indiancountrytoday.com/newscasts/it-s-hard-when-a-death-occurs-during-covid-19-BN8-9UeAqEa-UzDPGm4Lyw

Iyengar, S. (1996). Framing responsibility for political issues. *Political Behavior*, *12*(1), 19–40. https://doi.org/10.1007/BF00992330

James, C., Schwartz, K., & Berndt, J. (2009). *Race, ethnicity, and healthcare issue brief: A profile of Americans Indians and Alaska Natives and their health coverage*. National Resource Center on Native American Aging. https://www.kff.org/wp-content/uploads/2013/01/7977.pdf

Jarding, L. J. (2004). Native American and non-Indian newspaper coverage of land and resource issues in the self-determination era. *The Social Science Journal*, *41*(4), 559–573. http://dx.doi.org/10.1016/j.soscij.2004.08.011

Johnston, A., Friedman, B., & Sobel, M. (2015). Framing an emerging issue: How U.S. print and broadcast news media covered sex trafficking, 2008–2012. *Journal of Human Trafficking*, *1*(3), 235–254. https://doi.org/10.1080/23322705.2014.993876

Kaplan, E., & Davis, T. (2020, May 31). 'Huge disparity' in COVID-19 death rates for Native Americans in NM. *Albuquerque Journal*. https://www.abqjournal.com/1461218/huge-disparity-in-covid19-death-rates-for-native-americans-in-nm.html

Kerry. (2014). Sistergirls/brotherboys: The status of indigenous transgender Australians. *International Journal of Transgenderism*, *15*(3–4), 173–186. https://doi.org/10.1080/15532739.2014.995262

Kim, A. E., Kumanyika, S., Shive, D., Igweatu, U., & Kim, S. H. (2010). Coverage and framing of racial and ethnic health disparities in U.S. newspapers, 1996–2005. *American Journal of Public Health*, *100*(S1), 224–231. https://doi.org/10.2105/AJPH.2009.171678

Kristof, N. (2020, May 30). The top U.S. coronavirus hot spots are all Indian lands. *The New York Times*. https://www.nytimes.com/2020/05/30/opinion/sunday/coronavirus-native-americans.ht

Lam, S., Cunsolo, A., Sawatzky, A., Ford, J., & Harper, S. L. (2017). How does the media portray drinking water security in Indigenous communities in Canada? An analysis of Canadian newspaper coverage from 2000-2015. *BMC Public Health*, *17*(1), 1–14. https://doi.org/10.1186/s12889-017-4164-4

LaPoe, V., Carter Olson, C., & LaPoe, B. (2018). *Underserved communities and digital discourse: Getting voices heard.* Lexington Press.

LaPoe, V., & LaPoe, B. (2017). *Indian country: Telling a story in a digital age.* Michigan State Press.

Lippmann, W. (1922). *Public opinion.* Simon & Schuster.

London, S. (1993). *How the media frames political issues.* Scott. https://scott.london/reports/frames.html

McCallum, K., Meadows, M., Waller, L., Dunne Breen, M., & Reid, H. (2012). *The media and Indigenous policy: How news media reporting and mediatized practice impact on Indigenous policy.* University of Canberra.

McCombs, M. E., & Shaw, D. L. (1972). The agenda-setting function of mass media. *Public Opinion Quarterly, 36*(2), 176–187. https://doi.org/10.1086/267990

Morris, J. L. (2004). Textual analysis in journalism. In S. H. Iorio (Ed.), *Qualitative research in journalism: Taking it to the streets* (pp. 159–171). Routledge. https://doi.org/10.4324/9781410609557

Nagle, R. (2020, April 24). Native Americans being left out of U.S. coronavirus data and labelled as 'other.' *The Guardian.* https://www.theguardian.com/us-news/2020/apr/24/us-native-americans-left-out-coronavirus-data

National Congress of American Indians. (2020a). *Gaming.* https://www.ncai.org/policy-issues/economic-development-commerce/gaming

National Congress of American Indians. (2020b, July 31). *NCAI calls on the FCC to honor its trust responsibility to tribal nations during global pandemic.* http://www.ncai.org/news/articles/2020/07/31/ncai-calls-on-the-fcc-to-honor-its-trust-responsibility-to-tribal-nations-during-global-pandemic

Native American Journalists Association. (2019a, May 30). *NAJA urges journalism organizations to complete diversity survey.* https://najanewsroom.com/2019/05/30/naja-urges-journalism-organizations-to-complete-diversity-survey/

Native American Journalists Association. (2019b, August 12). *NAJA demands the Washington Post retract unreliable data sets and all associated reporting.* https://najanewsroom.com/2019/08/12/naja-demands-the-washington-post-retract-unreliable-data-sets-and-all-associated-reporting/

Native American Journalists Association. (2019c, November 1). *NAJA Calls for Audit on New York Times story.* https://najanewsroom.com/2019/11/01/naja-calls-for-audit-on-new-york-times-story/

Native American Journalists Association. (2020a). *NAJA media spotlight report.* https://najanewsroom.com/2020-naja-media-spotlight-report/

Native American Journalists Association. (2020b). *Bingo Card.* https://najanewsroom.com/bingo-card/

Native American Journalists Association. (2020c). *2020 NAJA NBC fellowships.* https://najanewsroom.com/2020/01/10/2020-naja-nbc-news-summer-fellowship/

Native American Journalists Association. (2020d). *Covering COVID-19 in Indian Country.* https://najanewsroom.com/2020/07/10/naja-to-host-first-covering-covid-19-in-indian-country-virtual-roundtable-july-23-2020/

Native American Journalists Association. (n.d.). *Reporting and Indigenous Terminology.* https://najanewsroom.com/wp-content/uploads/2018/11/NAJA_Reporting_and_Indigenous_Terminology_Guide.pdf.

O'Connor, C., & Joffe, H. (2020). Intercoder reliability in qualitative research: Debates and practical guidelines. *International Journal of Qualitative Methods, 19,* 1–13. https://doi.org/10.1177/1609406919899220

Oklahoma City Indian clinic continues to hire during COVID-19. (2020, June 24). *Cherokee phoenix.* https://www.cherokeephoenix.org/Article/Index/134908

Ortiz, E. (2020, May 24). As the coronavirus pandemic strains supplies, Native Americans fight food insecurity. *NBC News.* https://www.nbcnews.com/news/us-news/coronavirus-pandemic-strains-supplies-native-americans-fight-food-insecurity-n1213116

Pan American Health Organization & World Health Organization. (2020, July 15). *Epidemiological alert: COVID-19 among indigenous peoples in the Americas.* https://www.paho.org/en/documents/epidemiological-alert-covid-19-among-indigenous-peoples-americas-15-july-2020

Pevar, S. (2004). *The rights of Indians and tribes: The authoritative ACLU guide to Indian and tribal rights* (3rd ed.). New York University Press.

Romero, S., & Healy, J. (2020, May 11). Tribal nations face most severe crisis in decades as the coronavirus closes casinos. *The New York Times.* https://www.nytimes.com/2020/05/11/us/coronavirus-native-americans-indian-country.html

Rose, M., & Baumgartner, F. R. (2013). Framing the poor: Media coverage and U.S. poverty policy, 1960–2008. *The Policy Studies Journal, 41*(1), 22–53. https://doi.org/10.1111/psj.12001

Saguy, A. C., & Gruys, K. (2010). Morality and health: News media constructions of overweight and eating disorders. *Social Problems, 57* (2), 231–250. https://doi.org/10.1525/sp.2010.57.2.231

Schwitzer, G. (2004). A statement of principles for health care journalists. *The American Journal of Bioethics, 4*(4), 9–13. https://doi.org/10.1080/15265160490908086

Sottile, C., & Ortiz, E. (2020, April 19). Coronavirus hits Indian Country hard, exposing infrastructure disparities. *NBC News.* https://www.nbcnews.com/news/us-news/coronavirus-hits-indian-country-hard-exposing-infrastructure-disparities-n1186976

Spence, L. K. (2010). Episodic frames, HIV/ AIDS, and African American public opinion. *Political Research Quarterly, 63*(2), 257–268. https://doi.org/10.1177/1065912908330727

Starr, T. S., & Oxlad, M. (2020). News media stories about cancer on Facebook: How does story framing influence response framing, tone and attributions of responsibility? *Health: An Interdisciplinary Journal for the Social Study of Health, Illness and Medicine.* https://doi.org/10.1177/1363459320912817

Sunuwar, D. K. (2019, September 19). *Indigenous media caucus amplifies indigenous voices globally.* Cultural Survival. https://www.culturalsurvival.org/news/indigenous-media-caucus-amplifies-indigenous-voices-globally

The Department of Economic and Social Affairs of the United Nations. (2018). *State of the world's indigenous people: Indigenous people's access to health services.* https://www.un.org/development/desa/indigenouspeoples/wp-content/uploads/sites/19/2018/03/The-State-of-The-Worlds-Indigenous-Peoples-WEB.pdf

Walker, M., & Cochrane, E. (2020, May 2). Native American tribes sue treasury over stimulus aid as they feud over funding. *The New York Times.* https://www.nytimes.com/2020/05/01/us/politics/coronavirus-native-american-tribes-treasury-stimulus.html

Wang, H. L. (2015, January. 18). *Broken promises on display at native American treaties exhibit.* National Public Radio. https://www.npr.org/sections/codeswitch/2015/01/18/368559990/broken-promises-on-display-at-native-american-treaties-exhibit

World Health Organization. (2020a, April 27). *Archived: WHO timeline-COVID-19.* https://www.who.int/news-room/detail/27-04-2020-who-timeline—covid-19

World Health Organization. (2020b, July 20). *Coronavirus disease (COVID-19): Situation report-182.* https://www.who.int/docs/default-source/coronaviruse/situation-reports/20200720-covid-19-sitrep-182.pdf?sfvrsn=60aabc5c_2

Family Connections and the Latino Health Paradox: Exploring the Mediating Role of Loneliness in the Relationships Between the Latina/o Cultural Value of Familism and Health

Monica L. Gallegos and Chris Segrin

ABSTRACT

This study aims to understand Latina/o health from a social relationships perspective. Specifically, a major goal of the study is to explain how despite disadvantages (e.g., lower income and less education), Latinas/os in some cases have superior health compared to non-Latina/o whites, a phenomenon known as the Latino Health Paradox. Based on the central role of familial relationships in Latina/o culture, and utilizing Hawkley and Cacioppo's theoretical model of loneliness and health as a foundation for the study, the premise underlying this research is that the Latina/o cultural value of *familism* has a beneficial impact on health via reduced loneliness. Participants were 255 adults who identified as Latina/o (N = 139) or non-Latina/o white (N = 116), ranging in age from 19–88. Results indicate that being Latina/o predicted strong endorsement of familism, that predicted lower loneliness, and lower loneliness subsequently predicted better overall health, mental health, and health practices. These results suggest that the cultural value of familism provides health-related benefits for Latinas/os, which contributes to understanding the Latino health paradox. Results also underscore the value of including loneliness in studies examining the impact of cultural values on health, as only loneliness had statistically significant direct associations with all three health outcomes.

As of 2017, there were approximately 60 million Latinas/os[1] in the U.S., accounting for nearly 18% of the population (Noe-Bustamante & Flores, 2019). Compared to non-Latina/o whites, Latinas/os face a number of socioeconomic disadvantages. For example, Latinas/os are less likely to finish high school or have a college degree (Noe-Bustamante & Flores, 2019), have a lower median income compared to non-Latina/o whites (49,793 vs. $65,845, USD respectively), are more likely to live in poverty, and are the least likely of all ethnic minorities in the U.S. to have health insurance (Fontenot et al., 2018). Latina/o communities are also burdened with structural inequalities that negatively impact health, such as food insecurity (Potochnick et al., 2019, poor air quality (Yip et al., 2011), and unsafe drinking water (Schaider et al., 2019).

Despite these disadvantages that are linked to poor health outcomes in the general population (U.S. Centers for Disease Control and Prevention, 2013), Latinas/os have unique health-related advantages compared to their non-Latina/o white counterparts. For example, Latinas/os live on average 81.8 years; nearly three years longer than non-Latina/o whites (78.5 years), and the U.S. population overall (78.6 years; Arias & Xu, 2019). Moreover, despite high rates of cardiovascular disease and cancer mortality in general, compared to non-Latina/o whites, Latinas/os have better overall mortality, income-adjusted all-cause cancer mortality, and lower age-adjusted prevalence and mortality from cardiovascular disease (Abraido-Lanza et al., 1999; Arias et al., 2010; Balfour et al., 2016; Mozaffarian et al., 2016; Yanez et al., 2016). Better mental health outcomes exist for Latinas/os compared to non-Latina/o whites as well (Alegría et al., 2008). This phenomenon, often referred to as the *Latino health paradox* or *Hispanic health paradox* (Markides & Coreil, 1986), is documented in several national epidemiological studies (see Heron, 2015; Liao et al., 1998; Sorlie et al., 1993). Importantly, findings from a meta-analysis of 58 longitudinal studies not only support the existence of the Latino health paradox, but also identify a 17.5% lower overall mortality rate for Latinas/os (Ruiz et al., 2013); a health advantage that is considered "large [and] clinically meaningful" (Ruiz, Campos et al., 2016, p. 63).

Some scholars attempting to explain the Latino health paradox initially suggested that health and mortality advantages are due to immigration and emigration patterns based on health status (i.e., the healthy migrant hypothesis and salmon bias hypothesis), or methodological issues (i.e., the data misclassification and data artifact hypotheses), but these explanations have been rejected (see Abraido-Lanza et al., 1999; Arias et al., 2010). Instead, others suggest that various aspects of Latina/o culture provide protection against poor health outcomes (Abraido-Lanza et al., 1999). However, there is a substantial lack of empirical research on Latina/o health that includes measures of specific cultural values (Perez & Cruess, 2014).

One cultural value that may help explain the Latino health paradox is *familism*, also known as *familismo*. Familism is commonly described as a strong focus on caring for, and maintaining relationships with, both close and extended family members (Marin & Marin, 1991; Parsai et al., 2009; Ruiz,

2007). Familism impacts numerous aspects of interpersonal and family communication among Latinas/os. Generally, familism encourages individuals within the family to provide social support, advice (Sabogal et al., 1987), regular contact, and communication with close and extended family members (Keefe, 1984). Familism also impacts communication specifically related to health. For example, Latinas/os often care for family members by communicating reminders for medication and encouraging treatment adherence (Ashing-Giwa et al., 2004; Laroche et al., 2009). Latinas/os are also influenced by descriptive and injunctive norms established and modeled within the family. For example, Latinas are more likely to engage in physical activity and eat healthy when family members model and express positive opinions about these behaviors (Abraido-Lanza et al., 2017; Salvy et al., 2017). Furthermore, familism prescribes close relationships and interpersonal communication between parents and children that can help lower the risk of beginning harmful behaviors such as substance use (Lac et al., 2011), and encourage positive sexual communication (Gaioso et al., 2015). However, familism can also have a negative impact on health communication. For example, Latinas/os may avoid self-disclosure about some health issues due to fears of burdening the family or bringing shame to its members (Ashing-Giwa et al., 2004; Simoni et al., 1995).

Importantly, familism includes a commitment to sustaining emotional bonds with family members, remaining physically close to family in order to maintain mutual involvement in day-to-day life, an obligation to put family members' needs before one's own, and an inherent expectation of reciprocity for the provision of resources on both a daily basis and when challenging circumstances arise (Lugo Steidel & Contreras, 2003). As such, to a large extent, Latinas/os' personal identity is strongly tied to familial interconnectedness throughout the lifespan, which could provide long-term protection against loneliness. This benefit could be particularity advantageous, especially considering the significant negative impact loneliness has on both mental and physical wellness including depression, poor cardiovascular health, immune system deficiencies, and accelerated health decline with age (Hawkley & Cacioppo, 2010). Therefore, empirical research that examines links between the Latina/o cultural value of familism, loneliness, and health may help explain the Latino health paradox and fill the "significant" gaps (Ruiz, Campos et al., 2016, p. 62) that persist in our understanding of Latina/o health and well-being. Hawkley, Cacioppo, and colleagues' theoretical model of loneliness and health (see Hawkley & Cacioppo, 2007, 2010) is a viable framework for such a study.

Theoretical model of loneliness and health

Loneliness is a perceived discrepancy between desired and achieved levels of social contact (Peplau et al., 1979). Hawkley, Cacioppo, and colleagues' theoretical model of loneliness and health (see Hawkley & Cacioppo, 2007, 2010) highlights how loneliness impacts health and well-being through five primary mechanisms. Specifically, compared to non-lonely people, lonely individuals engage in poorer health behaviors, have increased stress exposure, engage in maladaptive stress appraisal and coping, experience less effective restorative processes (e.g., sleep), and tend to have an overactive physiological response to stress (see Hawkley & Cacioppo, 2003, 2010). As a result, lonely individuals experience significant health problems, including increased inflammation, poor metabolic functioning, increased risk for coronary heart disease, stroke, and other vascular diseases, as well as greater cardiovascular mortality and overall mortality (Hawkley & Cacioppo, 2010; Hawkley et al., 2006). Lonely people moreover, experience overactivation of systems that control immune function and regulation of hormones during stress (e.g., epinephrine and norepinephrine), resulting in increased wear and tear on physiological systems and accelerated physiological decline with age (Hawkley & Cacioppo, 2007). Loneliness has also been associated with mental health problems including schizophrenia, suicide, depression, anxiety, alcohol abuse, recreational drug use, eating disorders (Ernst & Cacioppo, 1999; Heinrich & Gullone, 2006), and increased risk for Alzheimer's disease. (Wilson et al., 2007). Overall, loneliness affects health in ways similar to obesity, smoking, and sedentary lifestyle (Holt-Lunstad et al., 2015; House et al., 1988). However, the presence of close relationships and lasting feelings of interconnectedness can help mitigate perceptions of loneliness (Hawkley et al., 2008) which can protect against the poor health outcomes associated with it (Hawkley & Cacioppo, 2010).

Familial relationships, loneliness, and health

Familial relationships can benefit health in a number of ways, that include reducing loneliness. The prophylactic effect of close, strong connections with others, including with family members, on health has been well-established (see Albrecht & Goldsmith, 2003; Cohen & Wills, 1985; Seeman & McEwen, 1996). A meta-analysis of 148 longitudinal studies reported a 50% reduced mortality risk for people with stronger relationships; an effect that is greater in magnitude than other risk factors such as obesity, and is comparable to cigarette smoking (Holt-Lunstad et al., 2010). Intimate, supportive, and reliable relationships are also essential to thwarting and reducing the experience of loneliness (Chen, 2012; Jones & Moore, 1987; Segrin & Passalacqua, 2010), which can protect health (Hawkley et al., 2003; Hawkley & Cacioppo, 2010). In fact, reducing perceptions of loneliness is a key mechanism through which relationships benefit health (Segrin & Domschke, 2011). For example, reduced loneliness afforded by social relationships is directly linked to a lower risk of mortality, and is stronger predictor than sheer number of relationships, even when controlling for other risk factors such as age, sex, chronic disease, and smoking (Phennix et al., 1997).

The relationships most consistently related to beneficial health outcomes are familial (Uchino et al., 1996). Indeed, the strong and dependable connections provided by family are associated with better immune, cardiovascular, and neuroendocrine functioning, as well as better health overall (Albrecht & Goldsmith, 2003). As such, the importance of family cohesion among Latinas/os (Marin, 1993), may provide benefits related to health and well-being. Specifically, numerous characteristics of the Latina/o cultural value of *familism* (or *familismo*) suggest that family provides lifelong feelings of connection and social integration for Latinas/os, which can reduce perceptions of loneliness.

For example, familism is characterized by lifelong familial obligations (Rodriguez et al., 2007), strong connections with both immediate and extended family, intergenerational solidarity, and a belief that the family's needs supersede one's own (Perez & Cruess, 2014). The value highlights that family is a key source for instrumental and emotional resources, as well as information for behaviors and attitudes (Marin & Marin, 1991; Parsai et al., 2009; Ruiz, 2007). An obligation to care for one's family and to take family into consideration when making decisions, including those about health, are also central tenets of familism (Davila et al., 2011). Furthermore, familism includes an assumption that older adults will be provided with care, specifically by their children, as they experience age-related physical and/or mental declines (Ruiz, 2007). Moreover, evidence suggests that compared to other ethnic groups, Latina/os more strongly perceive that they can rely on family members, even when actual contact is not greater (Ruiz, 2007), and that Latina/o family ties tend to be "close both psychosocially and geographically" (Mirowsky & Ross, 1984, p. 3). Collectively, these characteristics of familism may increase the likelihood that Latinas/os will have a network of close social connections that can effectively prevent or mitigate feelings of loneliness.

Finally, research has identified familism as a central Latina/o cultural value, and an important factor to consider when studying Latina/o health (Coohey, 2001; Davila et al., 2011). A review of studies that examines the relationship between familism and health among Latinas/os (Perez & Cruess, 2014) highlights numerous contexts in which the cultural value is beneficial and protective, including diabetes care, general health practices (e.g., exercise, smoking, and risky sexual behavior), and breast cancer treatment. However, the authors also note that in some cases familism may be problematic by causing detrimental outcomes such as feelings of increased stress, high felt obligation, reduced self-care routines when individual needs conflict with family needs, or delays in treatment due to family obligations (see also Mendez-Luck et al., 2016). Related research shows that Latinas with breast cancer are at risk of dropping out of vital treatment if they feel needed by their family (Ashing-Giwa et al., 2004), they sometimes conceal their diagnosis from family members to avoid becoming a burden (Gonzalez et al., 2005), and their distress may be passed on to family caregivers (Segrin et al., 2020). Moreover, the "familial honor" aspect of familism (see Lugo Steidel & Contreras, 2003) may be problematic for individuals with marginalized identities. For example, those who are HIV positive or LGBTQ may hide those aspects of their identity out of fear that they would bring shame or embarrassment to the family (Muñoz-Laboy, 2008; Simoni et al., 1995) and could be ostracized as a result. Considering the central role that familism plays in Latina/o culture, Latinas/os may be more sensitized to rejection from family, which could amplify perceptions of loneliness and the poor health outcomes associated with it. Importantly, Perez and Cruess (2014) noted that the majority of the studies on familism and well-being were "exploratory in nature" (p. 114) and call for more rigorous research in this area that includes direct measures of familism.

Overall, the key characteristics that comprise the cultural value of familism illustrate how closely Latinas/os' individual lives and identities are linked to strong familial connections that persist throughout their lifespan. Moreover, expectations of reciprocity for maintaining lifelong physical and emotional connections with one another; the requirement to prioritize familial needs above one's own; as well as an obligation to be available and responsive to the needs of family members, while knowing family members will do the same (Lugo Steidel & Contreras, 2003; Marin & Marin, 1991; Parsai et al., 2009; Rodriguez et al., 2007; Ruiz, 2007), provides Latinas/os with a cache of valuable relationships that are likely to be effective at reducing or preventing loneliness. Considering that the effects of loneliness accumulate over time in a "dose-response fashion" to accelerate physiological decline throughout the lifespan (Hawkley & Cacioppo, 2010, pp. 219, 221), the extended familial networks in place from birth through old age for Latinas/os can provide a continuous buffer against loneliness, thereby protecting against the deleterious health outcomes associated with it. Yet, there is a lack of empirical research in Latina/o populations examining the relationships among familism, loneliness, and health.

In addition, familism characteristics (Marin & Marin, 1991; Parsai et al., 2009; Perez & Cruess, 2014; Ruiz, 2007) are likely to address some of the key mechanisms through which loneliness impacts health (see Hawkley & Cacioppo, 2010). For example, familism can promote beneficial health behaviors, buffer the impact of stress on health, and provide resources that promote adaptive responses to stress (Corona et al., 2019; Perez & Cruess, 2014). Considering evidence that perceptions of close, reliable, high-quality family relationships predict lower loneliness (Shiovitz-Ezra & Leitsch, 2010), as well as the established deleterious links between loneliness and health (Hawkley & Cacioppo, 2010), it is conceivable that reduced loneliness stemming from endorsement of familism could protect health. Moreover, although the idea of taking care of and relying on one's family is not unique to Latinas/os (Coohey, 2001; Ruiz, 2007; Schwartz, 2007), there is evidence that Latinas/os tend to endorse filial support and obligations more strongly than non-Latina/o whites (Connell & Gibson, 1997), there is greater "participation in family networks within and across generations" for Latinas/os compared to non-Latina/o whites (Organista, 2007, p. 142), and Latinas/os are more likely to have a stronger orientation toward family (Gaines et al., 1997; Perez & Cruess, 2014).

The current study

In light of previously reviewed evidence, it is probable that being Latina/o will predict endorsement of familism. Testing this assumption is important, in order to distinguish the impact of ethnicity on health from the impact of cultural values on health (Gallo et al., 2009; Ruiz, Hamann et al., 2016). Also, considering that loneliness can negatively impact physical health, mental health, and health practices (Hawkley & Cacioppo, 2010), it is important to test the relationship between ethnicity, familism, and loneliness with multiple health outcomes. Thus, we hypothesize:

H1: Ethnicity (i.e., being Latina/o) will positively predict endorsement of familism; familism will have an inverse relationship with loneliness; and loneliness will have an inverse relationship with overall health.

H2: Ethnicity (i.e., being Latina/o) will positively predict endorsement of familism; familism will have an inverse relationship with loneliness; and loneliness will have an inverse relationship with beneficial health practices.

H3: Ethnicity (i.e., being Latina/o) will positively predict endorsement of familism; familism will have an inverse relationship with loneliness; and loneliness will have a positive association with depression.

The data used to test these hypotheses were collected as part of a larger study of social psychological determinants of health (Gallegos, 2013). In the present study, only the data from Latina/o and non-Latina/o white participants in the parent study were analyzed for the hypothesis tests. Findings from that parent study documented the Latino health paradox in this sample. Specifically, non-Latina/o white participants reported significantly higher income and education than Latina/o participants. Nevertheless, there were no significant differences between the two groups in terms of overall health or mental health. As predicted by the Latino health paradox, the Latina/o participants in this study face socioeconomic disadvantages that are typically associated with health disparities, yet their health is no worse than non-Latina/o white participants.

Table 1. Demographics: Latina/o and Non-Latina/o white participants.

	Non-Latina/o White	Latina/o
Average Income	$126, 670[†]	$49, 570
Average Age	48.59 (*SD* = 18.85)	48.60 (*SD* = 19.85)
Participants Per Age Category		
18–33	30	43
34–49	20	27
50–65	43	33
66+	23	36
Sex		
Male	35 (30.2%)	40 (28.8%)
Female	81 (69.8%)	97 (69.8%)
Education		
Completed Grade School or Jr. High	0 (0%)	11 (7.9%)
Completed a High School Degree	6 (5.2%)	17 (12.2%)
Completed Some College	36 (31.0%)	36 (26.0%)
Completed a 4-Year Degree	48 (41.4%)	27 (19.4%)
Advanced Degree (M.A., Ph.D., etc.)	17(14.7%)	20(14.4%)
Marital Status	68(58.6%)	61(43.9%)
Completed Online Survey	101 (87.1%)	84 (60.4%)
Completed Paper Survey	15(12.9%)	55(39.6%)*

Standard deviations and percentages are indicated in parentheses
[†]Does not include a response of $1 million
*Includes eight Spanish-language paper surveys

Method

Participants

The study included 139 Latina/o and 116 non-Latina/o white participants. The majority of participants were female (69.8%) and married (50.8%). The average age of participants was 48.6 years (*SD* = 19.36), and the average income after removing a response of 1 USD million was 82,247 USD (*SD* = 92,885 USD). For a small percentage of participants (9.0%) a high school degree was the highest level of education completed, while over half of the participants had either completed some college (28.2%) or a four-year college degree (29.4%). Separate demographics for Latina/o and non-Latina/o-white participants can be found in Table 1.

Measures

All measures were translated to Spanish by a professional, Ph.D.-level translator, using Marin and Marin (1991) criteria. Correlations for major study variables are in Table 2.

Familism

Familism was measured with a 28-item version of the 18-item scale by Lugo Steidel and Contreras (2003). The scale measures multiple dimensions of familism, including subjugation of self for family, familial interconnectedness, familial honor, and familial reciprocity. The original scale was augmented with ten mirrored versions of existing items (reverse-scored) to enhance the reliability of the measure. For example, participants respond to items such as, "A person should live near his or her parents and spend time with them on a regular basis" as well as "It is unimportant for a person to live near his or her parents and spend time with them on a regular basis." Response options range from 1 (*strongly disagree*) to 10 (*strongly agree*). An overall familism score is obtained by calculating the average of the scores for individual items. Higher scores indicate stronger endorsement of familism. The reliability of this scale was (α = .87).

Loneliness

The 20-item UCLA Loneliness Scale (Version 3, Russell, 1996) was used to assess loneliness. Participants respond to items such as, "How often do you feel left out?" Response choices range from 1 (*never*) to 4 (*always*). A total loneliness score is calculated by summing individual item scores. Higher scores indicate stronger perceptions of loneliness. The internal consistency reliability of this measure was α = .91.

Overall health

The Medical Outcomes Study (MOS) 36-Item Short-Form Health Status Survey (SF-36; Ware & Sherbourne, 1992) was used to measure overall health. The survey contains scales that measure eight domains of health that include physical functioning, limitations in role activities due to physical health, bodily pain, vitality, social functioning, limitations in role activities due to emotional health, general mental health, and general health perceptions (Perkins et al., 2006). Participants respond to items with a range of response choices on Likert scales. For example, for questions regarding physical limitations such as, "Does your health limit you in climbing one flight of stairs?"(physical functioning domain) responses range from 1 (*yes, limited a lot*) to 3 (*no, not limited at all*). For questions such as, "How true or false is the following statement for you: I seem to get sick a little easier than other people?" (general health domain) choices range from 1 (*definitely true*) to 5 (*definitely false*). Additional

Table 2. Descriptive statistics and correlations among major study variables.

Variable	*M*	*SD*	Scale Range	1	2	3	4	5	6
1. Ethnicity r_{pb}	.44	.50	0–1	–					
2. Familism	6.90	1.17	3.52–9.75	.17**	–				
3. Loneliness	37.03	8.48	20–61	.03	–.19**	–			
4. Overall Health	609.72	137.28	112–790	–.11	–.01	–.49***	–		
5. Health Pract.	4.37	.66	2.46–5.85	–.13*	–.04	–.30***	.33***	–	
6. Depression	3.20	2.74	0–17	.02	–.04	.61***	–.66***	–.35***	–

Health Pract. = Health Practices. $N = 255$ * $p < .05$. ** $p < .01$. *** $p < .001$.
Ethnicity coded as 0 = non-Latina/o white, 1 = Latina/o

sample items include, "During the past four weeks, did you accomplish less than you would like as a result of your physical health?" (role limitations due to physical health domain); and "How much bodily pain have you had during the past four weeks?" (pain domain). Response values are recoded to be on a 1 to 100 scale representing the percentage of total possible scores achieved (Hays et al., 1993; Perkins et al., 2006). Subscale scores are created by averaging the items from each of the eight subscales. An overall health score is calculated as the sum of all subscale scores. Higher scores indicate better health. The internal consistency reliability of the overall MOS-36 measure was α = .87.

Depression

The 7-item depression subscale of the Hospital Anxiety and Depression Scale (Zigmond & Snaith, 1983) was administered to measure depression. A sample item is, "I feel as if I am slowed down." Likert scale responses range from 0 (*not at all*) to 3 (*most of the time*). A total depression score is calculated as the sum of all items in the subscale. Larger scores indicate greater depression. Internal consistency reliability of this measure was α = .72.

Health practices

A 13-item subset from Jackson's (2006) 58-item Health Practices Scale was administered to measure health practices. Items were selected from each of the five subscales in the original measure, including substance use, sleep adequacy, medical adherence, regular exercise, and healthy diet. Items for the original scale were selected from valid and reliable measures of health practices (see Kulbok et al., 1999; National Center for Health Statistics, 1999; Williams et al., 1991). Participants respond to items that assess how often they engage in practices such as "eat healthy food" (healthy diet subscale); "smoke cigarettes" (substance use subscale); "get daily aerobic exercise" (exercise subscale); "discuss concerns with your doctor" (medical adherence subscale); and "sleep 7–8 hours per night" (sleep adequacy subscale). Responses are recorded on a Likert scale ranging from 1 (*never*) to 6 (*always*). Scores for each item are averaged to calculate a total health practices score. Higher scores indicate more frequent engagement in healthy practices. The internal consistency reliability of this scale was α = .75.

Demographics

Demographic variables including ethnicity, income, and education, were also measured.

Procedure

Participants in this study were taking part in a larger investigation of social relationships and health (Gallegos, 2013). After obtaining university IRB approval, participants were recruited through stratified sampling to enroll approximately equal numbers of Latinas/os and non–Latina/o white participants in four age categories (18–33, 34–49, 50–65, 66+), in order to represent individuals at different stages in the lifespan. The number of Latina/o and non-Latina/o white participants in each age category are presented in Table 1.

Informed consent was secured by asking participants to sign a written consent form that stated the purpose of the study and explained that no risks were involved, identifying information would not be associated with responses, participants could skip questions or quit, as well as the time commitment and compensation for participating. Extra credit was offered to undergraduate students at a university in the Southwestern United States to either complete the study, or recruit someone from another age category. Approximately 82% of non-Latina/o white participants were recruited in this way. Latina/o participants were from both undergraduate classes and their recruits, as well as community contacts (i.e., Latina/o club members, community center directors, etc.). Participants who were not university affiliated received a 15 USD gift card to a retail store as compensation for their time. Individuals were only allowed to participate in the study or recruit another participant, to ensure independence of the observations.

The questionnaire was offered in English or Spanish, and in online or paper format. Most participants (72.5%) completed an online version of the survey (in English; no Spanish surveys were completed online). Participants who completed a paper survey were older (*M*age = 64.01; *SD* = 16.60) than those who completed an online survey (*M*age = 42.93; *SD* = 17.11). Numbers of Latina/o and non-Latina/o white participants who completed online and paper surveys can be found in Table 1. In addition, a small number of individuals ($n = 10$) returned a paper survey via U.S. mail, using a self-addressed stamped envelope provided by the researchers. Contact information for some participants, including a mailing address, was collected solely for the purpose of compensation and was stored separate from surveys to safeguard confidentiality.

Power analysis

G-Power (Faul et al., 2009) was utilized to conduct an a-priori power analysis for a linear regression model that includes four predictors (i.e., the IV, two mediators, and the DV). Using a power standard of .80 with $\alpha = .05$ to detect a medium effect size of $f^2 = .15$ ($R^2 = .13$) or larger, the minimum sample size needed is $N = 85$.

Results

To test the hypothesized serial mediation in which Latina/o ethnicity would predict greater familism, that would predict lower loneliness, which would in turn would predict better health outcomes including overall health (H1), health practices (H2), and depression (H3), three serial mediation models were analyzed. These models were tested in the PROCESS 3.3 path analysis utility (Hayes, 2018) within SPSS 25. Specifically, model 6 in PROCESS was used to estimate the direct, indirect, and total effects. The 95% confidence interval around each indirect effect was estimated with a bias corrected bootstrapping procedure (Hayes, 2009) based on 5000 bootstrap samples. For all models, Latina/o ethnicity (dummy coded as 0 = nonLatina/o, 1 = Latina/o) was specified as the independent variable. Familism was specified as the first mediator and loneliness as the second. This process was repeated for each of the three dependent variables: overall health, health practices, and depression.

For the sake of brevity, the three direct effects and the serial mediation indirect effect are presented in Table 3. However, there are several other effects in this model that remain more or less constant across dependent variables that are important to understand as they are components of the serial mediation effects. First, the effect of ethnicity on familism was positive and statistically significant across the three models ($\beta = .34 - .36$, $p < .01$ across the three models). Second, the effect of familism on loneliness was negative and significant in all models ($\beta = -.20$, $p < .01$ in each model). In the model predicting overall health, only loneliness had a significant direct effect ($\beta = -.50$, $p < .001$). However, as predicted, there was a statistically significant serial mediation effect for Latina/o ethnicity→ familism→ loneliness→ overall health (partially standardized $\beta = .03$, $p < .05$). In the model predicting health practices, once again, only loneliness exhibited a significant direct effect ($\beta = -.32$, $p < .001$). As predicted, there was a statistically significant serial mediation effect from Latina/o ethnicity through familism and loneliness to health practices ($\beta = .02$, $p < .05$). Finally, in the model predicting depression, only loneliness had a statistically significant direct effect ($\beta = .63$, $p < .001$). Consistent with prediction, there was a statistically significant serial mediation effect from Latina/o ethnicity to depression, through familism and loneliness ($\beta = -.05$, $p < .05$).

Collectively, these results show that although Latina/o ethnicity did not have a direct effect on overall health, health practices, or depression, it did, as predicted, have an indirect effect on all three of these indicators of health and well-being through familism and loneliness. Also, in all three models, only loneliness had a statistically significant direct association with the various forms of health and well-being. Thus, all three hypotheses were supported.

Discussion

Results from tests of serial mediation models revealed that ethnicity (i.e., being Latina/o) positively predicts endorsement of familism, stronger endorsement of familism is associated with lower loneliness, and lower loneliness is associated with better overall health, more beneficial health practices, and lower depression. In all three models, only loneliness had a statistically significant direct association with the various forms of health and well-being. These findings suggest that familism may be a psychological resource in the Latina/o community that is associated with lower loneliness and, indirectly, with greater health.

The findings regarding direct effects are noteworthy for a number of reasons. First, the nonsignificant direct effects of Latina/o ethnicity on overall health, health practices, and depression, in contrast with the significant indirect effect of Latina/o ethnicity on all three health outcomes through familism and loneliness, highlights the importance of disentangling effects of ethnicity on health from the impact of cultural values on health; an approach suggested by previous research (Gallo et al., 2009; Ruiz, Hamann et al., 2016). In other words, results from all three hypotheses suggest that it is unlikely that the Latino health paradox is a manifestation of superior health outcomes intrinsically linked to Latina/o ethnicity, but rather the protective function of specific cultural values that are more likely to be strongly endorsed by individuals whose ethnic identity is Latina/o.

Second, the nonsignificant direct association between familism and all three health outcomes, juxtaposed with the significant serial mediation models, indicates that the health-related protection provided by familism stems in part from its ability to reduce perceptions of loneliness. Had the current study focused solely on examining the impact of familism on health, without hypothesizing loneliness as a statistical mediator in the relationship, this novel understanding of the relationship between familism and health would have been missed. This outcome highlights the importance of testing mediating variables that can provide specificity regarding the relationship between familism (or other cultural values) and health outcomes in Latina/o

Table 3. Direct effects of ethnicity, familism, and loneliness on health.

DV	IV Ethnicity	Mediator 1: Familism	Mediator 2: Loneliness	IV→Med1→Med2→DV indirect effect (95% c.i.)[a]	R^2
Overall Health	−.16	−.08	−.50***	.03* (.01, .08)	.25***
Health Practices	−.20	−.09	−.32***	.02* (.004, .05)	.11***
Depression	−.03	.08	.63***	−.05* (−.10, −.01)	.38***

[a]Coefficients for indirect effects are partially standardized indirect effects. All other coefficients are standardized effects unless otherwise noted. Confidence intervals around indirect effects are estimated with a bias-corrected bootstrapping procedure.
IV: Latina/o Ethnicity (0 = non-Latina/o white, 1 = Latina/o). * $p < .05$. ** $p < .01$. *** $p < .001$.

populations, especially within the context of understanding the Latino health paradox.

Furthermore, the central role of loneliness in establishing the relationship between familism and health for this sample emphasizes the importance of studying the association between cultural values and health from a social relationships perspective. Specifically, our results showed that a key benefit of familism–a Latina/o cultural value based on lifelong familial interconnectedness and mutual obligation among numerous close, reliable, relationships–is reducing perceptions of loneliness, which protects health. As such, communication scholars, particularly those who study the impact of interpersonal relationships on health, are in a prime position to address the "lack of direct evidence for specific cultural values ... linking Latina/o culture to advantageous [health] outcomes" (Ruiz, Campos et al., 2016, p. 64).

Moreover, while these findings support previous suggestions that some aspects of Latina/o culture protect health (Abraido-Lanza et al., 1999), results of the current study extend beyond existing research in a number of important ways. First, we address a major shortcoming of many studies on familism and health by directly measuring familism (Perez & Cruess, 2014). Second, we measured three different indictors of well-being including overall health, depression, and health practices. This approach highlights the relationship between familism and general perceptions of mental and physical well-being, as well as how familism is related to specific behaviors that can protect health. Third, we tested specific statistical pathways, including relationships between ethnicity and familism, familism and loneliness, and loneliness with overall health, depression, and health behaviors, in addition to the direct effects of ethnicity, familism, and loneliness on health. Consequently, the current study addresses three limitations of existing research on the relationship between cultural values (including familism) and health: a lack of empirical evidence that establishes relationships between specific cultural values and health outcomes among Latina/o populations, the mostly "exploratory nature" of existing studies (Perez & Cruess, 2014, p. 114), and the need for a better understanding of specific ways in which familism can safeguard health (Corona et al., 2019). Fourth, to our knowledge, no previous studies have examined loneliness as a key mediator in the relationship between familism and health, or tested associations among ethnicity, familism, loneliness, and health in the same statistical model. Moreover, our results were produced without controlling for demographic covariates that disadvantaged Latina/o participants, including income and education (see Table 1), which provides further support for the Latino health paradox. In other words, despite the presence of disadvantages in education and income that are typically associated with health disparities in the general population (U.S. Centers for Disease Control and Prevention, 2013), our results suggest that familism can play a protective role in Latina/o health by reducing perceptions of loneliness. Collectively, our novel approach to studying the role of familism and loneliness in the Latino health paradox contributes to a broader understanding of the phenomenon.

Overall, results from the current study indicate that although caring for and relying on family is not unique to Latinas/os (Coohey, 2001; Ruiz, 2007; Schwartz, 2007), compared to non-Latina/o whites, Latinas/os are more likely to endorse familism, which is associated with lower loneliness. Ultimately, this reduced loneliness is associated with lower depression, better overall health, and more beneficial health behaviors. As such, one possible explanation for the Latino health paradox is that stronger familism experienced by Latinas/os protects their mental and physical health by reducing loneliness.

Finally, the results from this study provide support for the utility of Hawkley and Cacioppo's (2007, 2010) theory of loneliness and health. In particular, it was the inclusion of loneliness as a statistical mediator that provided more specification regarding the relationship between familism and health than was previously known. The finding that only loneliness had a direct effect on all three health outcomes underscores the important role that loneliness plays in health and well-being, particularly for Latinas/os. Therefore, this theoretical framework will be useful for future research that aims to increase understanding of the Latino health paradox as well as the relationship between cultural values and health among Latina/o populations.

Limitations and future research

The results of the current study should be considered with some limitations in mind. First, cross sectional data does not allow for causal ordering of independent, mediating, and dependent variables. Future studies should employ longitudinal designs to address this issue. Second, the study did not include a random sample of participants; doing so would allow for more generalizable results. Third, the self-report nature of the study could have biased results regarding health issues. This includes the possibility that the sample included an overrepresentation of older adults in good health, as some older Latinas/os who were recruited from community centers were presumably healthy enough to be there. Older adults may have also assessed their own health using downward social comparison (Carstensen et al., 2003; Segrin & Domschke, 2011), resulting in more positive subjective assessments of health and well-being. It would be beneficial for future studies to include non-subjective measures of health, such blood pressure or salivary cortisol, although costs of such a study could be prohibitive.

Finally, although data related to ethnic subgroups (e.g., Cuban, Mexican) for Latina/o participants were collected, there was not sufficient data within each category to make meaningful statistical comparisons in our analyses. However, whereas differences among various subgroups do exist (Gallo et al., 2009), the core characteristics of familism appear to remain consistent (Perez & Cruess, 2014; Villarreal et al., 2005). Thus, while it is probable that our results apply across subgroups, future research should include sufficient numbers of Latinas/os from various subgroups so that comparisons can be made. In addition, Latina/o participants predominantly identified as Mexican-American, limiting the generalizability of our results.

Conclusion

Despite the growing Latina/o population in the U.S. (Noe-Bustamante, Lopez et al., 2020), the numerous health disparities they experience (Heron, 2019), and strong evidence that Latinas/os' health and well-being is no worse, and in some cases better, than more advantaged non-Latina/o whites (Heron, 2015; Liao et al., 1998; Ruiz et al., 2013; Sorlie et al., 1993), there is still a significant lack of empirical research aimed at understanding the unique characteristics of Latina/o health, including explaining the Latino health paradox, (Gallo et al., 2009; Perez & Cruess, 2014). Communication scholars are in a unique position to address this issue, particularly by applying well-established knowledge about the significant impact of social relationships, including families (Albrecht & Goldsmith, 2003; Cohen & Wills, 1985; Seeman & McEwen, 1996) and loneliness (Hawkley & Cacioppo, 2010) on health to new studies focused on understanding how cultural values–especially those based on interpersonal connections–can protect outcomes related to health and well-being. Perhaps if scholars can more clearly identify and explain the "bank of resilient resources" Latina/o populations appear to possess (Gallo et al., 2009, p. 1731), community interventions could be utilized to develop, cultivate, and/or maintain the characteristics that are so beneficial, that even in the face of significant disadvantages, they add years to Latinas/os' life expectancy.

Note

1. The term Hispanic, Latina, and Latino are often used interchangeably in research on the Latino health paradox and other health topics. See Gallo et al. (2009) for a more detailed explanation. The term Latinx has also been increasingly used; however, only about 3% of those who traditionally identify as Hispanic, Latina, or Latino use this term to self-identify (Noe-Bustamante, Mora, et al., 2020). Accordingly, Latina/o is used throughout the manuscript.

Acknowledgments

This work was supported in part by the Ford Foundation and by the University of Arizona Social and Behavioral Sciences Research Institute (SBSRI). Special thanks to Dr. Jaime Fatas, Associate Professor in the University of Arizona Department of Spanish and Portuguese, for help with English-to-Spanish translation of the survey and recruitment materials. The authors also wish to thank Dr. Jake Harwood and Dr. Steve Rains in the University of Arizona Department of Communication for comments on earlier versions of this manuscript.

Disclosure of potential conflict of interest

No potential conflict of interest was reported by the author(s).

Data availability statement

The data that support the findings of this study will be available on request from the corresponding author.

IRB approval

This study and its procedures were approved by the University of Arizona IRB (Human Subjects Protection Program). Please see supplemental file "Familism Loneliness and Health Study IRB Approval".

Funding

This work was supported by the Ford Foundation [Funding not specific to the study (broad use)]; University of Arizona [SBSRI Summer Dissertation Completion Fellowship].

ORCID

Monica L. Gallegos http://orcid.org/0000-0002-5435-1813
Chris Segrin http://orcid.org/0000-0003-1797-2503

References

Abraido-Lanza, A. F., Dohrenwend, B. B., Ng-Mak, D. S., & Turner, J. B. (1999). The Latino mortality paradox: A test of the "salmon bias" and healthy migrant hypotheses. *American Journal of Public Health*, *89*(10), 1543–1548. https://doi.org/10.2105/ajph.89.10.1543

Abraido-Lanza, A. F., Shelton, R. C., Martins, M. C., & Crookes, D. M. (2017). Social norms, acculturation, and physical activity among Latina women. *Journal of Immigrant Minority Health*, *19*(2), 285–293. https://doi.org/10.1007/s10903-016-0519-7

Albrecht, T. L., & Goldsmith, D. J. (2003). Social support, social networks, and health. In T. L. Thompson, A. M. Dorsey, K. I. Miller, & R. Parrott (Eds.), *Handbook of health communication* (pp. 263–284). Routledge.

Alegría, M., Canino, G., Shrout, P. E., Woo, M., Duan, N., Vila, D., Torres, M., Chen, C., & Meng, X. (2008). Prevalence of mental illness in immigrant and non-immigrant U.S. Latino groups. *American Journal of Psychiatry*, *165*(3), 359–369. https://doi.org/10.1176/appi.ajp.2007.07040704

Arias, E., Eschbach, K., Schauman, W. S., Backlund, E. L., & Sorlie, P. D. (2010). The Hispanic mortality advantage and ethnic misclassification on U.S. death certificates. *American Journal of Public Health*, *100*(s1), s171–s177. https://doi.org/10.2105/ajph.2008.135863

Arias, E., & Xu, J. (2019). *United States life tables, 2017* (National Vital Statistics Reports (Vol. 68, No. 7)). U.S. Department of Health and Human Services, Centers for Disease Control and Prevention. https://www.cdc.gov/nchs/products/life_tables.htm

Ashing-Giwa, K. T., Padilla, G., Tejero, J., Kraemer, J., Wright, K., Coscarelli, A., Clayton, S., Williams, I., & Hills, D. (2004). Understanding the breast cancer experience of women: A qualitative study of African American, Asian American, Latina, and Caucasian cancer survivors. *Psycho-Oncology*, *13*(6), 408–428. https://doi.org/10.1002/pon.750

Balfour, P. C., Ruiz, J. M., Talavera, G. A., Allison, M. A., & Rodriguez, C. J. (2016). Cardiovascular disease in Hispanics/Latinos in the United States. *Journal of Latina/o Psychology*, *4*(2), 98–113. http://dx.doi.org/10.1037/lat0000056

Carstensen, L. L., Fung, H. H., & Charles, S. T. (2003). Socioemotional selectivity theory and the regulation of emotion in the second half of life. *Motivation and Emotion*, *27*(2), 103–123. https://doi.org/10.1023/A:1024569803230

Chen, Y. (2012, May 24–28). *Social support, social strain, loneliness, and well-being: An investigation using the HRS national sample* [Paper presentation]. International Communication Association 62nd Annual Conference, Phoenix, AZ.

Cohen, S., & Wills, T. A. (1985). Stress, social support, and the buffering hypothesis. *Psychological Bulletin*, *98*(2), 310–357. https://doi.org/10.1037/0033-2909.98.2.310

Connell, C. M., & Gibson, G. D. (1997). Racial, ethnic, and cultural differences in dementia caregiving: Review and analysis. *The Gerontologist*, *37*(3), 355–364. https://doi.org/10.1093/geront/37.3.355

Coohey, C. (2001). The relationship between familism and child maltreatment in Latino and Anglo families. *Child Maltreatment*, *6*(2), 130–142. https://doi.org/10.1177/1077559501006002005

Corona, K., Campos, B., Rook, K. S., Biegler, K., & Sorkin, D. H. (2019). Do cultural values have a role in health equity? A study of Latina mothers and daughters. *Cultural Diversity & Ethnic Minority Psychology*, *25*(1), 65–72. http://dx.doi.org/10.1037/cdp0000262

Davila, Y. R., Reifsnider, E., & Pecina, I. (2011). Familismo: Influence on Hispanic health behaviors. *Applied Nursing Research*, *24*(4), e67–e72. https://doi.org/10.1016/j.apnr.2009.12.003

Ernst, J. M., & Cacioppo, J. T. (1999). Lonely hearts: Psychological perspectives on loneliness. *Applied and Preventative Psychology*, *8*(1), 1–22. https://doi.org/10.1016/s0962-1849(99)80008-0

Faul, F., Erdfelder, E., Buchner, A., & Lang, A. G. (2009). Statistical power analyses using G*power 3.1: Tests for correlation and regression analyses. *Behavior Research Methods*, *41*(4), 1149–1160. https://doi.org/10.3758/brm.41.4.1149

Fontenot, K., Semega, J., & Kollar, M. (2018). *Income and poverty in the United States: 2017* (Report prepared for United States Census Bureau). U.S. Department of Commerce Economics and Statistics Administration. https://www.minorityhealth.hhs.gov/omh/browse.aspx?lvl=3&lvlid=64

Gaines, S. O., Marelich, W. D., Bledsoe, K. L., Steers, W. N., Henderson, M. C., Granrose, C. S., Barájas, L., Hicks, D., Lyde, M., Takahashi, Y., Yum, N., Ríos, D. I., García, B. F., Farris, K. R., & Page, M. S. (1997). Links between race/ethnicity and cultural values as mediated by racial/ethnic identity and moderated by gender. *Journal of Personality and Social Psychology*, *72*(6), 1460–1476. https://doi.org/10.1037/0022-3514.72.6.1460

Gaioso, V. P., Villarruel, A. M., Wilson, L. A., Azuero, A., Childs, G. D., & Davies, S. L. (2015). A path analysis of Latino parental teenager and cultural variables in teenagers' sexual attitudes, norms, self-efficacy, and sexual intentions. *Revista Latino-Americana De Enfermagem*, *23* (3), 500–511. https://doi.org/10.1590/0104-1169.0398.2581

Gallegos, M. L. (2013). *Communication processes and the Latino health paradox: Exploring relationships among loneliness, cultural values, and health across the lifespan* [Doctoral dissertation, University of Arizona]. Proquest: The Humanities and Social Sciences Collection. (1436971150). https://libproxy.csun.edu/login?url=https://www-proquest-com.libproxy.csun.edu/dissertations-theses/communication-processes-latino-health-paradox/docview/

Gallo, L. C., Penedo, F. J., De Los Monteros, K. E., & Arguelles, W. (2009). Resiliency in the face of disadvantage: Do Hispanic cultural characteristics protect health outcomes? *Journal of Personality*, *77*(6), 1708–1746. https://doi.org/10.1111/j.1467-6494.2009.00598.x

Gonzalez, G., Gallardo, N. V., & Bastani, R. (2005). A pilot study to define social support among Spanish-speaking women diagnosed with a breast abnormality suspicious for cancer: A brief research report. *Journal of Psychosocial Oncology*, *23*(1), 109–120. https://doi.org/10.1300/J077v23n01_07

Hawkley, L. C., Burleson, M. H., Berntson, G. G., & Cacioppo, J. T. (2003). Loneliness in everyday life: Cardiovascular activity, psychosocial context, and health behaviors. *Journal of Personality and Social Psychology*, *85*(1), 105–120. https://doi.org/10.1037/0022-3514.85.1.105

Hawkley, L. C., & Cacioppo, J. T. (2003). Loneliness and pathways to disease. *Brain, Behavior, and Immunity*, *17*(1), S98–S105. https://doi.org/10.1016/S0889-1591(02)00073-9

Hawkley, L. C., & Cacioppo, J. T. (2007). Aging and loneliness: Downhill quickly? *Current Directions in Psychological Science*, *16*(4), 187–191. https://doi.org/10.1111/j.1467-8721.2007.00501.x

Hawkley, L. C., & Cacioppo, J. T. (2010). Loneliness matters: A theoretical and empirical review of consequences and mechanisms. *Annals of Behavioral Medicine*, *40*(2), 218–227. https://doi.org/10.1007/s12160-010-9210-8

Hawkley, L. C., Hughes, M. E., Waite, L. J., Masi, C. M., Thisted, R. A., & Cacioppo, J. T. (2008). From social structural factors to perceptions of relationship quality and loneliness: The Chicago health, aging, and social relations study. *Journals of Gerontology*, *63*(6), S375–S384. https://doi.org/10.1093/geronb/63.6.s375

Hawkley, L. C., Masi, C. M., Berry, J. D., & Cacioppo, J. T. (2006). Loneliness is a unique predictor of age-related differences in systolic blood pressure. *Psychology and Aging*, *21*(1), 152–164. https://doi.org/10.1037/0882-7974.21.1.152

Hayes, A. F. (2009). Beyond Baron and Kenny: Statistical mediation analysis in the new millennium. *Communication Monographs*, *76*(4), 408–420. https://doi.org/10.1080/03637750903310360

Hayes, A. F. (2018). *Introduction to mediation, moderation, and conditional process analysis: A regression-based approach* (2nd ed.). Guilford Press.

Hays, R. D., Sherbourne, C. D., & Mazel, R. M. (1993). The RAND 36-item health survey 1.0. *Health Economics*, *2*(3), 217–227. https://doi.org/10.1002/hec.4730020305

Heinrich, L. M., & Gullone, E. (2006). The clinical significance of loneliness: A literature review. *Clinical Psychology Review*, *26*(6), 695–718. https://doi.org/10.1016/j.cpr.2006.04.002

Heron, M. (2015). *Deaths: Leading causes for 2012* (National Vital Statistics Reports (Vol. 64, No. 10)). U.S. Department of Health and Human Services, Centers for Disease Control and Prevention. https://www.cdc.gov/nchs/data/nvsr/nvsr64/nvsr64_10.pdf

Heron, M. (2019). *Deaths: Leading causes for 2017* (National Vital Statistics Reports (Vol. 68, No. 6)). U.S. Department of Health and Human Services, Centers for Disease Control and Prevention. https://www.cdc.gov/nchs/data/nvsr/nvsr68/nvsr68_06-508.pdf

Holt-Lunstad, J., Smith, T. B., Baker, M., Harris, T., & Stephenson, D. (2015). Loneliness and social isolation as risk factors for mortality: A meta-analytic review. *Perspectives on Psychological Science*, *10*(2), 227–237. https://doi.org/10.1177/1745691614568352

Holt-Lunstad, J., Smith, T. B., & Layton, J. B. (2010). Social relationships and mortality risk: A meta-analytic review. *PLoS Medicine*, *7*(7), 1–20. https://doi.org/10.4016/19865.01

House, J. S., Landis, K. R., & Umberson, D. (1988). Social relationships and health. *Science*, *241*(4865), 540–545. https://doi.org/10.1126/science.3399889

Jackson, T. (2006). Relationships between perceived close social support and health practices within community samples of American women and men. *The Journal of Psychology*, *140*(3), 229–246. https://doi.org/10.3200/JRLP.140.3.229-246

Jones, W. H., & Moore, T. L. (1987). Loneliness and social support. *Journal of Social Behavior and Personality*, *2*(2, pt. 2), 145–156.

Keefe, S. E. (1984). Real and ideal extended familism among Mexican Americans and Anglo Americans: On the meaning of "close" family ties. *Human Organization*, *43*(1), 65–70. https://doi.org/10.17730/humo.43.1.y5546831728vn6kp

Kulbok, P. A., Carter, K. F., Baldwin, J. H., Gilmartin, M. J., & Kirkwood, B. (1999). The multidimensional health behavior inventory. *Journal of Nursing Measurement*, *7*(2), 177–195. https://doi.org/10.1891/1061-3749.7.2.177

Lac, A., Unger, J. B., Basáñez, T., Ritt-Olson, A., Soto, D. W., & Baezconde-Garbanti, L. (2011). Marijuana use among Latino adolescents: Gender differences in protective familial factors. *Substance Use & Misuse*, *46*(5), 644–655. https://doi.org/10.3109/10826084.2010.528121

Laroche, H. H., Davis, M. M., Forman, J., Palmisano, G., Reisinger, H. S., Tannas, C., Spencer, M., & Heisler, M. (2009). Children's roles in parents' diabetes self-management. *American Journal of Preventative Medicine*, *37*(6), S251–S261. https://doi.org/10.1016/j.amepre.2009.08.003

Liao, Y., Cooper, R. S., Cao, G., Durazo-Arvizu, R., Kaufman, J. S., Luke, A., & McGee, D. L. (1998). Mortality patterns among adult Hispanics: Findings from the NHIS, 1986 to 1990. *American Journal of Public Health*, *88*(2), 227–232. https://doi.org/10.2105/ajph.88.2.227

Lugo Steidel, A. G., & Contreras, J. M. (2003). A new familism scale for use with Latino populations. *Hispanic Journal of Behavioral Sciences*, *25*(3), 312–330. https://doi.org/10.1177/0739986303256912

Marin, G. (1993). Influence of acculturation on familialism and self-identification among Hispanics. In M. E. Bernal & G. P. Knight (Eds.), *Ethnic identity: Formation and transmission among Hispanics and other minorities* (pp. 181–196). State University of New York Press.

Marin, G., & Marin, B. V. (1991). *Research with Hispanic populations*. Sage.

Markides, K. S., & Coreil, J. (1986). The health of Hispanics in the Southwestern United States: An epidemiological paradox. *Public Health Reports*, *101*(3), 253–265. https://www.ncbi.nlm.nih.gov/pmc/articles/PMC1477704/

Mendez-Luck, C. A., Geldhof, G. J., Anthony, K. P., Steers, W. N., Mangione, C. M., & Hays, R. D. (2016). Orientation to the caregiver role among Latinas of Mexican origin. *The Gerontologist*, *56*(6), e99–e108. https://doi.org/10.1093/geront/gnw087

Mirowsky, J., & Ross, C. E. (1984). Mexican culture and its emotional contradictions. *Journal of Health and Social Behavior*, *25*(1), 2–13. https://doi.org/10.2307/2136700

Mozaffarian, D., Benjamin, E. J., Go, A. S., Arnett, D. K., Blaha, M. J., Cushman, M., Das, S. R., De Ferranti, S., Després, J.-P., Fullerton, H. J., Howard, V. J., Huffman, M. D., Isasi, C. R., Jiménez, M. C., Judd, S. E., Kissela, B. M., Lichtman, J. H., Lisabeth, L. D., Liu, S., Mackey, R. H., & Turner, M. B. (2016). Heart disease and stroke statistics–2016 update: A report from the American heart association. *Circulation*, *133*(4), e38–e360. https://doi.org/10.1161/cir.0000000000000350

Muñoz-Laboy, M. A. (2008). Familism and sexual regulation among bisexual Latino men. *Archives of Sexual Behavior*, *37*(5), 773–782. https://doi.org/10.1007/s10508-008-9360-y

National Center for Health Statistics. (1999). *Healthy people 2000 review, 1988–99*. Hayattsville, Maryland: Public Health Service, http://www.cdc.gov/nchs/products/hp_pubs.htm

Noe-Bustamante, L., & Flores, A. (2019). *Facts on Latinos in the U.S.* Pew Research Center. https://www.pewresearch.org/hispanic/fact-sheet/latinos-in-the-u-s-fact-sheet/

Noe-Bustamante, L., Lopez, M. H., & Krogstad, J. M. (2020). *U.S. Hispanic population surpasses 60 million in 2019, but growth has slowed*. Pew Research Center, https://www.pewresearch.org/fact-tank/2020/07/07/u-s-hispanic-population-surpassed-60-million-in-2019-but-growth-has-slowed/

Noe-Bustamante, L., Mora, L., & Lopez, M. H. (2020). *About one-in-four U.S. Hispanics have heard of Latinx, but just 3% use it*. Pew Research Center, https://www.pewresearch.org/hispanic/2020/08/11/about-one-in-four-u-s-hispanics-have-heard-of-latinx-but-just-3-use-it/

Organista, K. C. (2007). *Solving Latino psychosocial and health problems: Theory, practice, and populations*. John Wiley & Sons, Inc.

Parsai, M., Voisine, S., Marsiglia, F. F., Kulis, S., & Nieri, T. (2009). The protective and risk effects of parents and peers on the substance use attitudes and behaviors of Mexican American female and male adolescents. *Youth & Society*, *40*(3), 353–376. https://doi.org/10.1177/0044118x08318117

Peplau, L. A., Russell, D., & Heim, M. (1979). The experience of loneliness. In I. H. Frieze, D. Bar-Tal, & J. S. Carrol (Eds.), *New approaches to social problems* (pp. 53–78). Jossey-Bass.

Perez, G. K., & Cruess, D. (2014). The impact of familism on physical and mental health among Hispanics in the United States. *Health Psychology Review*, *8*(1), 95–127. https://doi.org/10.1080/17437199.2011.569936

Perkins, A. J., Stump, T. E., Monahan, P. O., & McHorney, C. A. (2006). Assessment of differential item functioning for demographic comparisons in the MOS SF-36 health survey. *Quality of Life Research*, *15*(3), 331–348. https://doi.org/10.1007/s11136-005-1551-6

Phennix, B. W., Van Tilburg, T., Kriegsman, D. M., Deeg, D. J., Boeke, J. P., & Van Ejik, J. T. (1997). Effects of social support and personal coping resources on mortality in older age: The longitudinal aging study Amsterdam. *American Journal of Epidemiology*, *146*(6), 510–519. https://doi.org/10.1093/oxfordjournals.aje.a009305

Potochnick, S., Perreira, K. M., Bravin, J. I., Castañeda, S. F., Daviglus, M. L., Gallo, L. C., & Isasi, C. R. (2019). Food insecurity among Hispanic/Latino youth: Who is at risk and what are the health correlates? *Journal of Adolescent Health*, *64*(5), 631–639. https://doi.org/10.1016/j.jadohealth.2018.10.302

Rodriguez, N., Mira, C. B., Paez, N. D., & Myers, H. F. (2007). Exploring the complexities of familism and acculturation: Central constructs for people of Mexican origin. *American Journal of Community Psychology*, *39*(1–2), 61–77. https://doi.org/10.1007/s10464-007-9090-7

Ruiz, J. M., Campos, B., & Garcia, J. J. (2016). Special issue on Latino physical health: Disparities, paradoxes, and future directions. *Journal of Latina/o Psychology*, *4*(2), 61–66. http://dx.doi.org/10.1037/lat0000065

Ruiz, J. M., Hamann, H. A., Mehl, M. R., & O'Connor, M. F. (2016). The Hispanic health paradox: From epidemiological phenomenon to contribution opportunities for psychological science. *Group Processes and Intergroup Relations*, *19*(4), 462–476. https://doi.org/10.1177/1368430216638540

Ruiz, J. M., Steffen, P., & Smith, T. B. (2013). Hispanic mortality paradox: A systematic review and meta-analysis of the longitudinal literature. *American Journal of Public Health*, *103*(3), e52–e60. https://doi.org/10.2105/AJPH.2012.301103

Ruiz, M. E. (2007). Familismo and filial piety among Latino and Asian elders: Reevaluating family and social support. *Hispanic Health Care International*, *5*(2), 81–89. https://doi.org/10.1891/154041507780978897

Russell, D. W. (1996). UCLA loneliness scale (Version 3): Reliability, validity, and factor structure. *Journal of Personality Assessment*, *66*(1), 20–40. https://doi.org/10.1207/s15327752jpa6601_2

Sabogal, F., Marín, G., Otero-Sabogal, R., Marín, B. V., & Perez-Stable, E. J. (1987). Hispanic familism and acculturation: What changes and what doesn't? *Hispanic Journal of Behavioral Sciences*, *9*(4), 397–412. https://doi.org/10.1177/07399863870094003

Salvy, S. J., Miles, J. N. V., Shih, R. A., Tucker, J. S., & D'Amico, E. J. (2017). Neighborhood, family, and peer-level predictors of obesity-related health behaviors among young adolescents. *Journal of Pediatric Psychology*, *42*(2), 153–161. https://doi.org/10.1093/jpepsy/jsw035

Schaider, L. A., Swetschinski, L., Campbell, C., & Rudel, R. A. (2019). Environmental justice and drinking water quality: Are there socio-demographic disparities in nitrate levels in U.S. drinking water? *Environmental Health*, *18*(3), 1–15. https://doi.org/10.1186/s12940-018-0442-6

Schwartz, S. J. (2007). The applicability of familism to diverse ethnic groups: A preliminary study. *The Journal of Social Psychology*, *147*(2), 101–118. https://doi.org/10.3200/SOCP.147.2.101-118

Seeman, T. E., & McEwen, B. S. (1996). Impact of social environment characteristics on neuroendocrine regulation. *Psychosomatic Medicine*, *58*(5), 459–471. https://doi.org/10.1097/00006842-199609000-00008

Segrin, C., Badger, T. A., Sikorskii, A., Pasvogel, A., Weihs, K., Lopez, A. M., & Chalasani, P. (2020). Longitudinal dyadic interdependence in psychological distress among Latinas with breast cancer and their caregivers. *Supportive Care in Cancer*, *28*(6), 2735–2743. https://doi.org/10.1007/s00520-019-05121-4

Segrin, C., & Domschke, T. (2011). Social support, loneliness, recuperative processes, and their direct and indirect effects on health. *Health Communication*, *26*(3), 221–232. https://doi.org/10.1080/10410236.2010.546771

Segrin, C., & Passalacqua, S. (2010). Functions of loneliness, social support, health behaviors, and stress in association with poor health. *Health Communication*, *25*(4), 312–322. https://doi.org/10.1080/10410231003773334

Shiovitz-Ezra, S., & Leitsch, S. A. (2010). The role of social relationships in predicting loneliness: The national social life, health, and aging project. *Social Work Research*, *34*(3), 157–167. https://doi.org/10.1093/swr/34.3.157

Simoni, J. M., Mason, H. R. C., Marks, G., Ruiz, M. S., Reed, D., & Richardson, J. L. (1995). Women's self-disclosure of HIV infection: Rates, reasons, and reactions. *Journal of Consulting and Clinical Psychology*, *63*(3), 474–478. https://doi.org/10.1037/0022-006x.63.3.474

Sorlie, P. D., Backlund, E., Johnson, N. J., & Rogot, E. (1993). Mortality by Hispanic status in the United States. *Journal of the American Medical Association*, *270*(20), 2464–2468. https://doi.org/10.1001/jama.1993.03510200070034

U.S. Centers for Disease Control and Prevention. (2013). *Morbidity and mortality weekly report: CDC health disparities and inequalities report–United States, 2013* (Vol. 62, No. 3). U.S. Department of Health and Human Services. https://www.cdc.gov/minorityhealth/CHDIReport.html

Uchino, B. N., Cacioppo, J. T., & Kiecolt-Glaser, J. K. (1996). The relationship between social support and physiological processes: A review with emphasis on underlying mechanisms and implications for health. *Psychological Bulletin*, *119*(3), 488–531. https://doi.org/10.1037/0033-2909.119.3.488

Villarreal, R., Blozis, S. A., & Widaman, K. F. (2005). Factorial invariance of a pan-Hispanic familism scale. *Hispanic Journal of Behavioral Sciences*, *27*(4), 409–425. https://doi.org/10.1177/0739986305281125

Ware, J. E., & Sherbourne, C. D. (1992). The MOS 36-item short-form health survey (SF-36): I. Conceptual framework and item selection.

Medical Care, *30*(6), 473–483. https://doi.org/10.1097/00005650-199206000-00002

Williams, R. L., Thomas, S. P., Young, D. O., Jozwiak, J. J., & Hector, M. A. (1991). Development of a health habits scale. *Research in Nursing Health*, *14*(2), 145–153. https://doi.org/10.1002/nur.4770140209

Wilson, R. S., Krueger, K. R., Arnold, S. E., Schneider, J. A., Kelly, J. F., Barnes, L. L., Tang, Y., & Bennett, D. A. (2007). Loneliness and risk of Alzheimer disease. *Archives of General Psychiatry*, *64*(2), 234–240. https://doi.org/10.1001/archpsyc.64.2.234

Yanez, B., McGinty, H. L., Buitrago, D., Ramirez, A. G., & Penedo, F. J. (2016). Cancer outcomes in Hispanics/Latinos in the United States: An integrative review and conceptual model of determinants of health. *Journal of Latina/o Psychology*, *4*(2), 114–129. http://dx.doi.org/10.1037/lat0000055

Yip, F. Y., Pearcy, J. N., Garbe, P. L., & Truman, B. I. (2011). *Morbidity and Mortality Weekly Report: Unhealthy air quality–United States, 2006–2009* (Vol. 60, pp. 28–32). U. S. Department of Health and Human Services Centers for Disease Control and Prevention, https://www.cdc.gov/mmwr/preview/mmwrhtml/su6001a5.htm?s

Zigmond, A. S., & Snaith, R. P. (1983). The hospital anxiety and depression scale. *Acta Psychiatrica Scandinavica*, *67*(6), 361–370. https://doi.org/10.1111/j.1600-0447.1983.tb09716.x

A Pilot Study of Latinx Lesbian, Gay, and Bisexual Adolescent Patients' Goal Prioritizations in Patient-Provider Sexual Orientation and Health Disclosures

Suzanne Burdick and Sarah Nicholus

ABSTRACT

This pilot study provides a theoretically-driven explanation of the dilemmas young Latinx LGB patients may experience surrounding disclosure of personal sexual orientation and sexual health information to a health care provider (HCP). The research team conducted face-to-face semi-structured interviews with LGB Latinx individuals (*N*= 29) ages 18–22 about their experiences, concerns, and preferences regarding divulging this type of information to an HCP. Interviews were thematically analyzed to identify (a) participants' instrumental, identity, and relational goals during the potential and real disclosures and (b) patterns of how the participants prioritized their goals. Thematic analysis revealed four distinct goal prioritization patterns detailed in this study. Participants' goals were shaped by (a) cultural upbringing, (b) beliefs about human sexuality, (c) perception of data leakage risk, (d) individual personality, (e) medical situation, and (f) the geographic location of clinic.

"There is kind of a stigma about it where I come from so it's not, like, talked about," Laura tells us in her interview. Laura is an 18-year-old bisexual Mexican-American woman from a small town in a conservative area. In another interview, Chad, a 21-year-old gay Guatemalan man asserts, "I just feel more comfortable with a Latino doctor … so, for Latino doctors, I would feel comfortable telling them my sexuality." Like many other lesbian, gay, and bisexual (LGB) youth of color in the United States, Chad and Laura experience multiple marginalization as they navigate a complex nexus of identity, stigma, and relationships that influence their disclosures of sexual orientation and sexual health in health care settings. First theorized by Black feminists and women of color (Crenshaw, 1991; Moraga & Anzaldúa, 2015; The Combahee River Collective, 2015), multiple marginalization refers to the exclusion and social disadvantage individuals experience at the intersection of multiple inequalities. This study aligns with an intersectional, critical health communication framework to investigate the multiple goals of Latinx LGB patients as they navigate disclosure in health care settings. It concerns itself with what motivates individuals such as Laura and Chad to choose to disclose or not disclose their sexual orientation and sexual health (SO/SH) information when visiting a health care provider (HCP).

A multiple goals framework allows us to consider the implications of multiple socio-cultural inequalities that can impact a patient's decision-making processes. Additionally, an intersectional, critical health communications framework allows us to consider the consequences of not feeling comfortable talking about sexual identity in health

care settings. We take into consideration not only individual sexual health behavior, but more importantly, we acknowledge how structural barriers to sexual health and sexual health disclosures disproportionately and doubly affect LGB Latinx youth. To address these concerns, we have conducted this pilot study to investigate the thought processes of Latinx LGB young people as they consider disclosing their SO/SH information. Sexual orientation and sexual health are not synonymous. We use the joint phrase "sexual orientation and sexual health" information as our unit of investigation in this study because we are aware that disclosure of one's sexuality and sexual orientation can occur directly (i.e., stating one's orientation) or indirectly by disclosing sexual health information (i.e., sharing sexual behavior information[1]) (Venetis et al., 2017). While we use the phrase SO/SH to speak to how both identity and behavior are at play, we have organized the demographic of this study around identity,[2] rather than behavior. As other critical health communication scholars argue, we need to interrogate power dynamics and structural barriers to health care in order to address issues of access, social inequality, and discrimination (Hudak, 2020; Hudak & Carmack, 2018). Identity not only takes into consideration the ways in which structural inequalities influence individual behaviors, but also addresses the ways in which identity shapes experiences (Hudak, 2020). Finally, a multiple goals framework allows us to consider how goals, like identities, are variable and dynamic; they may be in conflict with each other, yet they concurrently exist and influence individual decision-making processes regarding SH/SO disclosures in health care settings.

The organization of this report is as follows. First, we review health communication research on SO/SH disclosures while noting that much of the research has been done among White populations and that there is a need to conduct health communication research among nonwhite populations. Then, we consider intersectional barriers to health care and what makes young Latinxs an important group of people for this study. We next present the theoretical framework, research method, analyses, and results of the study. We then provide a discussion that situates our findings in the broader context of queer health disclosure studies and close by noting the study's practical implications and its limitations.

Queer health care disclosures, a literature review

Since it is now considered routine for HCPs to request SO/SH information due to the ways this information interfaces with major health outcomes (Marchalik, 2016), queer[3] health disclosures have become an area of much research (e.g., Goins & Pye, 2013; Law et al., 2015; Schrimshaw et al., 2016). Venetis et al. (2017) studied how LGBTQ adults enacted disclosure and found that many individuals prepare and are strategic about disclosing their sexual orientation to HCPs. These researchers also found that other individuals are burdened with the determining whether or not to correct HCPs' heteronormative assumptions by disclosing and providing accurate information. Indeed, there is extensive evidence that health disclosures are challenging and dependent on various factors (e.g., Bonvicini & Perlin, 2003; Caughlin et al., 2009; Farber, 2003; Fritz et al., 2020; Polek et al., 2008). Hudak and Carmack (2018) examined factors that influence LGB individuals' decision-making around disclosing their sexuality. Their participants reported that past experiences heavily influenced disclosure decisions. Additionally, their results indicated that LGB individuals felt more confident disclosing as they aged. Law et al. (2015) found that a solid therapeutic relationship between the HCP and the patient can mitigate some of the difficulty with disclosing SO/SH. They further noted that to establish such a relationship, it was important for HCPs to acknowledge heteronormativity as a social norm in medicine. Recognizing and addressing heteronormativity is important, concur Utamsingh et al. (2016). Their experimental study had LGB participants read vignettes of either heteronormative HCPs or non-heteronormative patient-provider interactions. "Participants were less likely to disclose health-relevant information to the doctor in the vignette and were less trustful of the doctor as compared to those in the non-heteronormative condition," they reported (2016, p. 566). The influential role of the HCP in facilitating disclosure was also noted in a systematic review of 31 studies on sexual orientation in health care involving 2,442 participants (Brooks et al., 2018). Venetis et al. (2017) reported four salient barriers and facilitators to disclosure: (a) patients' belief about the relevance of disclosure to their health, (b) the expected outcome of the disclosure, (c) the HCP themself, and (d) the setting or environment of disclosure. Notably, the majority of this research has focused on LGB individuals who are White. In contrast, this present study investigates queer health disclosures among Latinx individuals, specifically Latinx adolescents and young adults (AYAs).

Intersectional barriers to health care for an expanding Latinx AYA patient population

Talking about sexual health is a complex task rooted in communication and identity. As demonstrated by Laura and Chad in our introduction, Latinx LGB patients must navigate both heteronormative and White hegemonic structures while deciding whether or not to disclose SH/SO information in health care settings. In her interview, Laura expressed hesitancy in being open with others about her sexual identity due to the stigma surrounding it. Laura is not unique in this regard. Given the stigma attached to being a sexual minority (Haas & Lannutti, 2019; Herek, 2009), many LGB people feel afraid to disclose this information (Austin, 2013). As a bisexual Latina,[4] Laura's fear of stigma and discrimination is exacerbated given the White, heteronormative structures she must navigate in health care settings. Yet, these identities – bisexual and Latina – do not function independently. An intersectional, critical health communication framework allows us to better understand how they are mutually constituted. When Laura references the stigma surrounding her bisexual identity "where she comes from," she is also alluding to a place and a socio-cultural group. Disclosure may have significant consequences for her in her family and within her larger community.

The number of Latinx individuals in the United States has increased almost ninefold since 1960 (Pew Research Center, 2016). Latinx individuals have surpassed all other minority groups and number around 35.9 million. Nearly half of Latinx individuals born in the United Sates are under the age of 18 (Patten, 2016). Given these trends, it is important for HCPs to be cognizant of how to best meet the health needs of this population – especially since health care visits with Latinx patients have been measured as being less patient-centered with less psychosocial (i.e., socio-emotional) talk than visits with White patients (Beach et al., 2010). In our interview, Chad's preference for and comfortability with a HPC of the same race speaks to one of the structural barriers to SO/SH disclosures for people of color: a lack of diversity in the physician workforce. Without access to a Latinx HCP, Chad is less likely to disclose his SO/SH. Racial/ethnic identity can be a catalyst for establishing trust and communication; it encourages socio-emotional talk between patients and HCPs. Matching patients and doctors by race has proven to make a difference in health outcomes (Alsan et al., 2019; Hill et al., 2020; Vedantam, 2019).

There are complex health consequences of not feeling comfortable talking about sexual identity in health care settings beyond risk of STIs. However, many studies take a behavior-informed approach to discussing health disparities related to race and sexual orientation, focusing on STIs and HIV. Such a focus can further marginalize an at-risk population while eliding systemic racism, structural inequality, and exclusion in health care settings. To be sure, Latinx individuals are more at risk of contracting HIV and STDs than their White counterparts (Centers for Disease Control and Prevention, 2020). While acknowledging statistical disparities, we have based our demographic around identity (not behavior) in order to center structural inequalities as a main cause of these disparities. Identity not only takes into consideration the ways in which structural inequalities influence individual behaviors, but also addresses the ways in which identity shapes experiences (Hudak, 2020).

When compared to White individuals, Latinx individuals face a variety of structural barriers to receiving health care services of high quality (Escarce & Kapur, 2006). For example, as Tabler et al. (2018) note, inadequate access to quality health information results in limited knowledge about HPV and its role in cervical or other forms of cancer. Socio-economic conditions, such as lack of insurance is also a barrier for many (Juckett, 2013). Such barriers result in health disparities which are compounded by sexual orientation. Latinx lesbians and bisexual women, compared with Latinx heterosexual women, were found to have elevated risk for disparities in smoking and asthma (Kim & Fredriksen-Goldsen, 2012). Additionally, Latinx bisexual women showed higher odds of arthritis, acute drinking, poor general health, and frequent mental distress than Latinx heterosexual women (Kim & Fredriksen-Goldsen, 2012). Social discrimination experienced by gay and bisexual Latinx men in the forms of homophobia, poverty, and racism has been shown to result in negative mental health outcomes (Díaz et al., 2001). Given these disparities, it is just as important for Latinx AYA patients to feel comfortable discussing their health concerns with their HCPs as it is for HCPs to provide health services that address these barriers.

Finally, LGB Latinx patients must navigate a cultural identity which may be in tension with their sexual orientation. While misogyny[5] is omnipresent across cultural, racial, and ethnic difference, Baig et al. (2016) draw attention to the ways in which a Latinx cultural value of machismo can create heteronormative expectations that negatively impact Latinx LGB individuals. While machismo, an idealized form of masculinity, can be positive (e.g., assertiveness and courage) and negative (e.g., violence and sexual aggression toward women), identifying as a gay man may elicit stereotyped perceptions about gay men being less masculine (p. 336), and further marginalize gay Latinx men. Thus, LGB Latinx individuals may conceal their sexual identity and/or avoid medical care to evade additional stigmatization (García, 2009). Such avoidance of disclosure can exacerbate health disparities (Durso & Meyer, 2012), yet nondisclosure is, understandably, a strategy of stigma management used by minority individuals (Schrimshaw et al., 2016). There may be both benefits and risks to disclosure (Hudak & Carmack, 2018). Possible information leakage to third parties can cause additional negative socio-cultural effects (Kuo et al., 2014). Patients risk judgment and discrimination by their doctors (e.g., Mollon, 2012). Sometimes this discrimination is due to non-heteronormative sexual behavior, but sometimes it's due to sexual identity (Hudak, 2020). Identity is complex and nuanced. Elements of identity may seem to be in conflict with each other, yet they co-exist within individual patients. Identity reflects the socio-cultural and political nexus in which patients make decisions. To address the multiple ways in which identity shapes decision-making, this study uses a multiple goals framework to investigate a complex, nuanced, and salient communication construct.

A multiple goals framework

This theoretical approach focuses on individuals' motivations during communication situations in which disclosure could occur by considering how interpersonal interactions are shaped by the goals, or purposes, of the communicators. Foundational to this perspective is the idea that every interaction involves three types of goals: instrumental (or task) goals, relational goals, and identity goals (Clark & Delia, 1979). *Instrumental goals* refer to the task component of the communication (i.e., requesting or sharing information). *Identity goals* refer to how the speakers enact their own and each other's sense of identity through the communication (i.e., employing politeness when requesting information in order to express oneself as respectful or kind). *Relational goals* refer to the communicator's concerns about their relationship with the other communicator (i.e., employing certain message features to maintain the hearer's trust). O'Keefe (1988) assert that communication can be evaluated in its effectiveness to the extent that it successfully attends to all three goal types. Ideally, sophisticated communication is concerned not only with accomplishing the task at hand; it also sustains or enhances the identity and relational components as well.

A multiple goals perspective has been utilized by numerous scholars to examine communication in multiple contexts (e.g., Dillard et al., 1989; Edwards et al., 2014) including social support contexts between friends and family (Goldsmith, 2004) and health disclosures (e.g., Donovan-Kicken & Caughlin, 2010; Scott et al., 2013). A multiple goals approach applies to patient-provider disclosures because it emphasizes the constitutive power of communication "to shape our understanding of the situation" (Goldsmith, 2004, p. 45). How individuals communicate impacts what takes place during the situation (i.e., disclosure or concealment) and afterward, as a result of the situation (i.e., medical treatment, possible relational disruption, data leakage, etc.). To summarize, a multiple goals framework focuses on identifying individuals' motivations, or goals, which inform their communicative choices.

Identifying goal prioritizations in Latinx LGB AYA patients' SO/SH disclosures

A common assumption of a multiple goals perspective is that the goals involved in a communicative exchange may conflict. The more goals to which a message effectively attends, the more sophisticated the message is considered to be. Indeed, Caughlin (2010) names the creation of such sophisticated messages to be a main aim of interpersonal communication, reflection, and research. However, little theoretical development has moved beyond the assessment that goals may compete with one another to examine specifically how communicators might organize, or prioritize, these purposes. We consider it plausible that (a) communicators may order their goals in patterned ways and (b) communicating with these patterns in mind may produce effective disclosures. Think of the ordered pattern of individual wants and needs illustrated by Maslow's (1943) hierarchy of human needs. An individual must first satisfy the needs at the base of Maslow's pyramid (i.e., food, water, shelter) before moving up to achieve higher-level needs (i.e., intimacy, creativity, etc.). Similarly, perhaps there is an *order* of common Latinx LGB AYA patient concerns to which an HCP must speak – either literally, in conversation, or metaphorically, in the form and content of patient intake materials – to effectively elicit SO/SH disclosures. In this pilot study, we therefore aim to answer two questions: First, what instrumental, identity, and relational goals do Latinx

LGB AYA patients report when they are asked to disclose SO/SH information to their HCPs? Second, how do Latinx LGB AYA patients describe the prioritization patterns of their goals in SO/SH disclosures? In exploring these questions, we include both written and verbal forms of disclosure. Additionally, we define "HCP" to encompass not only the doctor but also their staff.

Methods

Participants

Given the sensitive nature of this study's inquiry, recruiting participants willing to be interviewed was initially a challenge. Following IRB approval, we secured funding to incentivize participation. Recruitment methods included posting paper flyers around the campus of a large university in Texas and posting an online announcement on the university's research opportunities listing page. Other recruitment methods in the broader community were initially used (i.e., posting paper flyers in local coffee shops, grocery stores, and bars); however all study participants reported hearing of the study either via postings on campus or by word-of-mouth from their friends who had participated.

The sample included 29 individuals, ages 18 years old (29%), 19 years old (29%), 20 years old (14%), 21 years old (18%), and 22 years old (10%). All participants identified as Latinx, though there was variation in the terms they utilized to describe their racial/ethnic identities. About half identified as Latina/Latino/Latinx; other terms included Chicana (*n*= 1), Uruguayan-American (*n*= 1), Mexican-American (*n*= 3), Venezuelan (*n*= 1), and Hispanic (*n*= 3). Some participants who identified as Latinx also expressed specific ethnic identities including Puerto Rican, El Salvadorean, Tejano, and Guatemalan. Though the study recruitment materials called for lesbian, gay, bisexual, or transgender (LGBT) individuals, all participants identified as cisgender; thus our findings reflect LGB perspectives. More than half of our participants identified as bisexual or pansexual women (46%) or bisexual men (7%). Roughly a third identified as gay men (29%); less than a fourth identified as lesbian women (10%) or queer women (7%).

Procedures

This project's procedures followed the participatory action research paradigm (Babbie, 2016). The data collection process consisted of one-on-one in-person conversations between a research team member and a participant. Qualitative interviewing allowed the researchers to immerse themselves deeply and broadly in the study area (Lindlof & Taylor, 2019). Interviews were conducted in a small university room that featured a table, two chairs, warm lighting, and international art. This room was selected for the interviews to create an inviting and comfortable space in which the participants might feel at ease. After the participant read and signed a bilingual consent form about the study and their rights to confidentiality and anonymity, the interviewer began a conversation with the participant about their experiences, feelings, and opinions regarding SO/SH disclosures to their HCP(s).

These conversations were guided by a list of open-ended questions that the research team had formulated using the multiple goals framework. The questions were aimed at eliciting participants' thoughts and feelings during real and hypothetical situations in which disclosure may occur. Sample interview questions included: What things do you think about or take into account as you consider whether or not to tell your health care provider information about your sexual identity or sexual health? What things would be most important to you to feel safe when sharing information about your sexual identity or sexual health with your health care provider? Have you ever disclosed your sexual identity or sexual health information to a health care provider? Why or why not? The interviewer was sensitive to the organic unfolding of the conversation, and the order of the questions varied so participants could provide detailed answers and researchers could ask follow-up questions (Wang & Yan, 2012). The conversations were conducted in Spanish and/or English, per the participant's preference. The interviews were audio-recorded and ranged from 8 to 37 minutes in length with an average of 18 minutes. The modest length of the interviews renders this a pilot study. At the end of the interview, each participant was given a 20 USD grocery store gift card and thanked for their time. The majority of the interviews were conducted by the project's first author (a White-presenting mixed-race heterosexual cisgender woman). The other interviews were conducted by a research team member (a Latinx gay cisgender man) who was trained in the interviewing procedures by the first author.

The interview recordings were translated from Spanish to English if the interviewee chose to speak in Spanish by an official Spanish-English translator. There was only one interviewee who chose to conduct the interview in Spanish. All interviews were then transcribed by the professional company GMR Transcription. This yielded 221 pages of single-spaced data which were thematically analyzed (Braun & Clarke, 2006). The data collection and data analysis processes were iterative (Tracy, 2010). Our thematic analyses involved the six phases outlined by Braun and Clarke (2006): (a) familiarizing ourselves with the data, (b) generating initial codes, (c) searching for themes, (d) reviewing themes, (e) defining and naming themes, and (f) producing the report. All coders and research team members received prior training in the multiple goals framework. Notes were taken during the interviews and more notes were recorded immediately after the end of the interviews. After one-third and two-thirds of the interviews were completed, the first author wrote out theoretical sketches of the latent themes and patterns that emerged from the interviews completed thus far. These sketches served to sensitize the interviewer in investigating similar themes and differing perspectives in upcoming interviews.

Next, research team members coded each interview for sections of text that appeared to reflect an identity goal, an instrumental goal, and/or a relational goal. This step was useful in identifying the kinds of identity, relational, and instrumental goals our participants had. Since inferences about an individual's goals based on recorded speech are somewhat subjective in nature, these initial codes were checked by another member of the research team to ensure validity. In the checking process, the additional research team member read over the transcripts. This team member met with the first author and discussed any instances in which they thought the initial coder had miscoded transcript segments. These instances, of which there were very few, were analyzed jointly by the first author and this team member to correctly assign the goal type. In the final step, members of the research team read through each interview in its entirety and looked for the overall latent goal prioritization pattern of each participant.

Findings

Types of goals

RQ 1 asked: What instrumental, identity, and relational goals do Latinx LGB AYA patients report when they are asked to disclose SO/SH information to their HCPs? Latinx LGB AYA patients reported a plethora of relational, identity, and instrumental goals that were shaped, largely, by participants' (a) cultural upbringing, (b) family members' beliefs about human sexuality, (c) awareness level of data leak risk when disclosing personal information to an HCP, (d), individual personality, (e) the medical situation, and (f) the geographic location of the clinic. Thematic analyses revealed seven identity goal themes, six relational goal themes, and five instrumental goal themes. These findings are displayed in Table 1.

Goal prioritization patterns

RQ2 asked: How do Latinx LGB AYA patients describe the prioritization patterns of their goals in SO/SH disclosures? The thematic analyses revealed four distinct prioritization patterns that showed which type of goals were more important to participants and why. The most common pattern (*n*= 15) was to prioritize relational and identity goals over instrumental goals to the extent that instrumental goals were not readily pursued. Other patterns included (a) prioritizing instrumental goals above relational or identity goals (*n*= 5); (b) valuing identity goals such as self-expression over relational or instrumental goals (*n*= 3); and (c) inconsistently prioritizing either relational or instrumental goals depending on each specific situation, due to the dilemma of risking social judgment through disclosure (*n*= 6). Each theme is described below by presenting participants' own voices wherever possible. The central aim of this project was to amplify our participants' voices to academic and health field audiences.

Pattern 1: Instrumental Goals as the Least Prioritized: "It's just not something I want written down on paper or, you know, to just bring up with my family."

About half of our participants (*n*= 15) employed this goal prioritization pattern in which relational and identity goals superseded motivations to accomplish plausible instrumental goals, such as asking for LGB-specific information or STI testing, while visiting an HCP. This pattern group included ten women and five men. These participants commonly expressed ambivalence, dilemma, and sadness as they explained their experiences of navigating and maintaining social relationships while being who they are. There tended to be a sense of struggle between relational goals (i.e., a desire to maintain closeness) and identity goals (i.e., a desire to be perceived as morally upstanding). There was commonly a painful dilemma of if/how to make their sexual identity known to their family members, relatives, community members, and – of course – their HCPs. This caused instrumental goals (i.e., seeking information) to recede in importance.

For some, their sense of sexual identity was so nascent and their sense of heteronormative expectations was so strong that they felt verbally expressing their SO might threaten relational rapport. This was most salient when interviewing Becca, a 19-year-old Latina woman:

> Becca: I say I'm straight, but like also I'm very open too because I've not only been with guys only.
>
> Interviewer: So, it sounds like – I just want to reflect back to make sure I'm hearing – so, it sounds like you've had like experiences that would be in the category of bisexual.
>
> Becca: Yeah.
>
> Interviewer: But that term is not one that you've used to identify yourself.
>
> Becca: Yeah. I mean I've never used it. I mean I've thought about it, but I'm still kind of unsure just because I don't know how to explain the label. It just feels weird.

At the close of the interview, Becca told the interviewer that their conversation was the first time she had verbalized her bisexual orientation to another person. She thanked the interviewer for providing a safe and confidential place in which to begin verbally exploring her sense of sexual identity. Unsurprisingly, she had not disclosed her SO/SH to an HCP. Other participants in this pattern group also indicated that their sense of their SO was so newly-formed, or in-flux since identities can change over time, that they were not ready to verbally claim that identity. For instance, participants who typically saw an HCP that had served their family for years expressed a concern about how disclosing their SO/SH information may impact their relational and identity goals in the context of their relationship with the doctor, as well as how that information might be passed along to the participant's family members. As Susi, a 19-year-old bisexual Venezuelan woman, explained:

> My doctor has always been a family friend and I'm not necessarily out to my family so I was always scared if I told him, even though there's doctor confidentiality stuff, it would somehow slip to them. So, I just didn't necessarily disclose it.

We hasten to clarify that there is nothing wrong with choosing to not disclose one's SO/SH information, particularly when one's sense of sexual identity is newly-formed or still in formation. Some participants' choice to not disclose appeared to be driven by a lack of awareness about why it may be pertinent for HCPs to know their SO/SH information and what instrumental goals they may be able to accomplish through disclosure. Nicolas, a bisexual 20-year-old Latino male, expressed: "If

Table 1. Multiple goals themes surrounding disclosure among LGB Latinx young adults.

Identity Goal Themes	
BBe seen as culturally "good"	"Latinx culture can be very conservative at times and Patriarchal, so being gay is seen as not a good thing. So, it's like you're scared to disclose that information." – Martín, 18-year-old gay Latinx male
BBe perceived as morally upstanding	"There's this culture, especially within the Hispanic community I would say, especially within my family as well, that because we're Catholic, to be abstinent, that is something that's preached strongly within my household. Also, a relationship should be between a man and woman. So, it was a challenge going to the doctor's office and trying to be healthy as far as my sexual health." – Gabriel, 19-year-old gay Latinx male
BBe respected & accepted	"I don't want to be judged or anything of that sort." – Lalo, 20-year-old gay Mexican-American male
MMaintain personal privacy	"For me, it's not entirely their business." – Mateo, 19-year-old gay Hispanic male
AAssert the right to choose when/how to come out to parents to come out to rest of family	"My biggest concern is that my parents might know ecause my parents don't know that I'm gay." – Chad, 21-year-old gay Guatemalan male the form, and I try to give the doctor very meaningful looks if any of my family is in the room, so they don't out me in front of my family." – Ana, 21-year-old pansexual Mexican-American female
EExpress identity fully & openly	"It's a part of my identity and so it should be a part of my conversations with HCPs." – Kate, 21-year-old bisexual Chicana female
Relational Goal Themes	
MMaintain parental closeness	"My dad would be, like, less accepting and there would be sort of, like, a rift." – Martín, 18-year-old gay Latinx male
MMaintain familial closeness	"Almost I'd be letting them down or would be the weird one in the family [if they knew I was bisexual]." – Citllali, 22-year-old bisexual Mexican-American female
MMaintain parental support	"They wouldn't support me financially anymore. Yeah, so it's hard." – Lili, 18-year-old bisexual Hispanic female
AAvoid awkward interaction with HCP	"What if that bothers them and then there's a sycho weird dynamic between us in the rest of the session?" – Sara, 18-year-old bisexual Latina female
AAvoid disrupting relationship with long-term HCP	"My primary HCP is a family doctor I've been seeing since I was 10, so it's weird ... I don't want to have that conversation with someone that has known me so long." – Susi, 19-year-old bisexual Venezuelan female
MMaintain Latinx community ties	"It's mostly fear of social isolation because I still do look up to these people since I grew up with them. It's just that one thing that I feel that if they knew, it would completely ruin this relationship we've had for life." – Monica, 18-year-old queer Latina female
Instrumental (Task) Goal Themes	
OObtain sexual health information	"I really want to be more open because I didn't take a sex ed class. Sex ed is very scary to me because there are still a lot of thing I still don't know and I'm unaware of and online stuff is even more scary because that's not a really reliable place to learn." – Samuel, 19-year-old queer Tejano male
OObtain STI testing	"There's an obvious risk in that being in the gay community, of course, regarding sexually-transmitted diseases. So, I think it's important for, like, the doctor to tell me, like, offer maybe certain tests whenever maybe I'm sick." – Lalo, 18-year-old gay Mexican male
OObtain sexual health treatment	"I would [disclose] because I think PrEP is something very important to be on." – Samuel, 19-year-old queer Tejano male
KKeep the interaction uncomplicated	"Getting regular checkups, I don't feel the need to disclose that." – Mateo, 19-year-old gay Hispanic male
EEducate others	"Some people don't know what pansexual is, so I like to educate people on it." – María, 18-year-old pansexual Mexican female

This table displays the results of RQ1 which asked, "What instrumental, identity, and relational goals do Latinx LGB AYA patients report when they are asked to disclose SO/SH information to their HCPs?"

I knew more about it – like what HCPs could do – I would be more inclined to know what to say to them." Others in this pattern group had a clearer sense that it mattered for their HCP to know their SO/SH information and expressed a desire to be more open with their HCP about their SO/SH information. Juan, a 19-year-old bisexual Latino man, said: "I'm not the most open, just because I'm still not that comfortable talking about it. But I wish I could be more open, just to learn more about any diseases that there are that are occurring, like HIV or AIDS, just to know how to prevent it." This is noteworthy since most of these same participants reported that they were not open with the HCP – which evidences the cognitive dissonance they may be experiencing as they would like to behave in a particular way yet do not enact that behavior due to prioritizing relational and identity goals above instrumental goals.

In listening to participants in this pattern group, it appeared their feelings of awkwardness toward disclosure partially stemmed from a perceived disconnect between cultural identity and sexual orientation within their familial and community contexts. Heteronormative expectations inhibited them from disclosing their SO/SH. This created a conflict between pursuing relational, identity, and instrumental goals simultaneously. Juan, a 19-year-old gay Latino male, avoided disclosure to maintain relational closeness. He stated: "It would be awkward, because they have their views, and I'm who I am. So, it's difficult." Similarly, 19-year-old Ida, who identified as a lesbian Latina woman, was reluctant to disclose for fear of how it would impact her relationship with her brother, stating: "I don't want to mess up the closeness that we have currently, because my brother does make a lot of gay jokes in terms of men. I don't know how he'd feel in regards to me being gay." Relational and identity goals relating to family and community members other than the HCP were paramount and often in tension as participants considered the relational ramification of making their identity known. For example, the relational goal of maintaining familial closeness conflicted with the identity goal of expressing one's identity fully and openly. The taboo was so strong for some such as 18-year-old Monica, who identified as a queer Latina woman, that it represented large threats to their emotional, mental, and physical wellbeing:

> They [my family] are just completely against it and I know because of the way my dad talked about people that are queer. I'm kind of scared of them completely rejecting me and disowning me because my dad had a conversation with my brother before saying, 'If you are gay, then you're not a part of our family.' I'm sorry, I'm getting a little emotional. [Participant begins to cry.]

In disclosing her SO to an HCP, Monica felt she ran a risk of that information getting back to her family. Participants perceived the greatest risk when visiting HCPs in their hometowns or in areas they suspected were not queer-friendly. The socio-political environment was a point for concern. For example, Laura shared: "I'm from El Paso. I mean, they're not gonna go and, like. attack LGBTQ people. It's just, like, it's not really out there and talked about. You know?" The geographic location and socio-political environment of the clinic was also a concern for Samuel, a 19-year-old queer Tejano male, who said:

> I really want to start on PrEP and I really want to be more open because I didn't take a sex ed class. Sex ed is very scary to me because there are still a lot of things I still don't know and I'm unaware of and online stuff is even more scary because that's not a really reliable place to learn. So, I want to be more open with my doctor about it, but I don't know how they would take it and I know that health care professionals have to be unbiased, but there are still people, where I'm from especially, who really don't particularly care.

All participants in this pattern group talked at length about the risk of social isolation, withdrawal of family financial support, and ostracization as a social punishment from non-LGB-friendly family members. Their hesitancy to disclose stemmed both from discomfort at their HCP knowing their SO/SH information, as well as from a fear that their information might be leaked to third parties. For some, the fear was a concern about what could happen. For others, such as Pat, the fear was based on a past negative experience:

> I don't know how it informed them, but she found out. I didn't put an address down for them to send me results and my phone number was the only one listed when I signed up to get tested. I tried to keep everything very towards me only. The only thing logically that I could think of was they informed her that it got charged to her insurance so it came up with something I guess. It's a service clinic and usually for people who go for like free condoms and free testing and stuff. So, I'm scared that if I continue to pursue something more medically for my sexuality that it will somehow end up getting back to her.

These participants considered disclosure to their HCP to potentially be a disclosure to others in their life, as well, either due to breaches in confidentiality practices or being on their parents' insurance. To illustrate these participants' dilemmas and honor their respective voices, here is a final quote from Gabriel, a 19-year-old gay Latinx male:

> You have to be understanding of the values and the cultures of what it means to be in a Hispanic family and that the most prevalent religion is Catholicism or just Christianity. Being abstinent and being in straight relationships is something that is definitely key to those cultures and something that many Latinx families do value. With acknowledging someone's sexuality, it's not as easy as just being open with it and having those open conversations with your family. It's something that has to be worked up towards. I feel like the easiest way to try to resolve the solution is to say like, 'Oh, just go tell your parents. It'll be all right.' But with the cultures and the standards of like your own community, your own family, it's not the easiest to just be blunt or outright with someone's sexuality.

In sum, these participants felt compelled to attend to their relational and identity goals to such an extent that disclosure was mostly avoided, and instrumental goals were left unpursued.

Pattern 2: Instrumental Goals as the Most Prioritized: "If it helped in their assessment of me at all, then I would be open about it."

This next goal prioritization pattern (*n*= 5) was marked by pragmatism. This pattern group included three women and two men. Whereas the interviews of the first pattern featured descriptions of the complex dilemmas they felt about navigating their relational and identity goals, the interviews of the second pattern were much simpler. From their comments it was apparent that these participants: (a) had a developed sense of their sexual orientation and identity, (b) had already come out to their family, and (c) either felt that their family supported their sexual identity or were able to access general relational support from their family by strategically underemphasizing their sexual identity when communicating with them.

To be clear, these interviews were not without dilemmas. These participants were still thoughtful and, at times, hesitant to volunteer personal information to their HCP for fear of discrimination or data leakage to third parties. However, these concerns were generally placed as secondary. They would disclose if they felt divulging their SO/SH information would secure them better medical care. For instance, 21-year-old Ana who identified as a pansexual Mexican-American woman reported: "I try to be honest on my medical forms just because that way I get the best care." Lalo, an 18-year-old gay Mexican male, shared: "There's an obvious risk in being in the gay community,[6] of course, regarding sexually transmitted diseases. So, I think it's important for the doctor to tell me – like offer certain tests whenever I'm sick." These participants had prominent instrumental goals that drove their interaction with their HCP.

If participants perceived information to be irrelevant to their care in a given medical encounter, they chose not to disclose their SO/SH information. Their choice of privacy in these situations served three functions. First, it minimized the risk of data leakage to third parties, such as insurance companies who may inadvertently commit a breach of privacy. For instance, Aetna suffered a lawsuit for accidentally divulging their clients' HIV status by printing confidential information in the viewable window of mailers (Gordon, 2018). These participants were sensitized to this risk. Ana explained: "I try to be honest on medical forms unless I think these forms will be turned into my insurance company." Second, avoiding disclosure kept the situation as uncomplicated as necessary. Ana continued sharing her reasoning: "If I think it's irrelevant to my care [I don't disclose]. I don't know if I've ever had to fill out something like that on a dentist form, but I know I just wouldn't because it's irrelevant to my care." Third, withholding disclosure avoided the risk of possible discrimination from the HCP. Nancy, a 22-year -old pansexual Latina woman, explained:

> There's no reason. And I think it can be a little uncomfortable to bring it up, and not just to a doctor, but like, you know, to anyone, because you don't know how they'll react and yeah, I mean, I don't – I wouldn't expect a doctor to, you know, respond in any particularly negative way because of it, but you wouldn't want that to affect anything or, you know, if there is any judgment on like sexual history or anything like that.

In situations where participants felt there was a high risk of discrimination, they chose not to disclose.

Finally, these participants were similar to the participants in the first prioritization group in two noteworthy respects. First, the geographical location of the clinic impacted the degree to which they felt inclined to openly discuss their SO/SH. It was important to participants in both groups that the HCP was in a socio-political area that was more accepting of LGB concerns. As Paula, a pansexual Mexican-American 21-year-old, explained:

> I actively allow myself to use inclusive language when I'm at the clinic at [name of university she attends that is located in a large metropolitan city]. I might use them or her referring to a past partner. Whereas I would watch my language if I were getting care in El Paso or anywhere else just because—I don't know. [This city] is really accepting, but I don't trust the rest of the world to be that accepting.

Ricardo, a 20-year-old gay Uruguayan American, echoed Paula's sentiment by stating, "If I were to go to a more conservative area, maybe I'd have issues." The location of the clinic was a factor in his disclosure decision-making.

Second, participants from both pattern groups expressed a desire to be more open with their HCP without risking judgment or discrimination. This indicates that both groups were concerned about social stigma due to their sexual identity.

Pattern 3: Identity Goals as the Most Prioritized: "Yeah, I'm happy. Like I said, I'm very open about it."

There were three participants for whom their approach toward the patient-provider conversation was different than the rest of the sample. This pattern group included three women. These participants conceptualized themselves, society, and health care in ways that caused them to highly prioritize identity goals – namely, the identity goal of verbally expressing their identities. For them, interactions with their HCP were not driven so much by a concern about being honest to receive the best care (i.e., an instrumental goal) or by a concern about concealing their SO/SH information to avoid judgment or relational awkwardness (i.e., relational goals). Rather, the impetus for what they said or did not say was a goal of asserting their identity.

These participants' reasons for valuing self-expression stemmed from two things. First, disclosing SO/SH information to an HCP was a natural choice for a participant who did not conceal her sexual orientation from anyone. Angela, a 22-year-old queer Latina woman, shared: "I've always been aware of it, and I don't think I've ever considered myself as being in the closet … I just have lived my life … That's just the kind of person I've always been." For Angela, disclosure was her norm. Concealing her sexual identity from her HCP would have felt strange.

Second, participants in this pattern group voiced a desire to show up with personal authenticity and thereby educate others. This was a motivator to disclose for Kate, a 21-year-old bisexual Chicana woman, who said: "It's a part of my identity and so it should be a part of my conversations with HCPs to find the best health care … I would like to just kind of let them know we're here – like we exist – and we're all looking for health care, like, proper health care." Kate prioritized her identity goal of self-expression and made sure her health care centered around who she is. Similarly, it was important to María, an 18-year-old pansexual Mexican woman, to express herself openly. She explained: "I'm very open about it … I like to educate. Some people don't know what pansexual is, so I like to educate people on it. That way, people can know there's more sexualities out there as well." Personal transparency during social interactions felt important to participants in this pattern group. This identity goal was linked to the instrumental goal of receiving personalized health care (i.e., relevant information, testing, and treatment). In the interviews of this pattern group, there was considerably less discussion of relational goals, such as seeking to maintain relational rapport with the HCP. Also absent from these participants' accounts was concern of the risk of third-party leakage. Either these participants were already out or did not fear the potential discrimination they might face through outing themselves to their HCP or third parties. Their desire to fully express their identity was paramount, regardless of the possible consequences.

Pattern 4: Vacillating Prioritizations of Relational/Identity and Instrumental Goals: "It might be nice" but "you never really know."

At first glance, this final pattern looked similar to the first: both groups of participants spoke frequently about prioritizing a confluence of relational and identity goals. However, upon closer investigation, it became apparent that these participants (n = 6) also highly prioritized instrumental goals, such as procuring health-related information from their HCP, and actively pursued these instrumental goals if certain situational conditions were met. This pattern group included three women and three men.

Participants of the first pattern group rarely brought instrumental goals to the forefront. Their instrumental goals remained "locked" behind a complicated layer of identity and relational goals. They expressed a desire to be more open with their HCP, however this desire was generally spoken of as a distant pining rather than a realizable intention. In contrast, the participants in the fourth pattern group's desire to be open with their HCP was tangible and attainable. They articulated practical steps HCPs could take to satisfy their relational and identity goals. In situations in which HCPs displayed behaviors that satisfied their relational and identity goals, they were ready and willing to voice their SO/SH information and satisfy their instrumental goal of seeking information tailored to their sexual identity and activities. This group's pattern was intrinsically malleable as they prioritized either relational/identity goals or instrumental goals based on their assessment of the interpersonal situation. As is shown in Figure 1, the satisfaction of certain goals appeared to facilitate the active pursuit of other goals. Similar to Maslow's hierarchy of needs in which lower-level needs must be met before the pursuit of higher-level needs, so the attainment of lower-level relational and identity goals was necessary before pursuing higher-level task goals.

For some participants in this group, such as 21-year-old Chad who identified as a gay Guatemalan man, the action needed to satisfy their lower-level needs was ensuring their SO/SH would be kept 100% confidential. He said: "My biggest concern is that my parents don't know I'm gay. And that's usually what comes up in my mind is because I might tell the doctor something and then my parents might wanna know and talk to the doctor." It was of utmost concern that their parents and Latinx community members would not find out to protect their relational and identity goals. For Chad, however, this reassurance of privacy was also paired with his personal level of comfort with seeing a Latinx HCP. He said, "I just feel more comfortable with a Latino doctor ... so, for Latino doctors, I would feel comfortable telling them my sexuality." The identity of the HCP was a variable in Chad's goal prioritization pattern.

For most, the salient relational and identity goals that needed to be met centered on feeling respected and accepted by their HCP. They began seeking to meet their goals before the office visit by vetting the HCP's website and professional bio. Lisa, a 21-year-old bisexual Latinx woman, said: "Just do as much as you can to took them up and see if there's anything that you can glean to see if you feel safe, and if you do then go for them." This is a practice that participants in other studies have also noted (e.g., Hudak & Bates, 2019; Martos et al., 2018). Then in the actual interaction with the HCP, they gingerly broached disclosure and incrementally disclosed (Petronio et al., 1996) while reading the HCP's nonverbal and verbal signals to assess whether this felt like an emotionally and mentally safe space for them. Lisa, a 21-year-old bisexual Latinx woman, explained:

> It's the body language. It's like they look at you. They go like oh, right, and then like step back a little bit. And you're like oh, okay, I see that's shocking to you, or like you don't feel comfortable around me, or that makes me feel uncomfortable, makes me feel like that you're judging me and that you might not give me the best quality of health care that I should get because you disagree with my lifestyle.

These participants made disclosure decisions based on the cues they received from their HCPs.

The fact that the HCP's behavior may or may not help participants satisfy their lower-level goals was echoed in other interviews of this pattern group. Monse, an 18-year-old lesbian Latina woman, commented: "Sometimes doctors tend to just assume that everyone that comes into their office is just straight and not really think about the fact that somebody might purposely not be telling them." These participants noted how the words, actions, or overall "vibe" they received from their HCP made a significant difference in whether or not they pursued instrumental goals.

HCPs' communication features such as tone of voice and voluntary use of inclusive language made a difference for some of these participants' goal prioritizations. Certain speech features cued participants to possible heteronormative assumptions. Rosa, a 20-year-old lesbian Mexican-American woman, reports:

> It just feels weird whenever you talk about sexual health or tiptoe around it and it's like, 'What do they think I am? Are there suggestions towards a hetero woman or a homosexual woman?' It's just kind of like maybe if doctors, nurse practitioners, nurses would really talk to you in the all-encompassing kind of way, that would be more freeing to openly communicate ... [because] to have them assume that heteronormative standard, a woman dates a man, it 'others' you in a sense and make you feel like you're not – like, you're supposed to be in this category but now you're in something else and they have to change how they're talking to

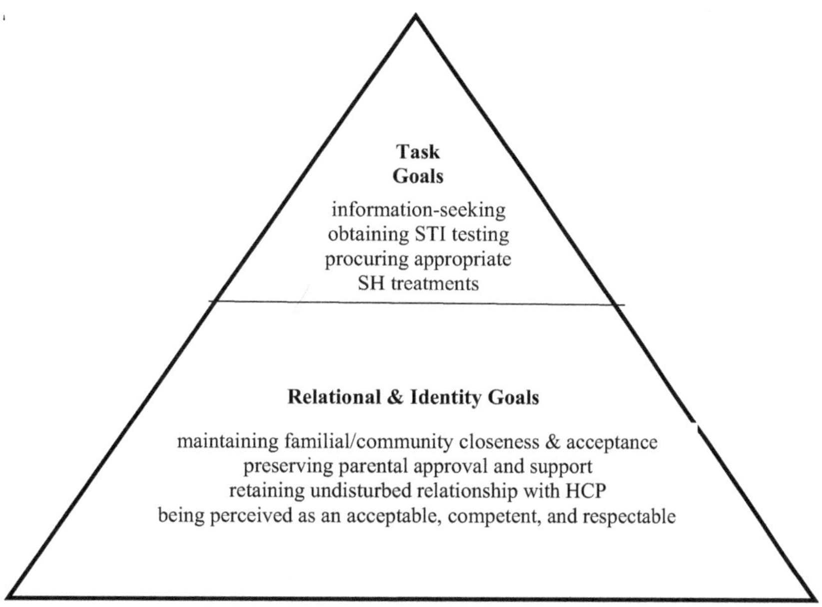

Figure 1. Goal prioritization pattern hierarchy of Fourth Participant Group. "Instrumental" and "task" are synonymous. This figure displays results to RQ2 which asked, "How do Latinx LGB AYA patients describe the prioritization patterns of their goals in SO/SH disclosures?"

> you to fit what they want. It's weird. As soon as you feel that weird, awkward vibe in the room, then you kind of shut down not just for that topic, but for other topics. It's like, 'Oh no, I'm already tiptoeing on the edge right now. I don't want to say any more out of the ordinary.'

Rosa assessed her HCP based on communication cues and decided accordingly whether or not to disclose. The practical steps of having intentionally welcoming language on one's website bio, using inclusive language when talking with patients, and being mindful of using an inviting and accepting tone of voice when discussing diverse sexualities with patients are three steps these participants highlighted that help met their identity and relational goals so they felt comfortable pursing task goals. Additionally, HCP's choice of décor and reading materials throughout the office was noted by these participants as impacting their feelings of comfort around disclosure. Mateo, a 19-year-old gay Hispanic man, suggested that HCPs post "rainbow flags or different other flags like the transgender flag or signs that say helpful things" to communicate that the clinic is welcoming to everyone.

However, even if the HCP appears professional and LGB-friendly, that is no guarantee that participants' relational and identity goals will be met during the interaction. Mateo, a 19-year-old gay Hispanic man, made this caveat: "I err on the side of not [disclosing] because I feel like you never really know how someone might absorb that information – even though they're not supposed to absorb that in any particular way. You just don't know." Clearly, these participants perceived that stigma toward LGB individuals is still societally pervasive.

Discussion

LGB Latinx individuals experience stigma and multiple marginalization which, in turn, exacerbate health disparities when compared to heterosexual White individuals (e.g., Walby et al., 2012). Disclosure of SO/SH information to an HCP is fraught with challenges (Greene et al., 2012), particularly for Latinx LGB individuals (Anhalt et al., 2020). To mitigate health disparities experienced by Latinx sexual minorities, this study was undertaken to understand their concerns and motivations surrounding disclosure by examining how LGB Latinx AYAs prioritize their interpersonal goals during interactions with their HCPs. Our findings are two-fold. First, our analyses about RQ1 reveal specific kinds of identity, relational, and instrumental goals experienced by our participants. Second, our RQ2 analyses suggest that participants did not all prioritize goals the same way. Rather, four patterns of goal ordering emerged from the data. In the first pattern, individuals were so strongly focused on identity and relational goals that instrumental goals were not actualized. Individuals in the second pattern exhibited the reverse: they focused primarily on attaining instrumental goals. Identity and relational goals were of secondary concern. In the third pattern, individuals were largely motivated by the identity goal of self-expression. For these individuals, relational and instrumental goals were secondary. Individuals in the fourth pattern vacillated between focusing on identity/relational goals or instrumental goals. If the HCP was perceived to be LGBTQ-friendly, these individuals tended to feel their identity/relational goals were met and felt freer to pursue their instrumental goals. If the HCP was perceived to be heteronormative, discriminatory, or untrustworthy, these individuals felt their identity/relational goals were not met, in which case they chose not pursue their instrumental goals. These goal prioritization patterns suggest that Latinx LGB individuals have differing motivations that influence their disclosure choices.

These findings extend prior work on multiple goals in two ways. First, our findings suggest that individual goals are not only differentiated as primary and secondary (Dillard et al., 1989) but may also be prioritized in various ways. Our analyses revealed four distinct goal prioritization patterns that appeared to vary based on individual differences, past experiences, and contextual factors such as the cues received HCPs. Second, whereas many prior studies using multiple goals focused on the experiences of heterosexual White populations (e.g., Caughlin et al., 2009; Donovan-Kicken & Caughlin, 2010), this present study focuses on the experiences of LGB Latinx individuals. Our study strengthens multiple goals as a theoretical framework by showing that its tenants are applicable and relevant to populations beyond White heterosexual individuals.

Our findings complement the findings of other queer health disclosure studies (e.g., Venetis et al., 2017). For instance, our RQ1 goal themes echo many of Hudak and Carmack (2018). In their study that they conducted with a predominantly White queer population on influencers of queer health disclosures, they found several factors to impact LGB patients' disclosure of sexuality, including experience with family, fear of gossip and connection, and level of trust with providers. In our study, we found experiences with family to shape participants' disclosures. Many of our participants also expressed the fear of gossip and questioned whether they could trust their HCPs to maintain confidentiality. Thus, the concern about whether the HCP can be trusted to not share the patient's information with others appears to be a concern for both White and Latinx study participants.

Additionally, our findings highlight concerns about how disclosure is conceptualized and how opportunities for disclosure are communicated to patients by HCPs (Larson & Chastain, 1990). Our participants understood disclosure in different and, at times, contradictory ways that indicate a need for greater clarity. For instance, multiple participants initially told us they had never disclosed their SO/SH information to an HCP yet later informed us that they accurately completed intake forms that requested SO/SH information. These participants did not consider such written or electronic reporting as "telling" an HCP their sexual identity. The distinction between verbally disclosing and filling out a form is valid. Revealing something vulnerable in conversation may feel different than checking a box on a form. Yet in both cases, the patient is sharing their SO/SH information with an HCP. This lack of awareness around non-verbal instances of disclosure raises concerns of consent (Worthington, 2002).

Moreover, our participants' experiences raise these questions: When does a patient's interaction with their HCP begin? Who is privy to the information on intake forms or information shared verbally with a doctor? Many of our participants feared that their data would be leaked to others. This is a concern that participants in other queer disclosure studies among non-Latinx populations have also reported (Goins & Pye, 2013; Hudak & Carmack, 2018). This suggests that sexual identity is salient in health care contexts. The participants in Goins and Pye (2013) study about LGBTQ health communication also voiced concerns about the immediate and long-term impacts of who views intake forms. A number of our participants – particularly those still in their late teens – displayed no awareness that their information might be shared with anyone other than the HCP physically present in the room. This is concerning since "new technological developments make widespread data collection and aggregation possible, increasing both the possibility and harms of disclosing sensitive data" (Kaplan, 2015, p. 260). De-identification of patients' data does not ensure their privacy is respected (Kaplan, 2015). Insurance company reporting, as noted by Samuel when his mother learned of his STI testing, is a legal way an individual's SH information might be shared with someone other than the HCP.

Although HIPPA legislation prohibits HCPs from sharing private data, our participants from socio-politically conservative cities and small towns where their HCP was a family friend wondered whether they could trust such protection. Notably, Hong et al. (2019) found that privacy concerns, trust in doctors, and the preference for control varied by race. The relational goals of our Latinx participants signaled concerns about their private information becoming known to others beyond the medical clinic. Our findings suggest that HCPs' confidentiality standards are currently unclear to LGB Latinx AYA patients. This, too, is a point prior research has outlined. Hudak and Carmack (2018) recommended HIPAA education for patients so they know their information is protected by law and communication training for HCPs to help communicate this to patients.

Our findings align with those of other sexual minority and health care researchers (e.g., Gessner et al., 2019; Schmitz et al., 2019; Whitehead et al., 2016) in emphasizing the need for reduction of LGB socio-cultural stigmatization. Such stigmatization influenced the relational and identity goals of our participants. The fear of discrimination commonly caused our participants to avoid pursuing instrumental goals such as seeking out sexual health information pertinent to the prevention and treatment of disease. Stigmatization and fear of homophobic discrimination are not unique to Latinx LGB individuals. Deciding whether to conceal or disclose one's sexual orientation involves considerable cost-benefit analysis for both White LGB individuals and LGB people of color alike (Moradi et al., 2010). However, as noted in our discussion on "Intersectional Barriers to Health Care for an Expanding Latinx AYA Patient Population," LGB people of color face additional barriers to receiving quality health care services that compound social and systemic inequalities.

Based on our study and prior research, we make several practical recommendations. First, we concur with Hudak and Carmack (2018) in their call for patient HIPPA education and provider training to allay patients' fears of data leakage. When multiple studies indicate that patients across varying racial/ethnic groups are afraid that the information they share at their HCP's office might reach third parties, it is time to craft effective and far-reaching patient education measures. This education needs to go beyond the proverbial HIPPA notice that is displayed at the office window, and it needs to be more reader-friendly than the legal notices patients are given upon arrival at the clinic. Possible education methods include creating informational videos shown in patient waiting rooms and brief click-through slides with meme segments included in pre-visit online health intake protocols illustrating how patient information is used and how it is not used. It goes without saying that providers should be acting according to HIPPA standards and should undergo refresher training to ensure their data usage practices comply with federal law. Additionally, education needs to include guidance for patients when and if they believe their HIPPA rights have been violated and resources for pursuing accountability of HCPs. Such efforts stand to diffuse tension around SO/SH disclosures.

Second, we call for provider heteronormativity awareness training that sensitizes HCPs to how their choice of language and nonverbals perpetuate or reduce the stigmatization experienced by LGB individuals. Our findings and Utamsingh et al.'s (2016) findings suggest that HCPs' words and behaviors impact patients' disclosure choices. Our participants in the fourth pattern group adjusted the extent to which they readily volunteered SO/SH information based on their perception of LGB-friendly or LGB-hostile cues. Many HCPs grew up in heteronormative cultural settings and may unwittingly act say or do things that communicate a threat to LGB patients. For instance, many HCPs may not have been initially trained to ask what pronouns a patient prefers or to inform the patient of their own preferred pronouns. Further, the development of Western medicine has historically suffered from a heteronormative bias. Thus, the training HCPs received in medical school likely contained this bias. For example, the standard questions HCPs were trained to ask a patient to gather information about the patient's sexual health may have been predicated on the assumptions that the patient's sex was (a) either male or female and (b) obvious due to the individual's physical appearance. Not only are these assumptions heteronormative, but also they are rooted in binary and reductionist sex categorizations; they exclude intersex, trans, non-binary, and gender-queer individuals while ignoring socially and relationally constructed sexuality and gender identity. HCPs need to be taught a new manner of going about their job that allows for and honors the breadth of human gender and sexual identities. This will take time and effort due to the tradition and repetition of heteronormative practices. Thus, intentional training is necessary to create significant change. These trainings must be substantial (i.e., more than a one-hour continuing education unit). A full-day or multi-day workshop format is likely to be most effective. The container of time and intention must be large and strong enough so that attendees can (a) reflect upon their most basic social and professional conditioning, (b) identify any internal resistance they may experience toward changing how and what they communicate to patients, and (c) develop strategies to overcome such resistance by establishing and practicing new communication habits.

In addition to training, we recommend that the office environment reflect LGBTQAI+ allyship, as well as provide bilingual educational materials. Waiting rooms and examination areas could have posters in multiple languages that provide information and address patient concerns. After completing training, HCPs could wear ally pins that signal that they are not only open to discussing LGBTQAI+ health concerns, but also qualified to do so.

Finally, in order to demonstrate accountability to their patients, health care facilities could request anonymous feedback from patients after a visit asking specific questions around diversity, equity, and inclusion. Feedback surveys provide an opportunity to gather further data on whether or not measures, such as HCP trainings, are an effective way to mitigate unconscious bias and inadvertent microaggressions. Health care systems would also need to implement fair and reasonable accountability measures for HCPs who may need additional education and training in order to serve all of their patients equally. This is no small task, but it will significantly change the quality of interactions between all patients and HPCs, notably Latinx LGB patients who face multiple inequalities.

Conclusion

This study makes several contributions. First, it extends multiple goals theorizing by demonstrating how Latinx LGB individuals may prioritize their communicative goals. Prior to this study, a multiple goals perspective had not been used to examine how disclosures function among Latinx LGB AYA patients. Second, this study extends multiple goals theorizing by highlighting that different goals may not only be in conflict with each other but that they may be prioritized in a meaningful fashion in relation to one another. This can also be said of the elements that make up a patient's identity. This finding has practical implications; by first attending to a patient's relational and identity goals, HCPs may be able to facilitate rather than hinder SO/SH disclosures. However, disclosure may not always be in the best interest of the patient, due to the risk of data leakage to third parties. Further research should explore the ethical and logistical complexities of communicating confidentiality standards to patients and ensuring that those standards are met, particularly when Latinx AYAs are concerned.

This study had its limitations. The relatively short average interview length indicates that the interview guide could have been better developed to elicit more detailed responses from the participants. Some participants naturally elaborated on the interview prompts, but others did not and could have used encouragement in the form of specific follow-up questions. The sample size was modest and consisted of LGB AYA patients currently living in the Texas. Further research could consider other geographical regions of the United States to test the validity of the proposed theoretical ideas. Because our study did not include transgender participants, future research could study, trans Latinx health care interactions. Additionally, these data could have been interpreted using a disclosure-specific theory such as Communication Privacy Management theory (Petronio, 2002). We may utilize such a theoretical frame for analyzing and interpreting other elements of this dataset and related datasets in future publications. Lastly, this study included the voices of Latinx LGB AYA patients who were willing to talk about their sexual minority status in an in-person interview format. We recommend that other methodologies, such as an anonymous online survey, be considered when developing future studies that explore this topic.

Notes

1. Disclosing SH information as it relates to behavior may or may not disclose LGB identity to a HCP. For example, disclosing frequency of sex or number of sexual partners is not related to identity. However, discussing contraception or what type of sex the patient engages in may reveal a non-heteronormative sexual orientation or a non-cis gender identity.
2. as it relates to race and sexual orientation
3. While our study focuses on LGB individuals, we use the term "queer" here as an umbrella term for LGBTQAI+ identities included in the previous studies we reference.
4. While gender is also an important variable in SO/SH disclosures, this study concerns itself with race/ethnicity and sexual orientation.
5. Misogyny – the dislike of, contempt for, and ingrained prejudice against women – applies broadly to all expressions of femininity.
6. Here we note that this participant has internalized harmful stereotypes of the gay community while being gay himself. "Being in the gay community" is related to identity, not behavior. It is not a risk. Having unprotected sex is a risk related to behavior. Many individuals engage in unprotected sex, regardless of sexual orientation.

Acknowledgments

The authors wish to thank Erin E. Donovan, Ph.D., for her guidance. They also thank McKenzie N. Castro, Carmen A. Gatrelle, and Lydia A. Medhanie for their assistance with coding. They thank Miguel Robles Marquez for his interviewing and recruiting assistance.

Funding

Data collection and analyses were supported by a grant from the Center for Health Communication's Health Scholars Program at the University of Texas at Austin. Portions of this material were presented at the 2018 Western States Communication Association annual meeting, San Jose, CA, United States and at the 2019 Health Communication: Barriers, Breakthroughs and Best Practices annual online conference, Urbana, Illinois, United States.

References

Alsan, M., Garrick, O., & Graziani, G. C. (2019). Does diversity matter for health? Experimental evidence from Oakland. *American Economic Review*, *109*(12), 4071–4111. https://doi.org/10.1257/aer.2018144

Anhalt, K., Toomey, R. B., & Shramko, M. (2020). Latinx sexual minority youth adjustment in the context of discrimination and internalized homonegativity: The moderating role of cultural orientation processes. *Journal of Latinx Psychology*, *8*(1), 41–57. https://doi.org/10.1037/lat0000134

Austin, E. L. (2013). Sexual orientation disclosure to HCPs among urban and non-urban southern lesbians. *Women & Health*, *53*(1), 41–55. https://doi.org/10.1080/03630242.2012.743497

Babbie, E. R. (2016). *The practice of social research*. Cengage Learning.

Baig, A. A., Lopez, F. Y., DeMeester, R. H., Jia, J. L., Peek, M. E., & Vela, M. B. (2016). Addressing barriers to shared decision making among Latino LGBTQ patients and healthcare providers in clinical settings. *LGBT Health*, *3*(5), 335–341. https://doi.org/10.1089/lgbt.2016.0014

Beach, M. C., Saha, S., Korthuis, P. T., Sharp, V., Cohn, J., Wilson, I., Eggly, S., Cooper, L. A., Roter, D., Sankar, A., & Moore, R. (2010). Differences in patient–provider communication for Hispanic compared to Non-Hispanic white patients in HIV care. *Journal of General Internal Medicine*, *25*(7), 682–687. https://doi.org/10.1007/s11606-010-1310-4

Bonvicini, K., & Perlin, M. (2003). The same but different: Clinician-patient communication with gay and lesbian patients. *Patient Education and Counseling*, *51*(2), 115–122. https://www.sciencedirect.com/science/article/abs/pii/S0738399102001891

Braun, V., & Clarke, V. (2006). Using thematic analysis in psychology. *Qualitative Research in Psychology*, *3*(2), 77–101. https://doi.org/10.1191/1478088706qp063oa

Brooks, H., Llewellyn, C., Nadarzynski, T., Pelloso, F., De Souza Guilherme, F., Pollard, A., & Juanes, C. (2018). Sexual orientation disclosure in health care: A systematic review. *British Journal of General Practice*, *68*(668), e187–e196. https://doi.org/10.3399/bjgp18x694841

Caughlin, J. P. (2010). Invited review article: A multiple goals theory of personal relationships: Conceptual integration and program overview. *Journal of Social and Personal Relationships*, *27*(6), 824–848. https://doi.org/10.1177/0265407510373262

Caughlin, J. P., Bute, J. J., Donovan-Kicken, E., Kosenko, K. A., Ramey, M. E., & Brashers, D. E. (2009). Do message features influence reactions to HIV disclosures? A multiple-goals perspective. *Health Communication*, *24*(3), 270–283. https://doi.org/10.1080/10410230902806070

Centers for Disease Control and Prevention. (2020). *Health disparities in HIV/AIDS, viral hepatitis, STDs, and TB: Hispanics/Latinos*. https://www.cdc.gov/nchhstp/healthdisparities/hispanics.html

Clark, R. A., & Delia, J. C. (1979). Topoi and rhetorical competence. *The Quarterly Journal of Speech*, *65*(2), 187–206. https://doi.org/10.1080/00335637909383470

Crenshaw, K. (1991). Mapping the margins: Intersectionality, identity politics, and violence against women of color. *Stanford Law Review*, *43*(6), 1241–1299. https://doi.org/10.2307/1229039

Díaz, R. M., Ayala, G., Bein, E., Henne, J., & Marin, B. V. (2001). The impact of homophobia, poverty, and racism on the mental health of gay and bisexual Latino men: Findings from 3 US cities. *American Journal of Public Health*, *91*(6), 927. https://ajph.aphapublications.org/doi/10.2105/AJPH.91.6.927

Dillard, J. P., Segrin, C., & Harden, J. M. (1989). Primary and secondary goals in the production of interpersonal influence messages. *Communication Monographs*, *56*(1), 19–38. https://doi.org/10.1080/03637758909390247

Donovan-Kicken, E., & Caughlin, J. P. (2010). A multiple goals perspective on topic avoidance and relationship satisfaction in the context of breast cancer. *Communication Monographs*, *77*(2), 231–256. https://doi.org/10.1080/03637751003758219

Durso, L., & Meyer, I. (2012). Patterns and predictors of disclosure of sexual orientation to health care providers among lesbians, gay men, and bisexuals. *Sexuality Research & Social Policy*, *10*(1), 35–42. https://doi.org/10.1007/s13178-012-0105-2

Edwards, L. L., Donovan-Kicken, E., & Reis, J. S. (2014). Communicating in complex situations: A normative approach to HIV-related talk among parents who are HIV+. *Health Communication*, *29*(4), 364–374. https://doi.org/10.1080/10410236.2012.757715

Escarce, J. J., & Kapur, K. (2006). Access to and quality of health care. In M. Tienda & F. Mitchell (Eds.), *Hispanics and the future of America* (pp. 410–446). National Academies Press. https://www.nap.edu/read/11539/chapter/11

Farber, B. A. (2003). Patient self-disclosure: A review of the research. *Journal of Clinical Psychology*, *59*(5), 589–600. https://doi.org/10.1002/jclp.10161

Fritz, Z., Griffiths, F. E., & Slowther, A. M. (2020). Custodians of information: Patient and physician views on sharing medical records in the acute care setting. *Health Communication*. Advance online publication. https://doi.org/10.1080/10410236.2020.1803553

García, L. (2009). "Now why do you want to know about that?" Heteronormativity, sexism, and racism in the sexual (mis)education of Latina youth. *Gender & Society*, *23*(4), 520–541. https://doi.org/10.1177/0891243209339498

Gessner, M., Bishop, M. D., Martos, A., Wilson, B. D., & Russell, S. T. (2019). Sexual minority people's perspectives of sexual health care: Understanding minority stress in sexual health settings. *Sexuality Research and Social Policy*, *17*(4), 607–618. https://doi.org/10.1007/s13178-019-00418-9

Goins, E., & Pye, D. (2013). Check the box that best describes you: Reflexively managing theory and praxis in LGBTQ health communication research. *Health Communication*, *28*(4), 397–407. https://doi.org/10.1080/10410236.2012.690505

Goldsmith, D. J. (2004). *Communicating social support*. Cambridge University Press.

Gordon, E. (2018). *Aetna agrees to pay $17 million in HIV privacy breach*. NPR. https://www.npr.org/sections/health-shots/2018/01/17/572312972/aetna-agrees-to-pay-17-million-in-hiv-privacy-breach

Greene, K., Magsamen-Conrad, K., Venetis, M. K., Checton, M. G., Bagdasarov, Z., & Banerjee, S. C. (2012). Assessing health diagnosis disclosure decisions in relationships: Testing the disclosure decision-making model. *Health Communication*, *27*(4), 356–368. https://doi.org/10.1080/10410236.2011.586988

Haas, S. M., & Lannutti, P. J. (2019). The impact of minority stress and social support on positive relationship functioning in same-sex relationships. *Health Communication*, *36*(3), 315–323. https://doi.org/10.1080/10410236.2019.1687130

Herek, G. M. (2009). Sexual stigma and sexual prejudice in the United States: A conceptual framework. In D. A. Hope (Ed.), *Contemporary perspectives on lesbian, gay, and bisexual identities* (Vol. 54, pp. 65–111). Springer. http://doi.org/10.1007/978-0-387-09556-1_4

Hill, A., Jones, D., & Woodworth, L. (2020). Physician-patient race-match reduces patient mortality. *Social Science Research Network, Available online*. https://doi.org/10.2139/ssrn.3211276

Hong, S. J., Drake, B., Goodman, M., & Kaphingst, K. A. (2019). Race, trust in doctors, privacy concerns, and consent preferences for biobanks. *Health Communication*, *35*(10), 1219–1228. https://doi.org/10.1080/10410236.2019.1623644

Hudak, N. (2020). Navigating publishing critical health communication research. *Frontiers in Communication*, *5*, 38. https://doi.org/10.3389/fcomm.2020.00038

Hudak, N. & Bates, B. R. (2019). In pursuit of "queer-friendly" healthcare: An interview study of how queer individuals select care providers. *Health Communication*, *8*(34), 818–824. https://10.1080/10410236.2018.1437525

Hudak, N. C., & Carmack, H. J. (2018). Waiting for the doctor to ask: Influencers of lesbian, gay, and bisexual identity disclosure for healthcare providers. *Qualitative Research in Medicine and Healthcare*, *2*(20), 20–29. https://doi.org/10.4081/qrmh.2018.7157

Juckett, G. (2013). Caring for Latino patients. *American Family Physician*, *87*(1), 48–54. https://www.aafp.org/afp/2013/0101/p48.html

Kaplan, B. (2015). Selling health data: De-identification, privacy, and speech. *Cambridge Quarterly of Healthcare Ethics*, *24*(3), 256–271. https://doi.org/10.1017/S0963180114000589

Kim, H. J., & Fredriksen-Goldsen, K. I. (2012). Hispanic lesbians and bisexual women at heightened risk or health disparities. *American Journal of Public Health*, *102*(1), e9–e15. https://doi.org/10.2105/AJPH.2011.300378

Kuo, K.-M., Ma, -C.-C., & Alexander, J. W. (2014). How do patients respond to violation of their information privacy? *Health Information Management Journal*, *43*(2), 23–33. https://doi.org/10.1177/183335831404300204

Larson, D. G., & Chastain, R. L. (1990). Self-concealment: Conceptualization, measurement, and health implications. *Journal of Social and Clinical Psychology*, *9*(4), 439–455. https://doi.org/10.1521/jscp.1990.9.4.439

Law, M., Mathai, A., Veinot, P., Webster, F., & Mylopoulos, M. (2015). Exploring lesbian, gay, bisexual, and queer (LGBQ) people's experiences with disclosure of sexual identity to primary care physicians: A qualitative study. *BMC Family Practice*, *16*(1), 175. https://doi.org/10.1186/s12875-015-0389-4

Lindlof, T., & Taylor, B. (2019). *Qualitative communication research methods* (4th ed.). SAGE.

Marchalik, D. (2016). *Yes, your doctor really needs to ask about your sexual orientation and gender identity. Slate*. http://www.slate.com/blogs/outward/2016/02/29/why_doctors_need_to_ask_Patients_about_sexuality_and_gender_identity.html

Martos, A. J., Wilson, P. A., Gordon, A. R., Lightfoot, M., & Meyer, I. H. (2018). "Like finding a unicorn": Healthcare preferences among lesbian, gay, and bisexual people in the United States. *Social Science & Medicine*, *208*(1), 126–133. https://doi.org/10.1016/j.socscimed.2018.05.020

Maslow, A. H. (1943). A theory of human motivation. *Psychological Review*, *50*(4), 370–396. https://doi.org/10.1037/h0054346

Mollon, L. (2012). The forgotten minorities: Health disparities of the lesbian, gay, bisexual, and transgendered communities. *Journal of Health Care for the Poor and Underserved*, *23*(1), 1–6. https://doi.org/10.1353/hpu.2012.0009

Moradi, B., DeBlaere, C., & Huang, Y.-P. (2010). Centralizing the experiences of LGB people of color in counseling psychology. *The Counseling Psychologist*, *38*(3), 322–330. https://doi.org/10.1177/0011000008330832

Moraga, C., & Anzaldúa, G. (2015). *This bridge called my back: Writings by radical women of color* (4th ed.). SUNY Press.

O'Keefe, B. J. (1988). The logic of message design: Individual differences in reasoning about communication. *Communication Monographs*, *55*(1), 80–103. https://doi.org/10.1080/03637758809376159

Patten, E. (2016). *The nation's Latinx population is defined by its youth*. Pew Research Center. https://www.pewresearch.org/hispanic/2016/04/20/the-nations-latino-population-is-defined-by-its-youth/

Petronio, S. (2002). *Boundaries of privacy: Dialectics of disclosure*. SUNY Press.

Petronio, S., Reeder, H. M., Hecht, M. L., & Mon't Ros-Mendoza, T. (1996). Disclosure of sexual abuse by children and adolescents. *Journal of Applied Communication Research*, *24*(3), 181–199. https://doi.org/10.1080/00909889609365450

Pew Research Center. (2016). *Statistical portrait of Hispanics in the United States*. https://www.pewhispanic.org/2016/04/19/statistical-portrait-of-hispanics-in-the-united-states-key-charts/#2013-hispanic-SP-int.

Polek, C. A., Hardie, T. L., & Crowley, E. M. (2008). Lesbians' disclosure of sexual orientation and satisfaction with care. *Journal of Transcultural Nursing*, *19*(3), 243–249. https://doi.org/10.1177/1043659608317446

Schmitz, R. M., Sanchez, J., & Lopez, B. (2019). LGB+ Latinx young adults' health autonomy in resisting cultural stigma. *Culture, Health & Sexuality*, *21*(1), 16–30. https://doi.org/10.1080/13691058.2018.1441443

Schrimshaw, E., Downing, M., & Cohn, D. (2016). Reasons for non-disclosure of sexual orientation among behaviorally bisexual men: Non-disclosure as stigma management. *Archives of Sexual Behavior*, *47*(1), 219–233. https://doi.org/10.1007/s10508-016-0762-y

Scott, A. M., Caughlin, J. P., Donovan-Kicken, E., & Mikucki-Enyart, S. L. (2013). Do message features influence responses to depression disclosure? A message design logics perspective. *Western Journal of Communication*, *77*(2), 139–163. https://doi.org/10.1080/10570314.2012.694007

Tabler, J., Mykyta, L., Schmitz, R., Kamimura, A., Martínez, D., Martínez, R., Flores, P., Gonzalez, K., Marquez, A., Marroquin, G., & Torres, A. (2018). Social determinants of sexual behavior and awareness of sexually transmitted infections (STI) among low-income HIV+ or STI at-risk Hispanic residents receiving care at the U.S.–Mexico border. *Journal of Community Health*, *44*(1), 127–136. https://doi.org/10.1007/s10900-018-0562-5

The Combahee River Collective. (2015). A Black feminist statement. In C. Moraga & G. Anzaldúa (Eds.), *This bridge called my back: Writings by radical women of color* (4th ed.; pp. 210–218). SUNY Press.

Tracy, S. J. (2010). Qualitative quality: Eight 'big-tent' criteria for excellent qualitative research. *Qualitative Inquiry*, *16*(10), 837–851. https://doi.org/10.1177/1077800410383121

Utamsingh, P. D., Richman, L. S., Martín, J. L., Lattanner, M. R., & Chaikind, J. R. (2016). Heteronormativity and practitioner-patient interaction. *Health Communication*, *31*(5), 566–574. https://doi.org/10.1080/10410236.2014.979975

Vedantam, S. Host. 2019. June 3. People like us: How our identities shape health and educational success [Audio podcast episode]. In *Hidden Brain*. NPR. https://www.npr.org/2019/06/03/729275139/people-like-us-how-our-identities-shape-health-and-educational-success

Venetis, M. K., Meyerson, B. E., Friley, L. B., Gillespie, A., Ohmit, A., & Shields, C. G. (2017). Characterizing sexual orientation disclosure to HCPs: Lesbian, gay, and bisexual perspectives. *Health Communication*, *32*(5), 578–586. https://doi.org/10.1080/10410236.2016.1144147

Walby, S., Armstrong, J., & Strid, S. (2012). Intersectionality: Multiple inequalities in Social Theory. *Sociology*, *46*(2), 224–240. https://doi.org/10.1177/0038038511416164

Wang, J., & Yan, Y. (2012). The interview question. In J. Gubrium, J. Holstein, A. Marvasti, & K. McKinney (Eds.), *The SAGE handbook of interview research: The complexity of the craft* (2nd ed., pp. 231–242). SAGE. https://dx-doi-org.ezproxy.lib.utexas.edu/10.4135/9781452218403.n16

Whitehead, J., Shaver, J., Stephenson, R., & Newman, P. A. (2016). Outness, stigma, and primary health care utilization among rural LGBT populations. *PLOS ONE*, *11*(1), e0146139–e0146139. https://doi.org/10.1371/journal.pone.0146139 Article

Worthington, R. (2002). Clinical issues on consent: Some philosophical concerns. *Journal of Medical Ethics*, *28*(6), 377–380. https://doi.org/10.1136/jme.28.6.377

When Engagement Leads to Action: Understanding the Impact of Cancer (Mis) information among Latino/a Facebook Users

Yonaira M. Rivera, Meghan B. Moran, Johannes Thrul, Corinne Joshu, and Katherine C. Smith

ABSTRACT

Latinos/as – the largest minority group in the U.S. – are avid Facebook users, making this an opportune tool to educate on the uptake of cancer prevention and screening behaviors. However, there is a dearth in scholarship exploring how Latinos/as engage with and act upon health content encountered on social media, which may be influenced by cultural values. This qualitatively-driven, mixed-methods study explores how Latinos/as engage with and act upon cancer prevention and screening information (CPSI) on Facebook. During one-on-one, in-depth interviews, participants (n = 20) logged onto their Facebook account alongside the researcher and discussed cancer-related posts they engaged with during the past 12 months. Interview questions included the reasons for engagement, and whether engagement triggered further action. Interviews were analyzed thematically. In parallel, a content analysis of the CPSI posts identified during the interviews was conducted. The majority of CPSI posts participants engaged with contained food-related content and visual imagery. Engagement was most common when individuals had personal relationships to the poster, when posts included videos/images, and when posts contained content promoting the curative properties of popular Latin American foods. Engagement often led to information-seeking and sharing, discussing content with others, and/or changing health behaviors. Findings highlight the importance of adequately contextualizing how cultural values influence the ways in which Latinos/as engage with and act upon CPSI on Facebook, which may lead individuals to bypass evidence-based procedures. Multi-pronged efforts are necessary to adequately leverage social media to empower Latinos/as to partake in behaviors that effectively reduce cancer health disparities.

Introduction

Cancer communication efforts play a pivotal role in improving health outcomes among vulnerable communities with a high burden of cancer, as is the case with Hispanics/Latinos/as (henceforth Latinos/as) – the U.S.'s largest minority group (U.S. Census Bureau, 2020a). Latinos/as face multiple structural, social, and individual barriers to the adequate uptake of cancer prevention and screening (American Cancer Society, 2018). These disparities contribute to cancer being the leading cause of death among this population (Miller et al., 2018). Furthermore, despite having lower incidence and mortality rates for breast, prostate, and colorectal cancers compared to non-Hispanic Whites (Miller et al., 2018), Latinos/as are more likely to be diagnosed with advanced stages of disease (National Cancer Institute, 2012); this has been partially associated with lower screening rates for these preventable and screenable cancers (American Cancer Society, 2018). These disparities are further evident among certain sub-ethnic groups, as is the case with prostate cancer incidence in Puerto Rico compared to non-Hispanic whites (Miller et al., 2018). It is thus instrumental to identify ways to effectively educate Latinos/as on how cancer prevention and screening efforts can reduce these disparities (National Cancer Institute, 2018).

Given the considerable evidence that media can promote cancer prevention and increase cancer screenings among Latinos/as (Baezconde-Garbanati et al., 2014; Davis et al., 2015; Murphy et al., 2015), it is important to explore how to best deliver effective, evidence-based cancer prevention and screening information (henceforth referred to as CPSI) on newer communication tools, such as social media. Latinos/as are avid social media users: 8 out of 10 Latinos/as in the U.S. are on at least one social media platform, and 73% of these are on Facebook (Smith & Anderson, 2018). Facebook's popularity is not limited to younger Latino/a audiences: 47% of U.S. Latinos/as 50 and older have reported using Facebook within the past 30 days (The Nielsen Company, 2018), and 74% of U.S. Latinos/as age 50 to 64 with smartphones actively used Facebook's mobile app (The Nielsen Company, 2015). Facebook, thus, presents a way to empower Latinos/as to actively participate in cancer control and prevention by fostering dialogical engagement via posts, pictures, videos, and other information sharing (Chou et al., 2013). This is particularly important among Latinos/as age 40–75, as they are eligible for breast, prostate, and/or colorectal cancers screenings per U.S. guidelines.

Yet, despite its importance in cancer control and prevention, little research has been conducted exploring CPSI on social media, with no known studies focusing on how Latinos/as engage with and act upon such content. Studies exploring cancer information on social media mainly target breast cancer survivorship via content analyses of online blogs, forums, and Facebook groups (Koskan et al., 2014), cancer information sharing (Abramson et al., 2015; Gage-Bouchard et al., 2017; Justice-Gardiner et al., 2012), and user engagement among national and state-level cancer prevention campaigns (Kapahi Theiss et al., 2016; Strekalova & Damiani, 2018; Strekalova & Krieger, 2017). Although analyzing content generated by or for cancer organizations provides insight to certain factors that may enhance engagement with cancer information, it fails to understand how individuals engage with general cancer-related content on Facebook – such as user-generated or shared content that may not come from a reliable source. This has become increasingly problematic in light of the abundance of potentially detrimental health misinformation currently online (Schmidt et al., 2018; Teoh, 2019).

Engagement on social media

Engagement with information on social media has been defined as the interaction with and creation and sharing of information with individuals and organizations within a person's network (McCay-Peet & Quan-Haase, 2016). In the context of Facebook, this is traditionally thought of as liking or reacting to a post, commenting on a post, or sharing a post. Understanding how and why social media users engage with CPSI is important because engagement is a precursor to multiple outcomes, such as increased awareness, knowledge, and health behavior change (Neiger et al., 2013; Yang, 2017). Information delivered on Facebook is generally disseminated through posts, which contain both message and source factors that may contribute to engagement (Figure 1). On Facebook, message factors include *post content* and *post features*. Post content refers to specific information about prevention and/or screening (such as the risk factors and relevant screening tests for colorectal cancer), while post features can include a post's language and how CPSI is conveyed (e.g., text, video, images). Engagement with CPSI can also be triggered by factors related to the source of the information. *Post sources* can be conceptualized in two ways: the source of the content within a post (*source type*, such as a news agency, health organization, or a blog), and the person or entity who created or shared a post so it appears on a user's News Feed (*Facebook poster*, such as a Facebook friend, group, or page). While these sources can be the same entity (e.g., NCI's Facebook Page sharing a link to an article on their website), they may be distinct (e.g., a Facebook friend sharing cancer prevention information from a third-party). Understanding the message and source factors that influence engagement with CPSI among Latino/a Facebook users may assist in developing better ways to expose this audience to online messages that promote cancer prevention behaviors, as well as tailoring cancer education interventions using social media to improve cancer screening rates.

The social media engagement model (SMEM)

A useful conceptual model to begin exploring how Latinos/as engage with CPSI on social media is McCay-Peet and Quan-Haase's social media engagement model (McCay-Peet & Quan-Haase, 2016), which explores the context of the experiences that motivate users to engage with content created, shared, or endorsed by people and organizations in their social network. This model partially stems from Uses and Gratifications Theory, which posits that individuals purposively utilize media sources to fulfill a myriad of needs that are influenced by individual, interpersonal, and social interests (Katz & Blumler, 1974). The SMEM specifically posits that engagement is influenced by multiple individual and contextual factors that interplay with each other (McCay-Peet & Quan-Haase, 2016). Among the individual factors included in this model are the *presentation of self* to others on the platform, the *uses and*

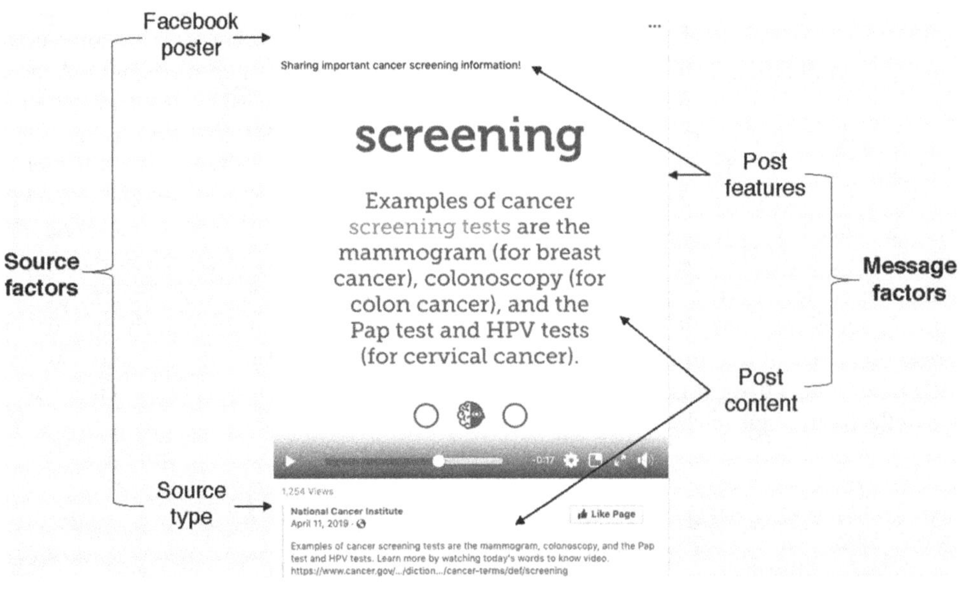

Figure 1. Factors within a Facebook post that may contribute to engagement.

gratifications for adopting a specific social media platform (e.g., using it for entertainment purposes), the *positive experiences* users have when interacting with others on the platform, and the ability to *act and participate* on the platform. Beyond these individual factors, the model suggests that the *social context* of an individual's social network within a social media platform also influences platform utilization and subsequent engagement, while a newer version of the model also acknowledges the role of *platform characteristics* in engagement (McCay-Peet & Quan-Haase, 2017). Examples of platform characteristics include features that enable users to communicate and share information with each other, while social context broadly refers to social, political, personal, and economic factors influencing platform usage.

The role of culture in CPSI engagement among U.S. Latinos/as

An important yet understudied contextual factor that may influence engagement with social media content is culture. Previous scholarship highlights that identity may act as an intermediary between a message and subsequent behavior (Comello, 2013; Flanagin et al., 2014). Taking this into account, we propose that elements of Latino/a cultural identity may influence how Latinos/as engage with CPSI on Facebook. These may include cultural heritage, language, and shared cultural values that are manifested through familial, religious, educational, and other social structures. While these elements are not intended to be prescriptive of all Latino/a identities in the U.S., Latin America's shared Spanish colonial history has influenced some common cultural values that may impact how and why Latinos/as from different sub-ethnic groups with different acculturation levels engage with and interpret CPSI.[1] This is an important first step in better understanding how Latinos/as from different backgrounds interact with health information disseminated in shared geographical and informational spaces (like social media) that expose them to content in multiple languages and from multiple sources.

Among the cultural values ascribed to many Latino/a communities are *machismo* (male gender identity roles fostering male superiority), *fatalismo* (beliefs that events are predetermined and cannot be prevented), *familismo* (strong familial ties), and *personalismo* (interpersonal relationships fostered by empathy, closeness, and warmth) (Abraído-Lanza et al., 2007; Flórez et al., 2009; Guilamo-Ramos et al., 2007; Marín & Triandis, 1985; Mindel, 1980; Torres, 1998; Yañez et al., 2016). These cultural values, which have been successfully incorporated into health communication efforts as a way to promote cancer prevention and screening uptake (Baezconde-Garbanati et al., 2014; Davis et al., 2015), may influence assessments of cancer information (Murphy et al., 2015) and whether Latinos/as participate in cancer control and prevention efforts (Erwin et al., 2010). Latinos/as may engage with CPSI containing specific types of message factors that resonate with Latino/a audiences. Beyond cultural values, language and cultural heritage are also strong cultural connectors for Latinos/as in the U.S., with 72% of Latinos/as speaking Spanish in their households and 73% believing their cultural heritage is an important part of their identity (The Nielsen Company, 2018). Therefore, CPSI shared on Facebook in Spanish or with content that speaks to Latino/a culture may also influence engagement, as these cultural connectors heavily influence digital content consumption – particularly among older generations who tend to be Spanish dominant (The Nielsen Company, 2018).

Cultural values may also influence how Latinos/as engage with content posted by different sources, particularly if it is shared by friends and family. Specifically, *familismo* and *personalismo* place a strong weight on interpersonal values tied to notions of trust, friendship, collectivism, and interdependence (Ayon & Aisenberg, 2010; Guilamo-Ramos et al., 2007). These values may therefore influence how Latinos/as engage with content shared by their friends or family, as recent research has found that trusting the sharer of an article on social media had higher effects on a person's trust and willingness to engage with it than did trusting the information source (Sterrett et al., 2018). This suggests that Latinos/as may place more trust in CPSI shared by Facebook friends than that shared by health organizations or outlets.

Taking into account the social context within which Latinos/as may engage with and interpret CPSI as influenced by relevant message and source factors, we ask:

RQ1. What message factors influence CPSI engagement among U.S. Latinos/as and why? This question specifically looked at message factors related to (1a) post content and (1b) post features.

RQ2. What source factors influence CPSI engagement among U.S. Latinos/as and why?

The role of engagement in subsequent action

Because engagement is an important precursor to behavior change, it is important to explore cases when engagement with CPSI can lead to improved outcomes (Neiger et al., 2013; Yang, 2017). Yet, to the best of our knowledge, models exploring engagement with content fail to address how engagement can lead to subsequent actions. The closest model that provides insights to how engagement may lead to subsequent action is Johnson's Comprehensive Model for Information Seeking (CMIS), which posits that cancer information seeking is triggered by communication channel utilities, characteristics, and individual antecedents – such as demographics, salience of cancer, beliefs about cancer, and personal experiences with cancer (Johnson, 1997; Johnson et al., 2001). CMIS has been used to understand how cancer survivors actively seek cancer information through various types of media (Johnson & Meischke, 1993). It has also been used to advance understanding of how individuals never diagnosed with cancer access cancer-related information (Johnson, 1997; Niederdeppe et al., 2007). However, CMIS only considers factors that may lead individuals to seek further information. While encountering CPSI on Facebook may contribute to further information seeking, it may also lead to other actions, such as talking about the cancer information with a friend or scheduling a cancer screening. Our final research question therefore asks:

RQ3. What actions does CPSI engagement among U.S. Latinos/as lead to, if any?

Materials and methods

Given the dearth of literature specifically exploring engagement with health information among Latino/a populations, this exploratory study sought to better understand general message and source features that may appeal to a heterogenous sample of Latinos/as. This study was conducted in the Tampa Bay area in Florida, which has a diverse Latino/a population that is higher than the national average (28% vs 17.8%) (U.S. Census Bureau, 2020b). Flyers, Facebook ads, and word-of-mouth were used to recruit participants through purposeful sampling methods (Patton, 2002) that stratified by language preference (English preferred, Spanish preferred, Bilingual). Twenty self-identified Latino/a Facebook users ages 40–75 without a history of cancer were interviewed during the summer of 2018 (average age = 54.2, sd = 7.4). Participants represented a myriad of Latin American sub-ethnic groups: 11 were from the Caribbean (7 Puerto Rican, 2 Dominican, 2 Cuban), 7 from Central/South America (2 Colombian, 2 Mexican, 3 Venezuelan), and 2 identified as being from the U.S. with Cuban and Spanish descent. Participants (n = 11) who were born outside of the U.S. or Puerto Rico had been living in the U.S. an average 23.4 years (sd = 17.4). Nine participants identified as fully bilingual, while five preferred English and six preferred Spanish; these preferences aligned with reported acculturation levels using Marin's 12-item Acculturation Scale (34.3, 46, and 23.2, respectively) (Marín et al., 1987). This study was approved by the Johns Hopkins Bloomberg School of Public Health Institutional Review Board (IRB8484).

Data collection

Participants began by completing a brief survey collecting demographic information, health and cancer information seeking behaviors, and Facebook utilization patterns, which was used to contextualize findings. Most participants self-identified as female (75%, n = 15), married (60%, n = 12), employed (80%, n = 16), and insured (85%, n = 17). There was a broad representation of household incomes and education levels. All participants reported having ever sought health information, while 55% (n = 11) reported seeking cancer information for themselves in the past year. Most participants (85%, n = 17) reporting checking their Facebook account at least once a day. The most common reasons to use Facebook were for social interactions (85%, n = 17), to share information (75%, n = 15), and to see what others were doing (60%, n = 12). Participants had an average 452.5 Facebook friends (range = 28–1,827) and followed 46.9 Facebook groups (range = 1–268). Only one participant followed cancer-related Facebook groups (23 total groups); this participant had a son who is a cancer survivor and described managing many "mommy cancer survivor" Facebook groups.

Participants then engaged in one-on-one, in-depth interviews (~2 hr) held in their preferred language (English and/or Spanish; led by YR). After first discussing general Facebook utilization, participants logged onto their Facebook account on a research laptop, typed "cancer" in the search bar, and scrolled-through 12 months of cancer-related posts that appeared on their News Feed (posts were sorted by "Most Recent" and posted by "Your Friends and Groups"). Engagement with a post (i.e. liking; commenting; sharing; recalling having clicked a link, read an article, and/or watched a video) prompted questions regarding the reasons for engagement, and whether engagement triggered further action. Any embedded videos/links were viewed to discuss the content and the process through which participants assessed the credibility of the post. This process was repeated with the search terms "cancer prevention" and "cancer screening"; when guided by the participant, additional search terms were used to find specific CPSI they recalled engaging with (e.g., "cancer guanábana" was used when a participant specifically recalled engaging with a post containing information about this Latin American fruit, commonly believed to have curative properties against cancer). A final search was performed using the term "cancer" and the filter "Posted By: You" to reveal any cancer information participants may have shared. A checklist was utilized during the interview to document engagement type and other features of each post discussed. Computer screen and audio were recorded during each interview. Participants received a $50 VISA gift card upon study completion.

Data analysis

Descriptive statistics were calculated for survey data using Stata version 14.2. Screen captures of posts discussed were saved and interviews were transcribed; both were de-identified prior to data analysis. MaxQDA PRO 2018.2 was utilized to manage and code captured posts and transcribed interviews.

Content analysis of CPSI posts

The cancer-related posts that participants engaged with on their Facebook accounts (n = 163) were extracted from the computer screen recordings taken during the interviews and their content was analyzed. Examples of posts are provided in Figure 2. A preliminary codebook was developed with codes from literature and additional codes and sub-codes that emerged from data collection using the interview checklist. The initial coding framework was applied to a sample of 10 publicly available cancer posts on Facebook by two bilingual members of the study team (YR and JM). Discrepancies were discussed and resolved, and a final codebook was developed. A list of main codes is provided in Table 1.

Using the codebook, YR and JM independently coded 20% of the sample, and intercoder reliability was calculated (Neuendorf, 2009). Final pooled Cohen's kappa coefficients ranged from 0.89–1.0. YR then proceeded to code remaining posts by first coding for *cancer content* and *CPSI sub-topic* (Table 1). This coding revealed that the majority of posts (n = 97) discussed cancer topics outside the scope of this study (e.g., survivorship, treatment, research). The remaining 66 posts specifically related to CPSI. The full set of codes was then applied to these 66 CPSI posts. Frequencies of each code were calculated upon completion of the analysis. Results of the content analysis are listed in Tables 2 and 3.

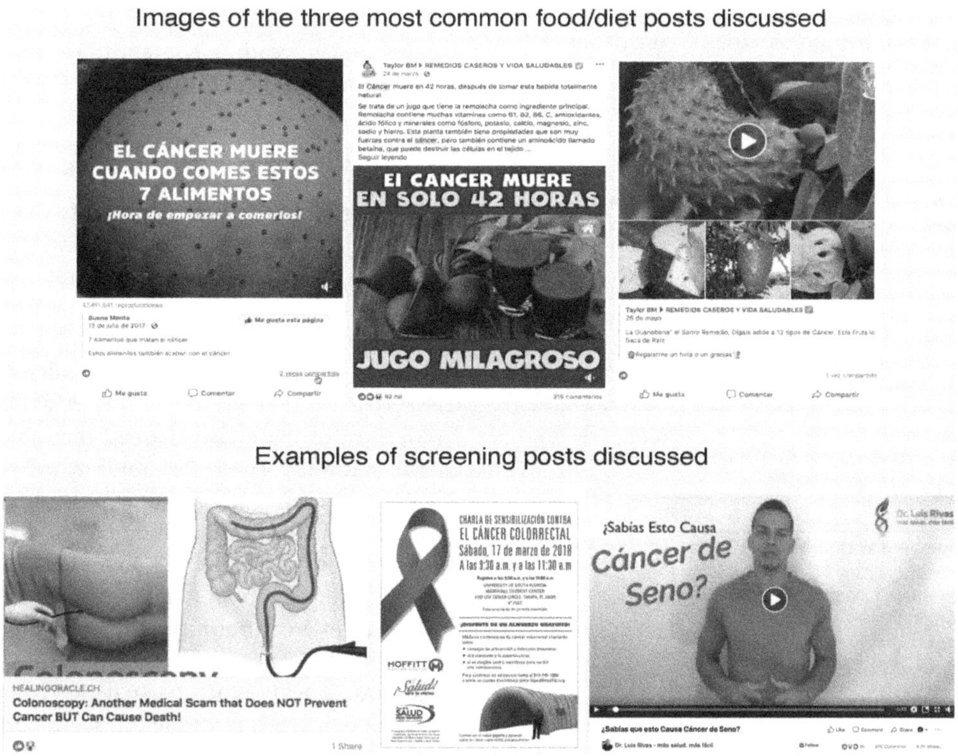

Figure 2. Examples of cancer prevention and screening posts that participants engaged with on Facebook.

Table 1. Summary of codes for content analysis of cancer prevention and screening information.

Topic	Codes[a]
Engagement	
	Like; Comment; Share; Read post; Watched video; Clicked on link; Read external content
Post content	
Post category	Health event; Informational[b]
Cancer content (general)	Prevention; Screening; Other cancer topic[b]
CPSI sub-topic	Food/Diet; Alcohol; Exercise; Obesity; Tobacco/E-cig; SPF; Vaccine; General prevention/healthy lifestyle; Natural remedy; Breast CS; Colon CS; Prostate CS; Other CS; General screening
Post features	
Post type	Text; Image; Video; Link to external content
Post language	Spanish; English
Sensationalism	Yes; No
Post sources	
Source type	News agency; Health or cancer organization; Community organization/nonprofit; Blog, personal or unofficial website; Special interest Facebook Group/Page; General user; Other
Facebook poster	Friend (shared or reposted); Public post liked by friend; Facebook Group/Page; User-generated (friend or self); Unclear/Unknown

[a]The only mutually exclusive codes were *source type, Facebook poster*, and *post category*; all other codes were not mutually exclusive; [b]Sub-codes listed in supplemental materials; CPSI = cancer prevention & screening information; CS = cancer screening.

Thematic analysis of interviews

A thematic analysis was conducted on all interview transcripts to capture why participants engaged with CPSI and subsequent actions. YR coded transcripts in their original language to ensure meanings were maintained. Transcripts were preliminarily coded

Table 2. Results of content analysis describing the message factors of cancer prevention and screening information participants (n = 16) engaged with on their Facebook accounts.

Message factors	Posts (n = 66)	%	Participants (n = 16)	%
Post content				
Cancer content*				
Prevention[a]	50	76%	15	94%
Screening	25	38%	9	56%
Cancer sub-topic*				
Prevention-related topics				
Food/Diet	35	53%	14	88%
Natural remedy	27	41%	12	75%
Other prevention	7	10%	4	25%
General prevention/healthy lifestyle	6	9%	5	31%
Screening-related topics				
Breast cancer screening	7	11%	7	44%
Colon cancer screening	9	14%	9	56%
Prostate cancer screening	5	8%	5	31%
Other cancer screening	9	14%	8	50%
Post category				
Informational	55	83%	16	100%
Health event	11	17%	6	38%
Post features				
Post type*				
Visual post (image and/or video)	60	91%	16	100%
Combination (e.g., text and image)	53	80%	16	100%
Post language*				
Spanish	39	59%	14	88%
English	28	41%	7	44%
Sensationalism (n = 51)[b]				
Contains sensationalist claim/ statement	33	65%	13	81%

*Codes in these categories were not mutually exclusive; [a]Includes 18 food/diet-related cancer posts discussed by participants as prevention; [b]Excludes health events and advocacy/fundraising information, as these do not include claims.

Table 3. Results of content analysis describing the source factors of cancer prevention and screening information participants (n = 16) engaged with on their Facebook accounts.

Source factors	Posts (n = 66)	%	Participants (n = 16)	%
Post source				
Facebook poster type				
Friend (shared or reposted)	36	55%	14	88%
Public post liked by friend	8	12%	4	25%
Friend (user-generated)	3	5%	3	19%
Group/Page	9	14%	7	44%
User-generated	3	5%	1	6%
Unknown	7	11%	4	25%
Source type				
Verifiable organization	26	40%	7	44%
Potentially unreliable source	40	60%	13	81%

Table 4. Emerging themes and sub-themes for the reasons Latinos engage with CPSI and subsequent actions, by research question.

Themes and sub-themes
RQ1. Reasons for engagement with message factors
1a. Post content
(1) General interest in prevention and/or healthy eating
(2) Salient chronic conditions
(3) Sociopolitical issues
(4) Personal experiences related to cancer
(5) Professional context
(6) Curiosity
1b. Post features
(1) Visual appeal
(2) Language
(3) Sensationalism
RQ2. Reasons for engagement with source factors
(1) Perceived topic expertise or authority
(2) Role of interpersonal relationships
(3) Alignment with identity
RQ3. Actions stemming from engagement
(1) Online actions
a. Information-seeking
b. Sharing content
(2) Offline actions
a. Discussing content
b. Behavior change/reinforcement
(3) Avoidance

using inductive and deductive codes; specifically, a round of open coding was performed, after which codes were grouped into broader categories that aligned with each aim. A final coding tree was developed to outline discovered themes and applied to all transcripts. Themes were identified and refined using a constant comparison method (Dye et al., 2000). Additionally, memos were composed with exemplary quotes for each theme and discussed with the research team to ensure dependability and credibility in theme development (Guba & Lincoln, 1989). A summary of the final themes and sub-themes that emerged for each aim is listed in Table 4.

Finally, data were triangulated to discuss what and why participants engaged with different types of CPSI. Triangulation allowed us to assess the kind of CPSI participants engaged with and connect that to their reasons for engaging with message and source factors, as well as how this engagement led to action.

Results

Overall, 16 of the 20 participants reported engaging with an average 4.1 posts containing CPSI in the previous 12 months; the remaining did not recall engaging with CPSI during this timeframe. Participants mainly engaged with CPSI content by viewing and/or reading content (73%, n = 48), rather than by liking, commenting, and/or sharing (27%, n = 18).

RQ1. Message factors contributing to CPSI engagement

There were multiple factors related to the content and features of a post that contributed to CPSI engagement. The following section first discusses post content, followed by post features.

1a. Post content

Results of the content analysis revealed that the majority of CPSI participants engaged with were about food/diet (n = 35, 53%); most of these also claimed these foods/diets could cure cancer naturally (n = 24) and/or provided recipes/dietary advice to prevent and/or cure cancer (n = 16). Participants engaged with screening content to a lesser degree (n = 25, 38%). Ten of these posts were advertising health events meant to educate about and/or provide free cancer screenings to the Latino/a community. The remaining posts were mainly about breast or colon cancer (n = 14). Table 2 describes the CPSI content with which participants engaged.

A thematic analysis of the interviews provides insights as to why participants engaged with CPSI, and why they predominantly engaged with food/diet-related content. In most scenarios, engagement with this content was not due to a direct interest in cancer prevention; rather, content appealed to other salient topics. Overall, six themes emerged discussing the reasons why participants engaged with post content. Emerging themes specific to engagement with food/diet posts included a general interest in prevention/healthy eating; other salient chronic conditions; and sociopolitical issues (Table 4). Additional reasons for engaging with any CPSI included personal experiences related to cancer; being in a professional context where cancer topics were salient; and curiosity. Reasons for engagement were not mutually exclusive, and most participants engaged with different content for multiple reasons.

General interest in prevention and/or healthy eating. Participants commonly engaged with food/diet-related content because they perceived eating healthy as preventive. As a Puerto Rican participant stated when discussing a video describing seven foods that "cure cancer": "It's true, all these are good for your health … [they] may not be specifically good for cancer – or do anything – but if you are healthy, it contributes to getting well faster" [Puerto Rican female, 60]. This statement further illustrates how messages claiming natural cures were generally associated with prevention, rather than treatment. Multiple participants clarified that they did not inherently believe in the curative claims within engaged posts. For example, when discussing whether she believed a post claiming that beet juice kills cancer in 42 hours, a female participant stated: "No, I don't believe in that [statement]. Does it help? It possibly helps, as prevention" [Colombian female, 45].

There was also consensus around the idea that "natural doesn't harm," suggesting that incorporating these foods into one's diet is not detrimental. When discussing the beet juice post, a Colombian male participant (age 56) said, "whether it works or not, it won't hurt me in any way." However, participants did at times believe the curative claims of the posts they engaged with. For some, having an affinity toward natural remedies stemmed from a respect toward Latin American Indigenous ancestors and their traditions. A native Colombian, one female participant stated: "As you can see, I have a lot of things [on my Facebook] about Indigenous peoples. [. . .] Indigenous peoples and our ancestors knew so much medicine, they really knew so much about what happens" [Colombian female, 45]. For others, religion played a strong role in why they embraced curative claims. In discussing his affinity toward natural remedies, a male participant stated:

> [W]hen God created the world, He made it perfect. And in the bible, it says that when He created the world, everything was good. So, everything [already] exists and must exist in what God created naturally, not in what man is inventing. [Cuban male, 61]

Nonetheless, these natural remedies were predominantly viewed as complementing, rather than replacing, Western medicine. For example, when discussing the curative properties of *guanábana*, a Colombian male (age 56) stated: "I see it as a complement, right? Obviously, it can't be a substitute to normal medicine, but it's definitely something that should be considered."

Salient chronic conditions. Some participants stated that their interest in food/diet-related content was related to having other chronic conditions. In these cases, the cancer claims were not regarded as essential to the message. For example, a Venezuelan female participant (age 67) recalled engaging with a post about papaya "as a preventive food, [rather] than for cancer, for your digestive tract." Later in the conversation, she also discussed a video of seven foods that "cure cancer," one of which was turmeric. She describes how she associated it with her frequent "joint" and "knee pain."

Sociopolitical issues. Sociopolitical issues also emerged as reasons for engaging with content claiming curative properties. An example of this pertained the current economic crisis in Venezuela, which has made it difficult for individuals to get access to medical care and cancer treatment. As such, a recent female Venezuelan (age 45) immigrant stated sharing information in hopes that it might benefit someone who cannot purchase medicine: "If it's a home remedy, it grabs my attention, because [right now] there's nothing in Venezuela. And that's why if there is something that can be planted and it works, then, that's useful [information]."

Personal experiences related to cancer. On occasion, engagement with food/diet-related content was due to previous experiences participants had with cancer survivors. There were multiple instances where participants' friends and/or family previously resorted to complementary and alternative medicine using traditional remedies from their countries of origin, making this content more salient. These individuals were more likely to consider both preventive and curative properties of the described foods. The most common example of this was *guanábana*, which is available in many Latin American countries. For example, although he didn't believe the curative claims in a beet juice post, the 56-year-old Colombian male explained that he sought alternative medicine for his mother when discussing engagement with a *guanábana* post. Some participants also engaged with screening information because of their personal experiences in dealing with cancer in their family. For example, a Venezuelan participant discussed engaging with a post about colonoscopies because this procedure helped diagnose her child with leukemia.

Professional context. Most participants engaging with content unrelated to food/diet did so because they were involved in professional or volunteer roles that made cancer a salient topic. As such, there were multiple instances where they engaged with posts sharing information about upcoming educational events and free screenings for members of the Latino/a community. For example, one participant frequently volunteered in cancer-related initiatives led by the local cancer center – particularly those related to breast cancer prevention and screening education. Therefore, she was aware of when this content appeared on her Facebook News Feed, sometimes sharing it with others. Such participants oftentimes engaged with posts that promoted health events via likes, comments, or shares as a way to show support.

Curiosity. Finally, there were times when participants were just curious about CPSI when they saw it as they leisurely scrolled through their News Feed. As one participant stated, "if there is a topic that's of interest to me, I look at it to see what it's about" [Colombian male, 56].

1b. Post features

Findings from the content analysis and interviews indicated that there were specific post features that consistently elicited more engagement. The three themes that emerged discussing the reasons why participants engaged with post features included visual appeal, language, and sensationalist titles/statements (Table 4). In most cases, these connected to cultural elements.

Visual appeal. The vast majority of posts (91%) included a visual component, such as embedded images and/or videos. Participants commented on the impact of videos and images in their engagement. One participant stated, "it's presentation more than anything else" and that "if it doesn't enter through your eyes, you don't get [the message]."

Visual elements appealed to culture and cultural values in different ways. Many participants commented on posts containing images or videos of foods common in Latin America, such as *guanábana*: "I do remember that [post] because it's a fruit that's very popular in Colombia. [. . .] It's supposed to be one of the best fruits to drink that prevents cancer. And it is a fruit from Colombia, from the Amazon" [Colombian male, 56]. Posts containing images of lemons/limes also garnered attention, although many stated not knowing the purported curative claims until having read/watched them on the platform. Rather, many saw these as dietary staples and commented on the ease of incorporating frozen lemon peel in their diet. Other visual elements of cultural connection included the presence of flags or someone from the same country. Videos were particularly attention-grabbing for some participants, especially if there were narrative elements that shared a testimony related to curative properties of foods.

Language. Another point of cultural connection was language. Although there was a similar language distribution among the posts discussed (58% were in Spanish), over half of the posts in English came from the same participant (a previous cancer educator who speaks both languages but prefers English). Instead, most participants (n = 9 or 56%) only engaged with CPSI in Spanish, while 5 (31%) engaged with CPSI in either language. Although participants did not explicitly discuss the role of language in engagement, one Puerto Rican participant (age 43) commented that "it's in Spanish, but I don't know if it's from Puerto Rico or Mexico or *whatever*," highlighting the transnational nature of content.

Sensationalism. Many posts participants engaged with contained sensationalistic titles or claims; the majority of these related to food/diet (n = 30) (e.g., "Cancer Dies in Only 42 Hours – Miracle Juice"). These titles seemed to be the main reason some individuals initially gravitated toward food/diet content. Yet, even then, some were apprehensive of the curative claims. For example, when discussing *guanábana* as a cancer cure, a participant said, "Well, if it cured [cancer], then EVERYONE would eat it! It would be in great demand! But whenever I go [to the supermarket], it's just a tiny corner with five or six fruit" [Mexican female, 52]. Others expressed concern about the impact these sensationalist claims may have on others who encounter them, but rarely did anything to correct them. This was generally due to the idea that it is not causing any harm for people to incorporate foods into their diet, so correcting the post was either futile or not in their best interest ("I don't feel that's my battle to fight for" [Puerto Rican female, 42]).

Some food/diet-related content with sensationalist titles also contained conspiratorial messages. These mainly supported the idea that the pharmaceutical industry does not want the general public to know that natural remedies can cure cancer for a fraction of the cost. Meanwhile, the only two screening-related posts that contained sensationalist titles were also conspiratorial. These posts claimed that current cancer screening methods could either cause cancer or death (e.g., "This Causes BREAST CANCER ... It's hard to believe and it will SURPRISE YOU"). These posts appealed to fear more so than did prevention-related posts, with one participant expressing a newfound concern that mammograms may cause breast cancer:

> I have had mammograms all my life, until I [watched] one of those things. And I start to make sense of it – and it makes sense! This guy from Puerto Rico – I don't know his name – he made a video and everything he says [...] He said so many things ... and I said, 'Oh my God ... !' [Puerto Rican female, 60]

RQ2. Source factors contributing to CPSI engagement

Post sources also contributed to engagement with CPSI (Table 3). Most participants engaged with CPSI that was shared or reposted by a Facebook friend (n = 36). Participants predominantly engaged with posts from unofficial sources discussing health topics (n = 40), almost all of which were related to food/diet (n = 32).

Participant interviews revealed three themes discussing the reasons a post's source contributed to engagement; these included perceived topic expertise or authority, the role of interpersonal relationships, and alignment with cultural identity (Table 4). Reasons were not mutually exclusive.

Perceived topic expertise or authority

Perceptions of expertise or authority about the topic within a post were an important reason for engaging with content. These perceptions could be related to the Facebook poster and/or source type. For example, one participant stated that she engaged with a post about colorectal cancer screening guidelines because it was from the American Cancer Society and was shared by a friend who works at the local health department. Perceived expertise was also important despite some sources not being formally trained in cancer prevention, as was the case for a participant who readily engaged with content related to eating healthy. Most of the content discussed during her interview came from the same person – a friend she described as being "like [her], she believes in a lot of natural stuff" [Puerto Rican female, 62]. Although her friend was not an expert, she deemed her very knowledgeable and would always engage with whatever content she posted.

At times, the source was the most important reason to engage with content, as was seen with content shared by a well-known Venezuelan community activist. This person was discussed in multiple interviews as being a trusted leader who is always present at community events and constantly shares important and relevant health information with community members. As one participant stated, "people [in the community] listen to him because he is in everything. [...] The truth is that he is very efficient, very collaborative and very proactive in all these things" [Venezuelan female, 67]. As such, several participants stated that they always pay attention to content he disseminates on his Facebook profile, local Facebook groups, and alternate social media platforms (specifically, WhatsApp).

Role of interpersonal relationships

There were several occasions where participants' relationships with those sharing a post contributed to engagement. These relationships were based on trust and appeared to either complement or supersede the relevance of the content within the post. For example, several participants highlighted that the interpersonal relationships of the aforementioned Venezuelan community activist further contributed to why participants deemed him a trusted and reliable person ("He calls everyone, and he goes to where the people are, and everyone receives him!"). Another example of source superseding content occurred with a Mexican participant who noticed that a family friend posted content describing five foods that can help prevent breast cancer. She described immediately paying attention to the content because the person who posted it has a family history of breast cancer.

Alignment with identity

Finally, engagement with CPSI was at times related to the how the source aligned with aspects of participants' identity (such as religion or country of origin). For example, one participant commented that she engaged with a breast cancer awareness video because it was shared by a religious group she follows. For others, engagement was triggered because the content was shared in a Facebook Group for people from specific countries in Latin America (e.g., Venezuelans in Tampa). Parasocial relationships with Latin American sources also contributed to CPSI engagement; these included celebrities or other influential persons. One video in particular appealed to two participants, both of whom expressed an affinity to the narrator also being Puerto Rican ("you kind of identify [with him]" [Puerto Rican female, 56]).

RQ3. Actions stemming from engagement

Engagement with CPSI oftentimes led to varying levels of online and offline actions (Table 4). Online actions included information-seeking or sharing content; offline actions included discussing content or behavior change/reinforcement. Finally, one participant discussed actively avoiding content after engaging with it.

Online actions prompted by CPSI engagement

Information-seeking. Engaging with content most often triggered participants to search for additional cancer information about the topic on the internet. Information-seeking mainly occurred outside of Facebook, on platforms such as Google or WebMD. As one participant stated, "I think Facebook is like a 'mouth-opener,' isn't it? It's obviously not going to give you everything you need, but it does wake up like a curiosity to keep investigating and keep informing yourself" [Venezuelan female, 45].

Sharing content. Participants were frequently prompted to share CPSI with others in their online networks. However, although some shared content by posting it on a Facebook profile, most did so via messaging apps (i.e. Facebook Messenger and/or WhatsApp). One participant highlights how this takes place:

> So, during the day I go on [to Facebook], I look and if there is anything there, I take it and share it on my page, and as I also receive things from other pages, from other applications, I copy and send [via] WhatsApp and [Facebook] Messenger – those two. [Puerto Rican female, 60]

Others shared information they engaged with because they saw it as a personal responsibility. A Venezuelan (age 49) participant spoke of her role in disseminating as much information as possible about cancer on Facebook, as this was an important source of information for her when her son was diagnosed with cancer. She described managing and sharing information on multiple Facebook groups tailored to mothers whose children have cancer. One of her shared posts linked to an article claiming that colonoscopies are deadlier than colorectal cancer (available at www.healingoracle.ch). She noted that while she did not agree with the content, it was her responsibility to share information *regardless* of her opinion about the content. In this scenario, she shared the information while stating that a colonoscopy "saved [her] son" at the top of the post. She further explains:

> There are always two sides to a coin. [. . .] Yes, there are risks, I will not deny it. But, in my son's case, that is what saved his life. So, how can I tell you that it is not effective? Every procedure has a risk. I am giving you my point of view. That is, 'ok, maybe this [article] is valid but, in my son's case, it's the opposite.' So, it's up to each person to discern, you know?

Offline actions prompted by CPSI engagement

Discussing content. Engaging with CPSI at times triggered participants to discuss the content with others – mainly friends and family. For example, a male participant explained that he regularly discusses food/diet-related content with his wife at home. He described that she normally shares content with him, which he then reads and decides which remedies they will incorporate into their diet. Meanwhile, another participant stated discussing a video claiming mammograms cause cancer with her daughter: "We were saying, 'how is it that something that prevents cancer will cause us cancer?' But I won't lie – [the video] left me with a lot of doubt . . . " [Puerto Rican female, 56]. These conversations appeared to clarify lingering doubt or were used to help make decisions about the content, further discussed below.

Behavior change/reinforcement. Some participants discussed making decisions informed by the CPSI with which they engaged. Many times, these included implementing new (or reinforcing current) dietary behaviors espoused by the post. This was common with food/diet-related posts containing recipes or dietary advice. For example, one participant described incorporating a cancer tonic into her diet:

> Supposedly if you drink this juice every day, it cures cancer . . . hehe. Well, do you know I was doing it every day, every week. I wrote it down on my notes, and every time I go to the natural food store, I say 'Hey, put this stuff in it.' Broccoli, ginger, apples, carrots, cauliflower, kale. I'll go and I juice it. I know that it's not 100% cure. I believe in prevention. I don't have cancer now, but if you start taking things that prevent it, I don't know . . . haha! [Puerto Rican female, 62]

As exemplified above, most dietary decisions were not evidence-based, but instead relate back to the concept of general prevention and "natural doesn't harm." However, other behaviors participants described were potentially harmful. The most extreme example of this was one of the participants who engaged with the video purporting mammograms cause cancer. After watching the video – which was shared by a source she deemed trustworthy – she decided to cancel her mammogram for the first time ever:

> So, [the guy in the video] is [either] a naturopath or a doctor, and he said so many things . . . [. . .] Well, I didn't get the mammogram. It was in February – and I've [had mammograms] all my life in February, which is my birthday – and this year I didn't do it. Well, I had the date and everything, and I called and canceled. I saw the video one day, and

> the appointment was the following week, and I called and canceled the appointment, hahaha! [Puerto Rican female, 60]

Avoidance after engagement. One participant discussed intentionally avoiding content after seeing it emerge on his News Feed. This Cuban male (age 61) spoke of purposefully avoiding topics and health events related to prostate and colorectal cancer screening:

> First you say: *solavaya* [a Cuban phrase to "chase away" death]. Prostate cancer, colon cancer. The best thing is not to know about it. Perhaps it's a Latin American custom to avoid looking. It's like when you were a kid and a dead man passed by and you said: "*Solavaya, solavaya*, never go by my house!" It's like not wanting to talk about it so it doesn't happen to me. As if just by talking about the topic, I put it in my cupboard. And it's a very bad Latin American custom. Very bad.

Discussion

In setting out to understand how and why Latinos/as engage with CPSI on social media, we discovered that cultural values and other cultural connectors (e.g., language and country of origin) play a salient role in how message factors and source factors influence engagement with CPSI among Latinos/as. Cultural values also appear to have an impact on how Latinos/as choose to act upon CPSI. These findings highlight the importance of adequately contextualizing how cultural values and other elements of cultural connection influence the ways in which Latinos/as engage with, interpret, and act upon CPSI on Facebook.

Consistent with literature highlighting the importance of tailoring content to Latino/a populations (Baezconde-Garbanati et al., 2014; Davis et al., 2015; Erwin et al., 2010), participants oftentimes engaged with visually appealing posts that contained features that provided connections to cultural identity. However, rarely did these posts come from verifiable health organizations (unless they were advertising a local health event). Rather, most participants engaged with CPSI from potentially unreliable sources that contained sensationalist titles and claimed cancer cures linked to foods popular in Latin American countries; these posts were mainly shared by Facebook friends. Most importantly, the interview portion of the study allowed participants to discuss the relevance of the offline relationships they shared with these individuals, which many times contributed to why they engaged with (and trusted) the content. While the importance of trusting the source of information is not unique to Latinos/as, *personalismo* and *familismo* are strong cultural values that tie notions of trust to core interpersonal and familial relationships (Ayon & Aisenberg, 2010; Guilamo-Ramos et al., 2007). The presence of these values appeared to reinforce messages being shared and consumed on social media, regardless of their accuracy.

Adding another layer of complexity is that there were multiple, co-existing reasons for Latinos/as to engage with CPSI shared by source factors. This was the case with multiple participants who discussed information shared by a Venezuelan community leader who they deemed a knowledgeable source of cancer information, was well-regarded in the Latino/a community, and shared their Latino/a identity. These findings highlight the significance of source factors, which appear to enhance engagement with – or be more important than – culturally-relevant content, an important consideration for public health efforts geared toward curtailing the spread of health misinformation on social media (Chou et al., 2018).

An interesting finding emerged when exploring the role of message factors in engagement: although most participants engaged with information related to cancer prevention, it was not due to a direct interest in cancer prevention. Rather, other salient topics – such as a general interest in healthy eating and maintaining a healthy lifestyle – commonly influenced engagement. It is noteworthy that a small subset of participants briefly discussed the role of God in providing remedies through such foods naturally. However, future research is needed to further explore the role of religiosity in engagement with such cancer prevention content. Nonetheless, the salience of other topics when compared to cancer may help explain why participants rarely engaged with prevention content beyond food/diet. It may also point to evidence-based cancer prevention content not reaching this audience, as the vast majority of this content promoted natural remedies with little to no empirical evidence.

Meanwhile, most participants who engaged with evidence-based CPSI did so because they had a role in cancer prevention/screening as an advocate, community leader, volunteer, or healthcare professional, making cancer topics generally more salient to them. Taking into consideration the role of source factors in why many participants engaged with CPSI, cancer communication interventions may benefit from leveraging trusted sources in Latino/a communities to adequately deliver cancer information on Facebook – an idea that supports using the well-established two-step flow of communication model in campaign and programmatic development (Katz, 1957).

This research highlights the need for more robust models that conceptualize social media engagement, particularly as it relates to issues relevant to Latino/a communities. Given the dearth of such models, we apply our findings to the SMEM in an effort to highlight areas for improvement. While the SMEM acknowledges that an individual's social context is an instrumental factor in social media engagement (McCay-Peet & Quan-Haase, 2016), its emphasis lies in outlining individual-level factors that contribute to engagement. This presents two important limitations. First, underlying the model's focus on individual-level factors that impact usage and activity counts is the operationalization of engagement through visible traces left on the platform (i.e. likes, comments, and shares). This excludes important factors that may not be seen by others on social media, yet still contribute to engagement. For example, 73% of the engagement reported in our study occurred by viewing or reading content, rather than liking, commenting, or sharing; this "passive" form of engagement still contributed to important actions, as was seen with the female participant who reported canceling her mammogram after watching a culturally-relevant video. In essence, source and message factors were instrumental in why Latinos/as engaged with CPSI that emerged on their Facebook accounts. Such external factors should be explicitly included in this and other social media engagement models. Similarly, a second limitation of the SMEM is that the model provides very little guidance as to what "social context" means and how it impacts engagement. Such a broad conceptualization risks important social factors being lost when exploring engagement, especially in communities where specific cultural values and other cultural connections explicitly influenced engagement and subsequent action. While we acknowledge social contexts are fluid, the SMEM would benefit from a more structured way to guide empirical research and model testing.

A particular strength of the current study is that it explores the implications of consuming cancer information on social media. Beyond providing further evidence that social media engagement is an important precursor to other outcomes (Neiger et al., 2013; Yang, 2017), results show that CPSI was acted upon in multiple ways. First, our findings support the notion of cancer information seeking as triggered by individual antecedents and the features of a communication channel (Johnson, 1997). They also suggest engagement can lead to offline behaviors, some of which were influenced by cultural values. Several participants reported discussing CPSI with other family members offline, highlighting the importance of *familismo* in offline interpersonal dynamics that stem from online interactions; this type of interpersonal communication may be an important mediator between online engagement and offline health behaviors. There was also evidence consistent with previous literature that shows *machismo* and *fatalismo* can act as barriers to cancer control and prevention efforts (Goldman et al., 2009; Hubbell et al., 1996; Powe & Finnie, 2003; Rivera-Ramos & Buki, 2011). This was best exemplified by the Cuban male participant who both spoke of his role in deciding what natural remedies he and his wife would incorporate into their diet (*machismo*), as well as intentionally avoiding content related to prostate and colorectal cancer out of fear that simply viewing it could bring him disease (*fatalismo*). Finally, not all actions were evidence-based, as demonstrated by the participant who canceled her mammogram after watching a video on Facebook. Combined, these findings provide important insight to the ways social media can both promote or hinder health outcomes, which merit further empirical and theoretical exploration.

Several limitations to the current study must be acknowledged. First, as an exploratory study, this study focused on individuals who have never had a cancer diagnosis. As such, their reasons for engaging with and acting upon CPSI may be different from cancer survivors. The ramifications of engaging with culturally-relevant cancer content that is not evidence-based may arguably have more immediate consequences among cancer survivors. Similarly, participants were predominantly female, which may have excluded important user-related experiences predominant among Latino men from our analysis. Although the themes that emerged were discussed among participants of both genders, future research should be expanded to include these voices. Another important limitation relates to potential recall bias. Our measure for exposure relied on recognition, rather than recall. Recognition measures ask participants to indicate whether they have seen a post before by first showing it to them (Niederdeppe, 2005), while recall measures rely on verbal cues only. Compared to recall, recognition tends to produce higher exposure estimates (Du Plessis, 1994), which may overestimate true engagement. However, recognition is preferred when measuring exposure after a long period of time has passed (Singh et al., 1988; Stapel, 1998). Future studies using this method on Facebook may limit these biases by incorporating the "Posts seen by you" feature, which was unavailable at the time of this study. Finally, only posts that contained search terms within the text were elicited during interviews. This inevitably excluded any posts that did not contain any text, such as image-only posts.

Despite these limitations, this work is – to the best of our knowledge – the first to explore how cultural values influence the ways in which Latinos/as engage with and act upon content they encounter on social media. Furthermore, findings highlight the complex and interrelated ways in which cultural values, source factors and message factors contribute to engagement with health content on social media. While the cultural values we discuss in this manuscript are not prescriptive of the multifaceted nature of Latino/a identities in the U.S., these are important contributions for current debates on how to best curtail the effects of health misinformation on social media platforms, as it may be harder to correct misinformation shared by a close friend with consonant cultural values. Cancer education interventions and communication campaigns must therefore consider delivering culturally-tailored content through trusted sources within the Latino/a community. Doing so may ultimately enable researchers to adequately leverage social media to encourage praxis and empower Latinos/as to partake in behaviors that reduce cancer health disparities.

Note

1. We would like to highlight that U.S. Latino/a identities are not monolithic, but complex and thus not easily encapsulated in this manuscript. Our work is not intended to be prescriptive of such identities, but a first step in exploring how Latinos/as may engage with and act upon information that is shared on platforms where different identities maybe be sharing content in the same spaces. This work is intended to be generative (not definitive) and to be used as a starting point to explore important within-group differences.

Acknowledgments

The authors would like to acknowledge Dr. Javier de la Maza assisting with content analysis coding; Dr. Asa Oxner for providing interview space; and the transcription services of Dr. Carlos Rodríguez Díaz's "Sex+ TEAM" at the Center for Evaluation and Sociomedical Research at the University of Puerto Rico's School of Public Health – Medical Sciences Campus (Ilia Otero Cruz, Ana Ruiz, Gabriel Pastrana, Jafet Sánchez, and Neishka Rodríguez). The main author also thanks Dr. João Carlos Magalhães for his instrumental feedback on earlier versions of this manuscript.

Funding

This project was supported by Johns Hopkins Bloomberg School of Public Health's Center for Qualitative Studies in Health and Medicine Dissertation Enhancement Award and by the National Cancer Institute Center to Reduce Cancer Health Disparities, [Award No. P30CA177558-05S3]. The first author was previously supported by the National Cancer Institute of the National Institutes of Health, Award No. [T32CA009314-36 (2015-2018) and F31CA224615 (2018-2020)]. The content is solely the responsibility of the author(s) and does not necessarily represent the official views of the National Cancer Institute.

ORCID

Yonaira M. Rivera http://orcid.org/0000-0002-5041-5250
Meghan B. Moran http://orcid.org/0000-0001-6745-6668
Johannes Thrul http://orcid.org/0000-0001-8929-9579
Corinne Joshu http://orcid.org/0000-0002-5100-172X
Katherine C. Smith http://orcid.org/0000-0003-2140-1690

References

Abraído-Lanza, A. F., Viladrich, A., Flórez, K. R., Céspedes, A., Aguirre, A. N., & De La Cruz, A. A. (2007). Commentary: Fatalismo reconsidered: A cautionary note for health-related research and practice with Latino populations. *Ethnicity & Disease*, *17*(1), 153–158. https://www.ethndis.org/priorarchives/ethn-17-01-153.pdf

Abramson, K., Keefe, B., & Chou, W. Y. S. (2015). Communicating about cancer through Facebook: A qualitative analysis of a breast cancer awareness page. *Journal of Health Communication*, *20*(2), 237–243. https://doi.org/10.1080/10810730.2014.927034

American Cancer Society. (2018). *Cancer facts & figures for Hispanics/Latinos 2018–2020*. https://www.cancer.org/content/dam/cancer-org/research/cancer-facts-and-statistics/cancer-facts-and-figures-for-hispanics-and-latinos/cancer-facts-and-figures-for-hispanics-and-latinos-2018-2020.pdf

Ayon, C., & Aisenberg, E. (2010). Negotiating cultural values and expectations within the public child welfare system: A look at familismo and personalismo. *Child & Family Social Work*, *15*(3), 335–344. https://doi.org/10.1111/j.1365-2206.2010.00682.x

Baezconde-Garbanati, L. A., Chatterjee, J. S., Frank, L. B., Murphy, S. T., Moran, M. B., Werth, L. N., Zhao, N., Amezola de Herrera, P., Mayer, D., Kagan, J., & O'Brien, D. (2014). Tamale lesson: A case study of a narrative health communication intervention. *Journal of Communication in Healthcare*, *7*(2), 82–92. https://doi.org/10.1179/1753807614Y.0000000055

Chou, W. Y. S., Oh, A., & Klein, W. M. (2018). Addressing health-related misinformation on social media. *JAMA*, *320*(23), 2417–2418. https://doi.org/10.1001/jama.2018.16865

Chou, W. Y. S., Prestin, A., Lyons, C., & Wen, K. Y. (2013). Web 2.0 for health promotion: Reviewing the current evidence. *American Journal of Public Health*, *103*(1), e9–e18. https://doi.org/10.2105/AJPH.2012.301071

Comello, M. L. N. G. (2013). Conceptualizing the intervening roles of identity in communication effects: The prism model. In D. L. Larosa & A. Rodríguez (Eds.), *Identity and communication: New agendas in communication* (pp. 186–206). Routledge. https://doi.org/10.4324/9780203557105

Davis, J. L., Ramos, R., Rivera-Colón, V., Escobar, M., Palencia, J., Grant, C. G., & Green, B. L. (2015). The Yo me cuido® program: Addressing breast cancer screening and prevention among Hispanic women. *Journal of Cancer Education*, *30*(3), 439–446. https://doi.org/10.1007/s13187-014-0710-2

Du Plessis, E. (1994). Recognition versus recall. *Journal of Advertising Research*, *34*(3), 75–92. https://psycnet.apa.org/record/1994-47302-001

Dye, J. F., Schatz, I. M., Rosenberg, B. A., & Coleman, S. T. (2000). Constant comparison method: A kaleidoscope of data. *The Qualitative Report*, *4*(1), 1–10. https://doi.org/10.46743/2160-3715/2000.2090

Erwin, D. O., Treviño, M., Saad-Harfouche, F. G., Rodriguez, E. M., Gage, E., & Jandorf, L. (2010). Contextualizing diversity and culture within cancer control interventions for Latinas: Changing interventions, not cultures. *Social Science & Medicine*, *71*(4), 693–701. https://doi.org/10.1016/j.socscimed.2010.05.005

Flanagin, A. J., Hocevar, K. P., & Samahito, S. N. (2014). Connecting with the user-generated Web: How group identification impacts online information sharing and evaluation. *Information, Communication & Society*, *17*(6), 683–694. https://doi.org/10.1080/1369118X.2013.808361

Flórez, K. R., Aguirre, A. N., Viladrich, A., Céspedes, A., De La Cruz, A. A., & Abraído-Lanza, A. F. (2009). Fatalism or destiny? A qualitative study and interpretative framework on Dominican women's breast cancer beliefs. *Journal of Immigrant and Minority Health*, *11*(4), 291–301. https://doi.org/10.1007/s10903-008-9118-6

Gage-Bouchard, E. A., LaValley, S., Mollica, M., & Beaupin, L. K. (2017). Cancer communication on social media: Examining how cancer caregivers use Facebook for cancer-related communication. *Cancer Nursing*, *40*(4), 332–338. https://doi.org/10.1097/ncc.0000000000000418

Goldman, R. E., Díaz, J. A., & Kim, I. (2009). Perspectives of colorectal cancer risk and screening among Dominicans and Puerto Ricans: Stigma and misperceptions. *Qualitative Health Research*, *19*(11), 1559–1568. https://doi.org/10.1177/1049732309349359

Guba, E., & Lincoln, Y. S. (1989). *Fourth generation evaluation*. Sage Publications, Inc.

Guilamo-Ramos, V., Dittus, P., Jaccard, J., Johansson, M., Bouris, A., & Acosta, N. (2007). Parenting practices among Dominican and Puerto Rican mothers. *Social Work*, *52*(1), 17–30. https://doi.org/10.1093/sw/52.1.17

Hubbell, F. A., Chavez, L. R., Mishra, S. I., & Valdez, R. B. (1996). Beliefs about sexual behavior and other predictors of Papanicolaou smear screening among Latinas and Anglo women. *Archives of Internal Medicine*, *156*(20), 2353–2358. https://doi.org/10.1001/archinte.1996.00440190107011

Johnson, J. D. (1997). *Cancer-related information seeking*. Hampton Press.

Johnson, J. D., Andrews, J. E., & Allard, S. (2001). A model for understanding and affecting cancer genetics information seeking. *Library & Information Science Research*, *23*(4), 335–349. https://doi.org/10.1016/S0740-8188(01)00094-9

Johnson, J. D., & Meischke, H. (1993). A comprehensive model of cancer-related information seeking applied to magazines. *Human Communication Research*, *19*(3), 343–367. https://doi.org/10.1111/j.1468-2958.1993.tb00305.x

Justice-Gardiner, H., Nutt, S., Rechis, R., McMillan, B., & Warf, R. (2012). Using new media to reach Hispanic/Latino cancer survivors. *Journal of Cancer Education*, *27*(1), 100–104. https://doi.org/10.1007/s13187-011-0267-2

Kapahi Theiss, S., Burke, R. M., Cory, J. L., & Fairley, T. L. (2016). Getting beyond impressions: An evaluation of engagement with breast cancer-related Facebook content. *mHealth*, *2*(41), 1–7. https://doi.org/10.21037/mhealth.2016.10.02

Katz, E. (1957). The two-step flow of communication: An up-to-date report on an hypothesis. *Public Opinion Quarterly*, *21*(1), 61–78. https://doi.org/10.1086/266687

Katz, E., & Blumler, J. G. (1974). *The uses of mass communications: Current perspectives on gratifications research*. SAGE Publications, Inc.

Koskan, A., Klasko, L., Davis, S. N., Gwede, C. K., Wells, K. J., Kumar, A., López, N., & Meade, C. D. (2014). Use and taxonomy of social media in cancer-related research: A systematic review. *American Journal of Public Health*, *104*(7), e20–e37. https://doi.org/10.2105%2FAJPH.2014.301980

Marín, G., Sabogal, F., Marín, B. V., Otero-Sabogal, R., & Pérez-Stable, E. J. (1987). Development of a short acculturation scale for Hispanics. Special Issue: Acculturation research. *Hispanic Journal of Behavioral Sciences*, *9*(2), 183–205. https://doi.org/10.1177%2F07399863870092005

Marín, G., & Triandis, H. C. (1985). Allocentrism as an important characteristic of the behavior of Latin Americans and Hispanics. In R. Díaz Guerrero (Ed.), *Cross-cultural and national studies of social psychology* (pp. 85–104). Elsevier Science Publishers.

McCay-Peet, L., & Quan-Haase, A. (2016). A model of social media engagement: User profiles, gratifications, and experiences. In H. O'Brien & P. Cairns (Eds.), *Why engagement matters* (pp. 199–217). Springer. https://doi.org/10.1007/978-3-319-27446-1_9

McCay-Peet, L., & Quan-Haase, A. (2017). What is social media and what questions can social media research help us answer? In L. Sloan & A. Quan-Haase (Eds.), *The SAGE handbook of social media research methods* (pp. 13–26). SAGE Publications, Inc. https://doi.org/10.4135/9781473983847.n2

Miller, K. D., Goding Sauer, A., Ortiz, A. P., Fedewa, S. A., Pinheiro, P. S., Tortolero-Luna, G., Martinez-Tyson, D., Jemal, A., & Siegel, R. L. (2018).

Cancer statistics for Hispanics/Latinos, 2018. *CA: A Cancer Journal for Clinicians*, *68*(6), 425–445. https://doi.org/10.3322/caac.21494

Mindel, C. H. (1980). Extended familism among urban Mexican Americans, Anglos, and Blacks. *Hispanic Journal of Behavioral Sciences*, *2*(1), 21–34. https://psycnet.apa.org/record/1981-12608-001

Murphy, S. T., Frank, L. B., Chatterjee, J. S., Moran, M. B., Zhao, N., Amezola de Herrera, P., & Baezconde-Garbanati, L. A. (2015). Comparing the relative efficacy of narrative vs nonnarrative health messages in reducing health disparities using a randomized trial. *American Journal of Public Health*, *105*(10), 2117–2123. https://doi.org/10.2105%2FAJPH.2014.302332

National Cancer Institute. (2012). *The national cancer program: Managing the Nation's research portfolio – An annual plan and budget proposal for fiscal year 2013.* NIH Publication No. 13-7957. http://www.cancer.gov/about-nci/budget/annual-plan/nci-plan-2013.pdf

National Cancer Institute. (2018, December 19). *Cancer health disparities research.* http://www.cancer.gov/research/areas/disparities#1

Neiger, B. L., Thackeray, R., Burton, S. H., Giraud-Carrier, C. G., & Fagen, M. C. (2013). Evaluating social media's capacity to develop engaged audiences in health promotion settings: Use of Twitter metrics as a case study. *Health Promotion Practice*, *14*(2), 157–162. https://doi.org/10.1177%2F1524839912469378

Neuendorf, K. A. (2009). Reliability for content analysis. In A. B. Jordan, D. Kunkel, J. Manganello, & M. Fishbein (Eds.), *Media messages and public health: A decisions approach to content analysis* (pp. 67–87). Routledge.

Niederdeppe, J. (2005). Assessing the validity of confirmed ad recall measures for public health communication campaign evaluation. *Journal of Health Communication*, *10*(7), 635–650. https://doi.org/10.1080/10810730500267662

Niederdeppe, J., Hornik, R. C., Kelly, B. J., Frosch, D. L., Romantan, A., Stevens, R. S., Barg, F. B., Weiner, J. L., & Schwartz, J. S. (2007). Examining the dimensions of cancer-related information seeking and scanning behavior. *Health Communication*, *22*(2), 153–167. https://doi.org/10.1080/10410230701454189

The Nielsen Company. (2015, October 13). *The new American vanguard – Latinos 50+: Healthy, wealthy and wise.* http://www.nielsen.com/us/en/insights/reports/2015/the-new-american-vanguard-latinos-50-are-healthy-wealthy-and-wise.html

The Nielsen Company. (2018, August 28). *Descubrimiento digital: The online lives of latinx consumers.* https://www.nielsen.com/us/en/insights/reports/2018/descubrimiento-digital-the-online-lives-of-latinx-consumers.html

Patton, M. Q. (2002). *Qualitative research and evaluation methods* (3rd ed.). SAGE Publications, Inc.

Powe, B. D., & Finnie, R. (2003). Cancer fatalism: The state of the science. *Cancer Nursing*, *26*(6), 454–467. https://doi.org/10.1097/00002820-200312000-00005

Rivera-Ramos, Z. A., & Buki, L. P. (2011). I will no longer be a man! Manliness and prostate cancer screenings among Latino men. *Psychology of Men & Masculinity*, *12*(1), 13. https://doi.org/10.1037/a0020624

Schmidt, A. L., Zollo, F., Scala, A., Betsch, C., & Quattrociocchi, W. (2018). Polarization of the vaccination debate on Facebook. *Vaccine*, *36*(25), 3606–3612. https://doi.org/10.1016/j.vaccine.2018.05.040

Singh, S. N., Rothschild, M. L., & Churchill, G. A., Jr. (1988). Recognition versus recall as measures of television commercial forgetting. *Journal of Marketing Research*, *25*(1), 72–80. https://doi.org/10.1177%2F002224378802500107

Smith, A., & Anderson, M. (2018, March 1). *Social media use in 2018.* Pew Research Center. https://www.pewinternet.org/2018/03/01/social-media-use-in-2018/

Stapel, J. (1998). Recall and recognition: A very close relationship. *Journal of Advertising Research*, *38*(4), 41–45. https://go.gale.com/ps/anonymous?p=AONE&sw=w&=00218499&v=2.1&it=r&id=GALE%7CA53176381

Sterrett, D., Malato, D., Benz, J., Kantor, L., Tompson, T., Rosenstiel, T., Sonderman, J., Loker, K., & Swanson, E. (2018). *Who shared it: How Americans decide what news to trust on social media.* NORC Working Paper Series WP-2018-001. NORC at the University of Chicago. http://www.norc.org/PDFs/Working%20Paper%20Series/WP-2018-001.pdf

Strekalova, Y. A., & Damiani, R. E. (2018). Message design and audience engagement with tobacco prevention posts on social media. *Journal of Cancer Education*, *33*(3), 668–672. https://doi.org/10.1007/s13187-016-1135-x

Strekalova, Y. A., & Krieger, J. L. (2017). A picture really is worth a thousand words: Public engagement with the National Cancer Institute on social media. *Journal of Cancer Education*, *32*(1), 155–157. https://doi.org/10.1007/s13187-015-0901-5

Teoh, F. (2019, January 28). *The most popular health articles of 2018, a scientific credibility review.* Health Feedback. https://healthfeedback.org/the-most-popular-health-articles-of-2018-a-scientific-credibility-review/

Torres, J. B. (1998). Masculinity and gender roles among Puerto Rican men: Machismo on the US mainland. *American Journal of Orthopsychiatry*, *68*(1), 16–26. https://doi.org/10.1037/h0080266

U.S. Census Bureau. (2020a, August). *ACS demographic and housing estimates: 2014–2018* [Data set]. American Community Survey 5-Year Estimates. https://data.census.gov/cedsci/table?q=hispanic%20&tid=ACSDP5Y2018.DP05&hidePreview=false

U.S. Census Bureau. (2020b, August). *Hispanic or Latino origin: 2014–2018* [Data set]. American Community Survey 5-Year Estimates. https://data.census.gov/cedsci/table?q=hillsborough%20county%20hispanic&g=0100000US&tid=ACSDT5Y2017.B03003&hidePreview=false

Yañez, B., McGinty, H. L., Buitrago, D., Ramirez, A. G., & Penedo, F. J. (2016). Cancer outcomes in Hispanics/Latinos in the United States: An integrative review and conceptual model of determinants of health. *Journal of Latina/o Psychology*, *4*(2), 114–129. https://doi.org/10.1037%2Flat0000055

Yang, Q. (2017). Are social networking sites making health behavior change interventions more effective? A meta-analytic review. *Journal of Health Communication*, *22*(3), 223–233. https://doi.org/10.1080/10810730.2016.1271065

Construyendo Conexiones Para Los Niños: Environmental Justice, Reproductive Feminicidio, and Coalitional Possibility in the Borderlands

Sarah De Los Santos Upton, Carlos A. Tarin, and Leandra H. Hernández

ABSTRACT

Familias Unidas del Chamizal is a community organization in El Paso, TX that works to increase awareness around the issues of education, environmental racism, development, and public health. In 2019, the El Paso Independent School District launched an initiative to close several schools due to low enrollment, forcing students in Barrio Chamizal to relocate to Frederick Douglass Elementary, which borders a designated industrial zone and is surrounded by two major recycling plants. In response, Familias Unidas has organized to reverse the decision and call attention to the discriminatory practices of the school district. We take the public advocacy efforts of Familias Unidas as an instrumental case study to trace the intersections of health communication, Latinx communication, and environmental racism along the U.S.–Mexico border. Utilizing an intersectional borderlands health communication approach, we draw on publicly available texts to trace the argumentative strategies employed by Familias Unidas to mobilize community members. Familias Unidas rhetorically constructs a public health crisis in the borderlands by connecting the school closures to larger coalitional struggles concerning the environment, citizenship, race/ethnicity, language, and class. We identify three rhetorical strategies – *familia, comunidad*, and *(in) justicia* – employed by Familias Unidas to shape their public argument(s).

Introduction

The El Paso Independent School District (EPISD) has a history of enacting classist and racist policies that marginalize children and families in El Paso, Texas. The most recent instance concerns the forced relocation of elementary school children to a campus that borders a designated industrial zone and creation of a bus hub next to a local high school. These actions expose children to high levels of pollution and, in the case of the elementary school, heavy metal contamination. While these environmental hazards would be concerning in any community, the number of kids in El Paso with chronic health issues is higher than the national average, with more than half of all children suffering from allergies and 17% diagnosed with asthma (Sadasivam, 2018). Exposure to higher levels of vehicle emissions for some children in EPISD has resulted in lower GPAs (Sadasivam, 2018), yet, community-driven requests for air quality testing at EPISD campuses have been denied by the district (Sadasivam, 2019). EPISD's policies have been particularly devastating in Barrio Chamizal, a predominantly low-income community with a population that is 97% Mexican/Mexican-American/Hispanic and 40% foreign-born (Sadasivam, 2018). As a result, the district now finds itself in an ongoing battle with Familias Unidas del Chamizal (FUDC), a community organization working to increase awareness around the intersections of education, environmental racism, and development (La Mujer Obrera, n.d.).

This essay centers the public efforts of FUDC as an instrumental case study to explore the intersections of health communication, environmental and reproductive justice, and Latinx communication studies. We draw on publicly available texts to trace the argumentative strategies employed by FUDC to mobilize community members. FUDC rhetorically constructs a public health crisis in the borderlands by connecting the school closures to larger coalitional struggles concerning the environment, citizenship, race/ethnicity, language, and class. By foregrounding our analysis in the broader constellation of borderland theory (Anzaldúa, 1987), we identify several key rhetorical appeals such as *familia, comunidad* and *(in) justicia* that are used by members of FUDC to advocate for equitable public health and social justice initiatives. These appeals, we argue, provide a nuanced view of how health communication scholarship can be inflected with culturally and geographically responsive meanings in fronteras tóxicas (Tarin, 2019).

Rationale

Utilizing an intersectional borderlands health communication approach, we address theoretical and population health communication gaps by focusing on Mexican/Mexican American/Chicano groups in El Paso, TX. From a critical health communication perspective, such an analysis fills an important gap in Latinx health communication research by focusing on how Latinx community epistemologies and activism combat structural racism and environmental injustice. As Hernández and De Los Santos Upton (2019) described, health communication research has provided valuable information on the interrelatedness of health experiences, behaviors, disparities, access, and more. However, traditionally, post-positivist health communication research is not well-equipped to untangle "the impacts of the historic, racialized, systemic injustices" (Hernández & De Los Santos Upton, 2019, p. 4) that characterize Latinx health disparities and experiences. Research has suggested that Latinx communities face higher levels of health disparities, particularly when compared to white communities. Such health disparities are elevated when environmental contexts are considered (Carter-Pokras et al., 2007; Quintero-Somaini et al., 2004). Latinx communities are disproportionately located in inner city areas and agricultural/rural communities, where they are routinely exposed to environmental pollutants. Representing one in six children in the United States, Latinx children "incur disproportionate exposures to air pollutants, pesticides, and toxic industrial chemicals" (Carter-Pokras et al., 2007, p. 307) and have higher rates of asthma, mercury and lead poisoning, and developmental and behavioral disorders.

Moreover, Latinx communities and health experiences have historically been underrepresented in health communication scholarship. Hernández and Martinez (2019) conducted a systematic review of health communication scholarship about Latina/o/x and Latin American populations in top health communication journals from 2014 to 2019 and found that Latina/o/x and Latin American populations were present in only 14% of health communication journal articles over the past 5 years (n = 257 out of 1,850 articles total). Moreover, from a sample perspective, Latina/o/x, and Latin American populations were the focus of 21% of all studies across health communication journals. At the outset, this percentage might appear slightly positive. However, Latina/o/x and Latin American populations comprised 0–5% of the article/study sample in 31.5% of all studies across health communication journals, meaning that "although Hispanic/Latino populations were present in these studies, their presence was marginal, given that they comprised less than 5% of the study sample" (Hernández & De Los Santos Upton, 2019, p. 5). Hernández and Martinez (2019) contend that scholars must intentionally foreground voices of the historically marginalized and minoritized, which undergirds the inspiration for this study. Our study contributes an important methodological and cultural case study about how Latinx families in El Paso have utilized community activism to advocate for environmental justice for themselves and their families.

This essay also builds upon previous research (Ross & Solinger, 2017) that has advocated for reproductive justice lenses, generally, and in health communication, in particular. Reproductive justice as an inclusive theoretical and praxis framework widens the pro-life/pro-choice binary to focus instead on reproductive equity and justice for women and families throughout the lifespan. It acknowledges that justice

> Can only be achieved when equitable and supportive healthcare is a reality for women of all backgrounds, including the ability and freedom to make their own informed decisions about whether or not to reproduce, free from intervention. … By extension, for women who do choose to have children, reproductive justice also includes the right to carry, birth, and raise children in safe cities free from toxic, environmental, and legal/governmental pollutants and intervention.". (Hernández & De Los Santos Upton, 2019, p. 6)

Our analysis of FUDC highlights the interconnected nature of reproductive and environmental justice struggles.

Environmental and reproductive justice on the border

The U.S.-Mexico border region is a toxic landscape. Following the initiation of the Border Industrialization Program by the Mexican government in the 1960s, hundreds of multinational corporations relocated manufacturing and assembly plants south of the border due to lax environmental regulations and inexpensive labor. The ratification of NAFTA in the early 1990s prompted a similar boom in commercial production and assembly plants in cities like Ciudad Juárez, Chihuahua (Tarin, 2019). The maquiladoras – large tax-free factories – have operated for decades with little oversight and, as a result, border communities must grapple with the environmental consequences that will persist for generations. Tarin (2019) argued "the complexity of environmental problems requires attentiveness to the historical legacy of coloniality and its contemporary manifestation in the Borderlands" (p. 44). Environmental degradation caused by maquiladoras represents only one facet of a complex constellation of toxicity that permeates the U.S.-Mexico border. Given the shared ecocultural landscape of the Borderlands (Tarin et al., 2020), environmental problems must be understood as fragmentary and multidirectional; as fronterizas we breathe the same air, drink the same water, and walk the same land that has been impacted by years of industrialization.

The ongoing conflict between FUDC and EPISD provides an opportunity for understanding the intersection of health communication and environmental communication, particularly through the lens of environmental justice. According to Sandler and Pezzullo (2007), the environmental justice movement calls for a recognition of the disproportionately harmful conditions placed on poor and minority communities, which typically have limited institutional recourse due to their exclusion from the decision-making process. Sowards (2012) argued that the El Paso, TX-Ciudad Juárez, Chihuahua region faces several unique environmental justice challenges stemming from a history of industrial development such as maquiladoras and the lingering effects of the ASARCO copper smelting facility. These challenges are particularly vexing because, as Pezzullo (2007) argued, contamination of air, soil, and water is ubiquitous in many low-income communities populated by people of color, but collective organizing is difficult because health impacts are often invisible until it is too late. Moreover, language barriers, high legal fees, and unfamiliarity with decision-making protocols often mean that traditionally marginalized groups are relegated to the margin due to their inability to engage in the deliberation process. By taking an environmental justice approach to analyzing the efforts of FUDC, our goal is to highlight the intersectional nature of their arguments as they draw attention to linkages between public health and the environment.

In understanding environmental justice as a concern for health communication scholars and practitioners, we also recognize that environmentalism is part of the larger reproductive justice framework. Environmental degradation and toxicity creates myriad conditions that affect children ranging from birth defects to stunted learning outcomes and are, thus, a vital component of reproductive health advocacy. For instance, in her analysis of metaphors used to link climate change and reproductive justice, de Onís (2012) explained, "Within this framework, recognition of the intersecting issues inhibiting environmental degradation mitigation and the advancement of women's rights is growing, as climate change disproportionately impacts women living on the margins" (p. 309). FUDC advocates for healthy communities on behalf of lower-income, Spanish-speaking, Latinx immigrants in the El Paso, TX region and, consequently, is invested in the struggle for reproductive and environmental justice.

We deploy a *reproductive feminicidio* approach to utilize health communication and feminist theories created by us for us to explore the intersectional nature of our experiences. Reproductive feminicidios are defined as acts of gendered violence against women on the reproductive spectrum, spanning from a structural limitation of reproductive options to the murdering of women because of their reproductive capabilities (Hernández, 2019; Hernández & De Los Santos Upton, 2019). We assert that this particular public health crisis *is* a reproductive feminicidio case because of its impacts on family health, children's health, and its relation to health disparities. In earlier research, Hernández and De Los Santos Upton (2019) analyzed reproductive (in)justice in contexts such as news framing of reproductive choice, (in)voluntary sterilization of Latin American women, and the murder of pregnant women in Mexico. With the FUDC case, we extend earlier research on reproductive feminicidios to focus specifically on environmental justice and activism driven by culture and family. In this context, by addressing the intertwined nature of familia, culture, and environmental concerns, we uncover how structural racism, environmental policy, and state legislation have led to institutional discrimination with detrimental health impacts. Such structures have created a toxic environment that we assert has led to reproductive feminicidios in El Paso. The FUDC organization, however, has illustrated the power of community alliances and activism, highlighting the importance of critical health communication activism informed by a community's particular needs and cultural backgrounds.

Borderlands theory & health communication

As fronterizas, or those who dwell within and cross borders, we understand that the border is much more than the militarized line that divides us; the border is the space that emerges around that line, the way we make sense of ourselves, and the consciousness that emerges as we learn to navigate the contradictions of artificial binaries (De Los Santos Upton, 2019). Those who inhabit physical, sociocultural, and psychological borderlands may find themselves in the in-between, a state which Anzaldúa (1987) calls nepantla. Necessitated by the borders they navigate in their daily lives, fronterizas develop what Anzaldúa calls *conocimiento*, a way of thinking that is transformative and draws from la facultad and mestiza consciousness. La facultad is a way of perceiving that stems from the body, much like a gut reaction or sixth sense, and mestiza consciousness is a way of understanding and being in the world which emerges from existing in a constant in-between state of the border (De Los Santos Upton, 2019). The nepantla state is also impacted by unique ecocultural circumstances for fronterizas in El Paso, Texas and Ciudad Juárez, Chihuahua, namely the desert landscape, the Rio Grande, human-made canals and walls that disrupt the movement of humans and non-human animals, and environmental injustices, including but not limited to our current case study. Navigating these tensions creates unique border ecocultural identities for fronterizas in the Paso del Norte region, as the border enables us to understand how "seemingly oppositional tensions can conflict and converge in order to (re)create a transformational praxis" (Tarin et al., 2020, p. 53). The borderland identities of the members of FUDC are thus sites of resistance in and of themselves.

Anzaldúa (2015) argued that fronterizas or neptantleras are uniquely positioned for alliance building and activism through the concept of new tribalism, meaning that while the affirmation of our own identity positions is important, we also align ourselves with larger social movements, building coalitions "to envision diverse futures" (Anzaldúa, 2015, p. 85). This coalitional work often emerges in spaces and moments where seemingly unrelated movements are brought together around a social issue. However, Chávez (2013) reminds us that these alliances are not self-sustaining and we must be willing to continuously nurture coalitions if we wish for them to endure. Residents of Barrio Chamizal demonstrate what this sustained process of coalition building looks like in practice, working for the right to live in and prosper in their community for more than half a century, and more recently bringing together movements for environmental, migrant, and reproductive justice.

The practice of building alliances does more than just strengthen social movements, it also contributes to the overall health and healing of communities. Anzaldúa (2000) illuminates the ways in which alliances are intertwined with health:

> Alliance making is therapeutic. You're trying to heal a community, or a culture while healing yourself. That's all alliance work is: you're trying to heal the wounds. You're trying to bring in justice, human rights, to people who have been wounded and disadvantaged in their lives–whether it's monetary, health, disease, mental illness, whether it's lack of knowledge, education, or training for higher-paying jobs. These are wounds–emotional and psychological as well as political wounds. Becoming allies with people is really about helping each other heal. (p. 199)

Through their work to build alianzas, FUDC is doing more than just fighting for the environmental health of the community. Their solidarity with other movements sends a ripple of healing energy throughout the frontera, attending to economic and cultural wounds as well. This activism, largely led by mothers, follows a tradition of women healing their communities (Delgadillo, 2011). These fronteriza approaches to healing are not just physical and communal, but are intertwined with the spirit as well.

In Anzaldúa's theorization of the borderlands, health is holistic; she moves beyond the body to include not only the community, but also the spirit, encouraging us to recognize that "our flesh is spiritualized" (Anzaldúa, 2000, p. 151) and therefore our spirituality is deeply interconnected with our health. Viewing health from a fronteriza perspective allows for the transcendence of binaries between the body and spirit, instead privileging spiritual mestizaje, the "transformative renewal of one's relationship to the sacred through a radical and sustained multimodal and self-reflexive critique of oppression in all its manifestations and a creative and engaged participation in shaping life that honors the sacred" (Delgadillo, 2011). The health of our bodies and spirits are deeply intertwined with the health of our communities, and approaching health communication from an Anzaldúan perspective illuminates not only FUDC's approach to health advocacy, but, we argue, encourages us to think about health activism as essential to healing bodies, minds, spirits, and communities. Because we, along with FUDC, are fronterizas, we understand that the border shapes every aspect of our daily lives. We argue that it is imperative to ground this essay in the borderlands to understand activism at the intersections of reproductive, migrant, and environmental justice.

Case study: Familias Unidas del Chamizal

Barrio Chamizal in El Paso, Texas is a community built on a legacy of struggle and resistance. The Chamizal Tract and Córdova Island were two parcels of land at the center of a century-long land dispute between the U.S. and Mexico regarding the ever-changing course of the Rio Grande/Rio Bravo. The river, which serves as the international boundary between the two countries, was ultimately cemented in place following the 1963 Chamizal Convention, and as result, families who lived on this land were forcibly displaced with minimal compensation (Tarin et al., 2020). The cementing not only disciplined the fluidity of the river and inhabitants of the region, but limited the movement of human and non-human animals, the growth of plants, and even seed disbursement (Tarin et al., 2020). Compounding the devastating social, economic, and environmental impact of the Chamizal Convention on the Barrio Chamizal neighborhood, the ratification of NAFTA in 1994 disproportionately affected its residents as well. NAFTA's trade policies resulted in the movement of El Paso factories across the border to Ciudad Juárez, taking with them many of the manufacturing jobs held by Chicanas (Navarro, 2002), and as result, many residents of Barrio Chamizal lost their jobs.

Legacies of racism and classism continue to impact the community and influence every aspect of daily life, as historic injustices are compounded by environmental racism. The neighborhood is bordered by an international bridge where trucks line up for miles, crossing goods back and forth across the border and smothering Barrio Chamizal in a "blanket of haze" (Sadasivam, 2018, para. 1). In 2018, the El Paso Independent School District proposed a plan to add yet another source of pollution to the neighborhood: a facility to refuel, service, and house 124 district school buses (Sadasivam, 2018). The proposed bus hub would be built adjacent to Bowie High School, one of the oldest schools in El Paso, which is situated 100 feet from the Mexico-U.S. border and international bridge. Hilda Villegas, founder of FUDC, has called the EPISD's decision a civil rights violation and example of environmental racism, pointing out that "EPISD didn't propose [the bus hub] anywhere else because other communities wouldn't have accepted it" (Sadasivam, 2018, para. 5). FUDC has organized numerous protests at Bowie High School and City Hall and filed a civil rights complaint arguing that building the bus hub at Bowie High School is "unlawful because it will cause disproportionate impacts based on race and national origin" (Sadasivam, 2018, para. 6).

In January of 2019, the El Paso Independent School District voted to close four elementary schools. As part of the "Rightsizing for the Future Initiative," district officials cited declining enrollment and concerns for fiscal responsibility as key determinants in their decision. It is worth noting, however, that an analysis by the *Texas Observer* found that the four schools targeted for closure had a significantly higher number of low income students when compared to the rest of the district (Sadasivam, 2019). One of these schools, Beall Elementary, is located in Barrio Chamizal and students are being forced to relocate to Frederick Douglass Elementary, which borders a designated industrial zone and is surrounded by two major recycling plants. At the request of FUDC, a research team from the University of Texas at El Paso studied the soil surrounding Douglass Elementary and found potentially harmful levels of heavy metal contamination (Sadasivam, 2019). Villegas has seen firsthand how these environmental hazards can have long-term health impacts on children in the Chamizal neighborhood, and she argues that the bus hub and school closures may lead to a forced displacement of families in the neighborhood, who are confronted with the decision to leave or put their children's health at risk (Sadasivam, 2018).

On June 15, 2020 FUDC filed another lawsuit against the district, demanding that they be held accountable for their discriminatory practices and "ensure equal access to safe, clean and accessible schools in Chamizal" (FUDC Por La Educación v. El Paso Independent School District, 2020). They argue that students in the Chamizal neighborhood are being targeted because the community is low-income and predominantly Mexican/Mexican-American/Chicano, and this argument is grounded in a historic legacy of racism and segregation, as many of the public schools that serve Barrio Chamizal were originally built to segregate Hispanic and African-American students (Sadasivam, 2018). FUDC explain that their ongoing demands for environmental and health assessments in the area, as well as protests against the bus hub and school closures, are part of an ongoing battle against EPISD's pattern of discrimination against families in Barrio Chamizal.

Analysis

As we have discussed thus far, a key contribution of this essay is an Anzaldúan approach to health communication, a spiritual, biopsychosocial, culturally informed approach that epistemologically recognizes the importance of alliances, spirituality, culture, and justice to advocate for better health experiences and outcomes. A central component of such an approach blends Anzaldúan borderlands theories and concepts such as nepantla and alianzas with reproductive justice. In what follows, we trace the public argumentative strategies employed by FUDC del Chamizal to advocate for safer environments. Our analysis is informed by an intersectional borderlands health communication approach that aims to represent these argumentative threads holistically and within an appropriate cultural context. Following Banerjee and Sowards' (2020) call for adecolonial bricolage approach to qualitative inquiry, our analysis is grounded by contextual, local meanings that aim to center the "complicated, nuanced aspects" (p. 17) of research that can also serve to amplify community-based advocacy. In working to develop this essay, we began by collecting avariety of publicly available texts created by FUDC as part of their public advocacy including: Facebook posts, speeches at public meetings, signage and chants used at rallies and protests, opinion editorials published in local newspapers, and lawsuits filed on behalf of (and in collaboration with) the organization. We reviewed these materials individually and engaged in first-cycle, descriptive-level coding (Saldana, 2013). After materials were reviewed, we engaged in conferencing to tease out significant, recurring themes and patterns in the data. Next, we reviewed the data again and engaged in aclose textual reading (Leff, 1992) of these materials that sought to highlight connections between FUDC' public arguments and Borderlands theory. The final stage of stage of our analysis involved additional conferencing that sought to reconcile the hierarchical umbrella codes (Tracy, 2013) and our own experiences with/in the local community.

This analysis was informed by our positionality as Latinx researchers (two of whom currently live along the U.S.-Mexico border). I, Sarah, am a queer Chicana feminist and my identity is shaped by the border I call home. My familia and I engage with FUDC's umbrella organization, La Mujer Obrera, in various ways. I, Carlos, am a queer Mexican-American who has lived in the El Paso region for almost my entire life. My childhood home was located in the Lower Valley, one of El Paso's traditional agricultural neighborhoods, less than a mile from the border. I, Leandra, also identify as a queer Mexican-American Chicana feminist who was born and raised in Houston. My regional identity as a Tejana and familial activist roots inspired my reproductive justice health activism efforts in Texas and California. Following Anzaldúa (1987), we draw on our *conocimiento* (e.g., a knowledge of body, self, and others) to understand this collective struggle in ways that also encompass body, feeling, and spirit. Our analysis here is inextricably linked to our lived experiences as fronterizas. Three dominant strategies emerged from our analysis of Familia Unida's public advocacy: familia, comunidad, and (in)justicia. Below, we explore each of these strategies to explain how a Borderlands consciousness is used for public health advocacy.

Familia

In their organizing efforts, both in-person and online, FUDC use familia as a rhetorical strategy to call attention to the reproductive and environmental injustices taking place in Barrio Chamizal and to hold those responsible accountable. Familia is frequently used in public argument because it offers affective resonance with audiences who may not be immediately linked to the particularities of a given situation. For instance, Sowards (2019) describes how Dolores Huerta used familia as a rhetorical strategy in her activism and organizing with the United Farm Workers (UFW), both including her biological family in activist efforts and rhetorically constructing the union as a family. Huerta often referenced her children during speeches, breastfed her babies during negotiations, and encouraged her children to participate alongside her in picket lines, marches, and protests; rather than being constrained by her motherhood, Huerta's use of familia enabled her to gain control of the rhetorical situation, which facilitated her negotiation of contracts and created awareness around her broader activist efforts (Sowards, 2019). Much like Huerta's use of familia as a rhetorical strategy, FUDC centers motherhood and children in their environmental activist efforts, powerfully invoking familia in new ways to highlight the impact of reproductive feminicidio and environmental racism in their community. FUDC utilizes the rhetorical strategy of familia in two distinct but intertwined ways. First, motherhood is privileged as a catalyst for activism as activists show up as their full madre-selves. Second, FUDC use familia as a rhetorical strategy to center children's rights and nurture children themselves as active agents of protest.

Motherhood is a driving force behind the activism of FUDC. First, the organization's activist efforts were born out of concerns that mothers have for their children, namely the desire to keep them safe. In an interview with the *Texas Observer*, Hilda Villegas, the founder of FUDC, explained that both of her older children developed health issues after attending Frederick Douglass Elementary, a school contaminated by a nearby metal recycling facility (Sadasivam, 2019). She described her assumption that school was a safe place to send her children, and the "horrible" realization that it could instead be having a negative effect on their health (Sadasivam, 2019, para. 2). After her youngest child's school was recently closed and he was expected to transfer to Douglass, Villegas began fighting to spare him the same fate. Second, in addition to motherhood driving their activism, this activism is performed with that very motherhood front and center. The madres that drive FUDC's activists efforts can be seen pushing strollers, babywearing, and holding the hands of young children at protests, marches, and press conferences. While this may not immediately seem significant, women are often expected to maintain the separation of public and private spheres, including leaving children at home when they enter workplaces or do the public work of marching at a protest or speaking at a press conference. Engaging in activist work as publicly visible madres is thus a meaningful act of protest that follows a long legacy of Chicana activism (Sowards, 2019).

The madres of FUDC are fighting back against reproductive feminicidio by leading the fight for reproductive justice in Barrio Chamizal, which includes the freedom to decide when and whether to have children, and the right to raise those children in safe cities, specifically free from toxic environmental hazards (Hernández & De Los Santos Upton, 2019). We argue that the El Paso Independent School District's decision to transfer children to a school next to a metal recycling facility, exposing them to high levels of lead, and to construct a dangerous bus hub next to a high school is a manifestation of reproductive feminicidio, as it denies families the right to raise their children in a safe space where they will have access to a quality education. From a reproductive injustice perspective, it also infringes on the rights of children to grow, learn, and thrive in healthy communities and denies them the personhood and agency that they so rightfully deserve.

As the rights of children are directly targeted by educational and environmental policy in Barrio Chamizal, another way that FUDC del Chamizal uses familia as a rhetorical strategy is by centering the rights of children and children themselves as active agents of protest. Anzaldúa (2009) argued that people do not really see children, but instead view them as little people who have no rights. This view of children (especially Black and Brown children) is pervasive and subjects them to violence at the hands of their parents, school systems, police, and in the streets (Patton, 2017). While reproductive feminicidio and environmental injustice is a problem for the entire Paso del Norte region, FUDC use the elementary and high schools attended by neighborhood children as a way to illuminate how the broad injustices facing the border target neighborhood children specifically. The protests at Bowie High School and Beall Elementary School are about more than just a bus hub and a school closure, they are about a legacy of environmental racism and FUDC center the experiences of children at these schools to highlight specific health disparities of individual children while demonstrating the interconnectedness of individuals, schools, the EPISD, and the city. Because Bowie and Beall are both schools in the El Paso Independent School District, FUDC can effectively demonstrate who is infringing upon the rights of children and the district becomes an entity that can be held accountable legally.

The madres are not the only ones who speak on behalf of neighborhood children, these children are also active agents in demanding their rights to an education free from a toxic environment. For example, on September 20, 2019, shortly after her graduation from Bowie High School, Katherine Villegas spoke at the El Paso Climate Strike, part of the Global Climate Strike that took place the same day. While opening her speech, Villegas thanks everyone for coming to the event. However, she is quick to add that this should not be interpreted as praise, because "when actions like these are committed on a daily basis, it is expected of us to come together as a community because it is our responsibility" (Familias Unidas del Chamizal, 2019). She describes how her high school used to have a beautiful baseball field surrounded by trees, but it now houses 150 buses and a parking lot. She explains that her little brother's elementary school was closed because "a white man with power decided it was cheaper to stuff 351 students into a toxic school." When describing lead contamination on the playground at her brother's new school, she reminds the audience that "no amount of lead is safe for a developing child" (Familias Unidas del Chamizal, 2019). Finally, she closes out her speech by calling out the hypocrisy of some of the attendees of the El Paso Climate Strike: "there's been families fighting and fighting against people who, people who shame on you have the nerve to show up, to show their faces at places like this when they clearly know that they caused this" (Familias Unidas del Chamizal, 2019). Her speech serves as an explicit example of the power of familia as a rhetorical strategy. While her mother, Hilda Villegas, evokes motherhood as the driving force behind her activism, Katharine Villegas brings her first hand experiences of the aftermath of environmental racism in Barrio Chamizal, effectively demonstrating how these policies have impacted her childhood, education, and life.

As Katherine Villegas delivered her speech, three children stood behind her holding a sign that said "Education Yes Contamination No," and this is one of many examples of neighborhood children using images to demonstrate their proximity to environmental racism. On the Facebook page for FUDC, children appear in photographs and videos holding banners and signs with messages such as "this school is not safe for children to learn" and "Justice for barrio students" In one image, children hold a banner that reads "no a la contaminación, si a la educación" as they stand atop a pile of rubble. One photograph shows children playing on the playground of their new school, a toxic recycling plant packed with mountains of scrap metal in clear view behind them, while another shows families standing in front of the same recycling plant wearing medical masks (pre-Covid) to demonstrate the dangers of the site. Finally, the children of FUDC produce their own protest images. A video called "Barrio Chamizal" on the group's Facebook page features a child's drawing of the school and recycling plant (Familias Unidas del Chamizal, 2020a). In the drawing, children stand in front of the school building, thought bubbles forming above their heads. One says "stop the pollution," another simply says "stop," and the third is just a sad face. To the left of the children is a chain link fence surrounding two buildings and a construction site. Underneath the word "gas" on one of the buildings is a drawing of a skull. The other building has the word "silver" written above it, accompanied by several towers with plumes of smoke coming out of them. This image showcases the dangers facing children in the neighborhood, and captures their emotional reactions to these dangers.

By utilizing familia as a rhetorical strategy, mothers and children work together to push back against reproductive feminicidio and environmental racism in their community. By centering motherhood and including children in activist efforts, children become empowered to advocate on behalf of themselves. In a collectivist culture such as our own, women are oftentimes compelled culturally to take care of children, handle childrearing, and take care of private sphere matters. However, the collective organizing of FUDC is significant because it is homegrown, home led, and spotlights the power of madres and niñxs in the community to extend their labor and efforts past the private sphere and toward the betterment of the community. From an activist perspective, this analysis also highlights an often-overlooked context of activism, that which stems from local, grassroots community efforts. FUDC uses a culturally centered, culturally responsive approach to reproductive justice organizing in direct response to community violence. Such an approach not only highlights the power of maternal, women-based organizing, but also demonstrates a how a passion for social justice can be passed to the next generation. As Sowards (2019) argued, "the connections between emotion, familia, and motherhood cannot be separated" (p. 103). Familia functions to foster communal, intergenerational connections around a common problem.

Comunidad

The members of FUDC recognize the need to build coalitions across multiple, intersectional concerns through the rhetorical strategy we identify as comunidad. Comunidad as a rhetorical strategy enables FUDC to work holistically toward building a healthy community. Rather than focusing on EPISD's plans to close schools as a single issue, they work together to heal various harms facing the community by weaving together environmental stewardship, education, food, art, and ancestral knowledge. The rhetorical strategy of comunidad recognizes the collective, interrelated relationships among various types of violence the community faces and allows the community to address different forms of outreach together

Comunidad's collectivist grounding also recognizes the significant role women play in the community as a central force underlying activist efforts, which is also representative of larger reproductive justice activist efforts led by women to improve the reproductive health and lifespan health of their communities. As described in the case study above, FUDC is part of a legacy of resistance and activism in Barrio Chamizal. In addition to the fight for housing and education, FUDC is linked to a larger struggle for reproductive justice in Barrio Chamizal as a program under the umbrella organization La Mujer Obrera (LMO). LMO was founded by Chicana feminist garment workers displaced by NAFTA, drawing on the conocimiento of these workers to envision and create communities defined by women (La Mujer Obrera, n.d.). We argue that LMO meets the call of reproductive justice feminists to ensure that families are able to raise their children in safe environments by organizing their programs around what they deem basic human rights, including employment, housing, education, nutrition, health, peace, and political liberty (La Mujer Obrera, n.d.). Together, they have built a collective practice centered on cooking, raising children, working the land, commerce, artisanry, and cultural celebrations because these practices are needed to "safeguard our ancestral knowledge and apply it to the present" (La Mujer Obrera, n.d., para. 2). Their work centers women, families, and future generations, as they will inherit the sacred space the women of LMO are working tirelessly to create.

In addition to FUDC and their fight against environmental racism, LMO has four other programs that work simultaneously to preserve traditional foodways and arts, document the history of Barrio Chamizal, organize cultural festivals, and reclaim ancestral food growing practices. One such program, Proyecto Verde, places value on the inherently healthy traditional practices of making food and creating art, and centers the wisdom of elders in Barrio Chamizal because, they argue, these cultural traditions are necessary for the embodiment and expression of Mexicanidad. Another program, Museo Mayachen, documents the history of Barrio Chamizal, namely the historic struggle of Mexican garment workers in the neighborhood. They argue that preserving this history serves an important function for sustaining their projects today, because "Being connected to history allows us to see parallels of systemic prejudice and community resilience between the past and the present" (La Mujer Obrera, n.d., para. 3). Through their Plaza Cultural program, LMO hosts community events such as festivals, ancestral health fairs, book and poetry readings, and other cultural events that feature artists who work at the intersections of art and resistance (La Mujer Obrera, n.d.). Finally, the Tierra es Vida Community Farm is a space where LMO members work together to grow food for Barrio Chamizal and the broader El Paso community, and in doing so work toward the health of their households and communities while connecting to the environment. They explain:

> Throughout human history, women have been the household stewards of good health and good eating. Growing food and cooking are sacred spaces in which we develop our love for the land and for our families, maintaining that critical connection to our nature as human beings and pillars of our family unit. (La Mujer Obrera, n.d., para. 11)

LMO approaches the health of individuals and the community holistically, not only ensuring access to healthy food that nourishes bodies, but also access to ancestral knowledge that feeds the soul. As Anzaldúa (2000) argues, the health of our bodies, minds, spirits, and communities are intertwined, and so by centering food, art, history, the land, and ancestral ways of knowing, LMO is working to ensure that families are able to live and thrive in a healthy Barrio Chamizal.

Informed by histories of oppressive capitalist policies, such as NAFTA, and their lasting impact on Barrio Chamizal, LMO has chosen to fund the above mentioned programs through social enterprises that, in addition to raising money, contribute to the health of the bodies, minds, and souls of the community. The largest of these enterprises is Café Mayapán, a restaurant that serves as a job and food employment training center and prepares food with respect for ancestral knowledge as a way to respect not only customers but also the employees themselves. Another enterprise is Lummetik Trading Co., a fair-trade import company that sells artesanias like textiles, toys, and home goods crafted by cooperatives of indigenous women across Mexico. Understanding all too well the harm NAFTA has caused from communities on both sides of the border, this enterprise also supports "the right of people to remain in their communities if they choose, to not be displaced from their lands by forced migration," thus mindfully raising money for community programs while acting in solidarity with other women en la lucha (La Mujer Obrera, n.d., para. 6). Finally, Rayito de Sol Daycare and Learning Center is LMO's third social enterprise, founded in 2000 to create jobs for NAFTA-displaced garment workers while addressing community needs for childcare. Rayito de Sol serves primarily low-income children of Mexican descent, using a Spanish-immersion curriculum to instill not only language, but also celebrate Mexican cultural heritage. In addition to providing childcare and education, Rayito de Sol fosters connections to the natural environment through lessons, activities, and weekly visits to Tierra es Vida. Understanding that "children naturally see themselves as part of nature," Rayito de Sol works to support the curiosity and creativity they innately possess, and foster a healthy, reciprocal relationship with the environment (La Mujer Obrera, n.d., para. 7).

FUDC and LMO recognize that Barrio Chamizal's fight extends beyond the EPISD. While they have organized to prevent school closures and environmental harms such as the bus hub, they continue to do the multifaceted reproductive justice work of ensuring that families in Barrio Chamizal are able to raise their children in a safe and sustainable community. The coalitional work of LMO across environmental justice, education, food, art, and history employs a rhetoric of comunidad to enact an approach to health envisioned by Anzaldúa that transcends binaries between body and spirit, between nos and otros, and privileges our connections to nature and each other. This approach to health is not only holistic, it is activist in nature. The connections made between loving the earth, accessing education as a right, working and raising families with dignity, and artistic expression as integral to health and community-building showcase what it takes to create and sustain "a creative and engaged participation in shaping life that honors the sacred" (Delgadillo, 2011).

(In)Justicia

In addition to organizing and coalition building, FUDC also recognizes the importance of pursuing corrective measures through a third rhetorical strategy we identify as (in)justicia. (In)Justicia, then, is an approach employed by the group that seeks to bring the past into the present by showing how ongoing efforts of reform are connected to ongoing injustices and white supremacy along the U.S.-Mexico border. For several years, FUDC has sought a reversal of EPISD's school closing plans through a series of lawsuits aimed at highlighting the discriminatory nature of the decision-making process. Additionally, the organization has filed several complaints claiming that the city of El Paso has consistently violated federal ozone standards, contributing to poor air quality in the area (Perez, 2020). Although these lawsuits are still being litigated, we turn to the complaints to highlight how FUDC is seeking justicia through state-sanctioned avenues. Any appeals for justice must inevitably be filtered through the legal system, making an analysis of legalistic arguments appropriate for understanding how FUDC is seeking state-sanctioned recourse. The lawsuits filed to stop the school closures were developed in collaboration with FUDC and, in a sense, represent a formal articulation of the larger constellation of meaning(s) the group draws on in their public advocacy. Litigation for these lawsuits is currently pending, with a preliminary trial scheduled to begin in late 2021. The lawsuits on behalf of FUDC broadly argue that the school closures follow a repeated pattern of discrimination that has persisted since the creation of the school district in 1883. If, as Anzaldúa (1987) argued, the border "es una herida abierta where the Third World grates against the first and bleeds" (p. 25), the ongoing conflict can be understood as a lingering specter of colonialism that plays out in the lives and livelihoods of residents of the Chamizal neighborhood. The legal complaint frames arguments primarily through a corrective lens meant to right injustices caused by EPISD.

In their lawsuit against EPISD, FUDC centralizes patterns of discrimination to highlight that the school closures are part of a more concerted effort to disenfranchise marginalized students and families. The plaintiffs argue, "EPISD has demonstrated a repeated and consistent history of purposeful discrimination ... [that] have required the intervention of this Court, the United States Court of Appeals for the Fifth Circuit, and various federal and state agencies" (Familias Unidas Por La Educación v. El Paso Independent School District, 2020, p. 4). The school closure controversy is the latest chapter in a storied history that has frequently sought to marginalize Chamizal community members. The tract of land where the Chamizal neighborhood is located was previously the site of an international dispute between the United States and Mexico that ended in 1964 (Tarin et al., 2020). The plaintiffs reference the agreement and its consequences noting, "The dispute, and associated lack of law enforcement authority, made the area a haven for slumlords who sought to obtain the most rent from the most vulnerable populations with the least government oversight" (Familias Unidas Por La Educación v. El Paso Independent School District, 2020, p. 6). The lawsuit draws a historical parallel by noting that the precedent that disenfranchised residents in the Chamizal neighborhood is being extended by EPISD leaders who consistently ignore the concerns of parents and arbitrarily apply standards to justify school closures. This injustice is compounded by the demographic makeup of the region as the plaintiffs argue, "El Paso is one of the most impoverished cities in the United States, and the Chamizal neighborhood is one of the poorest, most Hispanic, and most Mexican-American neighborhoods in El Paso (Familias Unidas Por La Educación v. El Paso Independent School District, 2020, p. 6). FUDC draws on a justicia framework to highlight how current patterns of discrimination are informed a legacy of disenfranchisement.

FUDC also asserts that the EPISD systematically engaged in practices that were meant to limit public participation from Spanish-speaking parents living in the Chamizal neighborhood. Anzaldúa (1987) argued that identity is inextricably linked to language and the policing of language (i.e. English-only mandates) is a form of linguistic terrorism that creates hierarchies. We argue that FUDC draws on the theme of (in)justicia to highlight how the public proceedings have enacted linguistic terrorism. For instance, the plaintiffs explain that "EPISD repeatedly provided the public with incorrect information concerning the meeting times and rescheduled the meetings, creating confusion and scheduling difficulties for parents and severely limiting the ability of the interested public to comment on the closures" (Familias Unidas Por La Educación v. El Paso Independent School District, 2020, p. 21). The lack of clarity surrounding public commentary periods presented problems for working-class parents who were unable to plan to attend meetings based on a constantly changing scheduling. Additionally, the school district limited speaking time to 1.5 minutes per person at these hearings, despite the fact that Board Operating Procedures allocate three minutes per speaker (Familias Unidas Por La Educación v. El Paso Independent School District, 2020, p. 21). For parents who were able to attend these meetings and speak in disagreement, their message went unheard. The plaintiffs explain that President of the EPISD Board of Trustees, Robert Geske, was present at the meetings but "does not speak Spanish and was not provided with a translator. As a result, Spanish-speaking parents were not able to provide any input to their elected representative" (Familias Unidas Por La Educación v. El Paso Independent School District, 2020, p. 25). District officials consistently limited opportunities for Spanish speakers and by privileging the comments of English-speakers, tacitly endorsed a hierarchy that further disenfranchised the residents of the Chamizal neighborhood. As the plaintiffs conclude, "This limitation almost exclusively targets Hispanic and Mexican-American families and operates as a proxy for race and national origin" (Familias Unidas Por La Educación v. El Paso Independent School District, 2020, p. 27).

FUDC also draws on the language of pain and suffering to make an explicit appeal for justicia. Anzaldúa (1987) argued that pain and vulnerability are necessary for healing and transformation on the path to conocimiento. In formal legal appeals, FUDC makes a similar argument by suggesting that school closures have inflicted a form of trauma that has consequences for both the physical and psychic wellbeing of students in the neighborhood. The plaintiffs argue that school closures have caused "nightmares, difficulty sleeping, anxiety attacks, drops in grades, and emotional outbursts such as crying in students who ... did not experience such problems before the closures" (Familias Unidas Por La Educación v. El Paso Independent School District, 2020, p. 36). Student safety is also raised as an argument against the school closures as the plaintiffs suggest being relocated presents both environmental and physical risks. For instance, Douglass elementary school is located less than 300 feet from an industrial site and "Students in the Chamizal are regularly required to make dangerous commutes to school, including walking across bridges over dangerous highways ... [that] are littered with glass, garbage and debris ... and experience significant amounts of criminal activity" (Familias Unidas Por La Educación v. El Paso Independent School District, 2020, p. 36). The lawsuits filed by FUDC draw on pain to argue that transformation via legal recourse is one way of achieving justicia.

Reimagining coalitional possibility in health contexts

FUDC is an exemplar case study for interrogating how marginalized communities are rendered invisible in analyses of public health issues. Latinx communities are underrepresented in health communication research generally, and this is especially true for border communities which are often populated by lower-income, non-English speaking residents. The environmental injustices facing residents of Barrio Chamizal extend understandings of how reproductive feminicidio operates through a "spectrum of experiences and webs of oppression that characterize modern reproduction for brown women, particularly at the Mexico-U.S. border" (Hernández & De Los Santos Upton, 2020, p. 3). While Hernández and De Los Santos Upton (2019) have explored the ways in which governments, religion, and healthcare professionals enact violence on the bodies of Black and Brown women, the actions of the El Paso Independent School District highlight the role that schools can and do play in endangering children, thus denying families the right to raise children in safe, healthy communities. In drawing our attention to the struggles of FUDC, our goal has been to highlight how their efforts have been successful in drawing on cultural meanings such as familia, comunidad, and (in)justicia to anchor public messaging about environmental racism, health inequities, and injustice.

A recent victory for FUDC demonstrates the power of these rhetorical strategies for organizing at the intersections of environmental and reproductive justice. On November 20, 2020, FUDC announced that the entrance of the Bridge of the Americas, also known as the "free bridge," would be permanently closed by the Texas Department of Transportation. For Barrio Chamizal, this means that semi-trucks headed for maquiladoras will no longer block the entrance to Bowie High School, and diesel trucks will no longer speed through or pollute the neighborhood with noisy horns and toxic gas (Familias Unidas del Chamizal, 2020b). While this victory has tangible implications, it demonstrates that familia, comunidad, and (in)justicia work hand in hand. Legal action to remedy these environmental and reproductive injustices is important. However, FUDC demonstrates that the act of showing up and protesting in familia is also an important way to raise awareness for the cause and demand action via other avenues. The strategy of comunidad illustrates that while the organization works to create change through protest and legal action, they do not wait idly for these structural changes to occur. To be certain, there are no easy solutions for FUDC because the problems they are addressing are multi-layered and deeply ingrained in the cultural and political landscape of the Borderlands. Yet, we argue that their efforts are a form of collective, embodied resistance that assembles diverse coalitions to achieve health equity and transformation.

The ongoing hardships caused by the Covid-19 pandemic also present scholars with a unique opportunity for understanding the intersection of health and marginalization, especially in times of crisis. Although over 50 million Americans have filed for unemployment benefits since the pandemic began in March (Jones, 2020), the economic realities of the virus are likely to inflict the most harm on already vulnerable populations such as those residing in Barrio Chamizal. For instance, the Rayito de Sol Daycare and Learning Center has been shuttered since mid-March 2020, cutting off an important community resource that many in Barrio Chamizal relied on for childcare. Many working class families are now being forced into an untenable decision: stay at home to care for children and risk being laid off or go to work without securing childcare. Because many parents in Barrio Chamizal community work in service or manufacturing industries, opportunities for stay-at-home work are limited and they may be forced to work in unsafe conditions (i.e. factories with poor ventilation), further risking viral spread. Additionally, after closing the dining room as a safety precaution to limit the spread of Covid-19, Café Mayapán is now at risk of closing permanently, adding to the economic hardship facing Barrio Chamizal. The Covid-19 pandemic underscores the importance of maintaining cultural assets such as comunidad and familia because, in many cases, these are the only forms of social support for marginalized populations.

Our analysis of the organizing efforts of FUDC highlights how issues affecting marginalized communities are frequently obfuscated in health communication literature. Many mainstream communication theories do not adequately reflect the lived realities of people of color, immigrants, LGBTQ+ people, the poor, etc. Issues pertaining to comunidad, familia, or (in) justicia may not be readily apparent in traditional post-positivist health communication analyses, underscoring the need for new ways of studying and writing about minoritized populations. Scholars such as Davis (2015), whose Strong Black Woman

Collective framework provides a culturally sensitive way of understanding racial and gendered experiences, have been instrumental in (re)shaping scholarly conversations about minoritized groups and their communication practices. Yet, these perspectives remain far too uncommon, even with calls from communication scholars to decolonize the communication discipline. Earlier scholarship by scholars such as Zoller and Dutta (2009), Dutta (2010, 2018), and Sastry et al. (2017) has advocated for the importance of recognizing community-based, community-owned interventions and the urgent need to recognize the necessity of critical/cultural health communication epistemologies. However, #[Health]CommunicationSoWhite persists. Even in writing this essay, we struggled with how to frame our analysis in ways that represented the cultural nuance of the borderlands while adhering to terse scholarly conventions regarding tone and (re)presentation. This struggle to tame our wild tongues (Anzaldúa, 1987) is relevant because telling the story of this rich cultural context requires us to attend to non-traditional ways of knowing and communicating that do not fit neatly into the dominant scholarly order. Thus, we have worked to tell cuentas about FUDC (y los héroes y heroínas del movimiento) in a voice that we feel might act as a corrective for the disciplining of our culture, its people, and its language(s).

Finally, our work emphasizes the importance of challenging dominant research paradigms as they pertain to marginalized communities. In drawing on Anzaldúa's (1987) theoretical corpus, we have attempted to maintain fidelity to the cultural meanings and messages espoused by the fronterizas engaged in this struggle. Following Dutta (2015), we are interested in pursuing decolonial research that centers those at the margins. The recent controversies involving #CommunicationSoWhite (Chakravartty et al., 2018) and the National Communication Association's distinguished scholars (Rodriguez et al., 2019) highlight that much work needs to be done in broadening our scholarly conversations, especially as they pertain to race and ethnicity. This exigency is greater than just topical interest; it requires a fundamental rethinking of the dominant theories and methods that permeate the discipline. In a field like health communication that is overwhelmingly saturated with post-positivist analyses (Hernández & Martinez, 2019; Hudak, 2020), we urge scholars to consider the possibility and potential of "delinking" (Mignolo, 2006) from Western, Eurocentric epistemologies to destabilize the canonical approach to studying health. For instance, drawing on conocimiento to make sense of environmental and reproductive justice issues in Barrio Chamizal was a deliberate move to account for esthetic, affective, and psychic dimensions of health that often pervade health communication research. We are hopeful that future research will begin challenging the dominant Western research paradigms that reify marginalization.

Disclosure of potential conflict of interest

We have no known conflict of interest to disclose.

ORCID

Sarah De Los Santos Upton http://orcid.org/0000-0002-7934-3764
Carlos A. Tarin http://orcid.org/0000-0002-5818-7942
Leandra H. Hernández http://orcid.org/0000-0002-0996-6456

References

Anzaldúa, G. (1987). *Borderlands: La frontera: The new mestiza.* Aunt Lute.

Anzaldúa, G. (2000). *Interviews/entrevistas* (A. Keating, Ed.). Routledge.

Anzaldúa, G. (2009). *The Gloria Anzaldúa reader* (A. Keating, Ed.). Duke University Press.

Anzaldúa, G. (2015). *Light in the dark/luz en lo oscuro: Rewriting identity, spirituality, reality* (A. Keating, Ed.). Duke University Press.

Banerjee, P., & Sowards, S. K. (2020). Working across languages/cultures in international and environmental communication fieldwork. *Journal of International and Intercultural Communication.* https://doi.org/10.1080/17513057.2020.1850844

Carter-Pokras, O., Zambrana, R. E., Poppell, C. F., Logie, L. A., & Guerrero-Preston, R. (2007). The environmental health of Latino children. *Journal of Pediatric Health Care, 21*(5), 307–314. https://doi.org/10.1016/j.pedhc.2006.12.005

Chakravartty, P., Kuo, R., Grubbs, V., & McIlwain, C. (2018). #CommunicationSoWhite. *Journal of Communication, 68*(2), 254–266. https://doi.org/10.1093/joc/jqy003

Chávez, K. R. (2013). *Queer migration politics: Activist rhetoric and coalitional possibilities.* University of Illinois Press.

Davis, S. (2015). The "Strong Black Woman Collective": A developing theoretical framework for understanding collective communication practices of Black women. *Women's Studies in Communication, 38*(1), 20–35. https://doi.org/10.1080/07491409.2014.953714

De Los Santos Upton, S. (2019). Nepantla activism and coalition building: Locating identity and resistance in the cracks between worlds. *Women's Studies in Communication, 42*(2), 135–139. https://doi.org/10.1080/07491409.2019.1605232

De Onís, K. M. (2012). "Looking Both Ways": Metaphor and the rhetorical alignment of intersectional climate justice and reproductive justice concerns. *Environmental Communication, 6*(3), 308–327. https://doi.org/10.1080/17524032.2012.690092

Delgadillo, T. (2011). *Spiritual mestizaje: Religion, gender, race, and nation in contemporary Chicana narrative.* Duke University Press.

Dutta, M. J. (2010). The critical cultural turn in health communication: Reflexivity, solidarity, and praxis. *Health Communication, 25*(6–7), 534–539. https://doi.org/10.1080/10410236.2010.497995

Dutta, M. J. (2015). Decolonizing communication for social change: A culture-centered approach. *Communication Theory, 25*(2), 123–143. https://doi.org/10.1111/comt.12067

Dutta, M. J. (2018). Culture-centered approach in addressing health disparities: Communication infrastructures for subaltern voices. *Communication Methods and Measures, 12*(4), 239–259. https://doi.org/10.1080/19312458.2018.1453057

Familias Unidas del Chamizal. (2019, September 20). Katherine Villegas representing Barrio Chamizal [video]. *Facebook.* https://www.facebook.com/comitedefamiliasunidas/posts/656759038152461.

Familias Unidas del Chamizal. (2020a, February 19). *BARRIO CHAMIZAL [Video].* Facebook. https://www.facebook.com/comitedefamiliasunidas/videos/2101724996640619

Familias Unidas del Chamizal. (2020b, November 20). El Paso families celebrate closure of free bridge to truck traffic. *KRWG.* https://www.krwg.org/post/el-paso-families-celebrate-closure-free-bridge-truck-traffic?fbclid=IwAR18M6VP7N6bAIXHl6ppfZSqeFKltOpcrjyfAAe-2CqoIHFLoeEZfLJy3NI

Familias Unidas Por La Educación v. El Paso Independent School District. (2020). *Case No. 3:20-cv-170.*

Hernández, L. H. (2019). Feminist approaches to border studies and gender violence: Family separation as reproductive injustice. *Women's Studies in Communication, 42*(2), 130–134. https://doi.org/10.1080/07491409.2019.1605213

Hernández, L. H., & Martinez, A. R. (2019). Latinidad, heterogeneity, and health communication scholarship: A literature review analysis of Latina/o/x representation. In L. H. Hernández, D. I. Bowen, S. De Los Santos Upton, & A. R. Martinez (Eds.), *Latina/o communication studies: Theories, methods, and praxis* (pp. 97–115). Lexington Books.

Hernández, L. H., & De Los Santos Upton, S. (2019). Critical health communication methods at the U.S.-Mexico border: Violence against migrant women and the role of health activism. *Frontiers in Communication*, *4*(34), 1–12. https://doi.org/10.3389/fcomm.2019.00034

Hernández, L. H., & De Los Santos Upton, S. (2020). Insider/outsiders, reproductive (in)justice, and the U.S.-Mexico border. *Health Communication*, *35*(8), 1046–1050. https://doi.org/10.1080/10410236.2019.1602819

Hudak, N. (2020). Navigating publishing critical health communication research. *Frontiers in Communication*, *5*(38), 1–5. https://doi.org/10.3389/fcomm.2020.00038

Jones, C. (2020, August. 27). 1M apply for unemployment as economy remains in limbo amid COVID-19 pandemic. *USA Today*. https://www.usatoday.com/story/money/2020/08/27/unemployment-claims-58-m-apply-unemployment-less-than-6-months/5624465002/

La Mujer Obrera (n.d.). *La Mujer Obrera*. http://www.mujerobrera.org/

Leff, M. C. (1992). Things made by words: Reflections on textual criticism. *Quarterly Journal of Speech*, *78*(2), 223–231. https://doi.org/10.1080/00335639209383991

Mignolo, W. D. (2006). Citizenship, knowledge, and the limits of humanity. *American Literary History*, *18*(2), 312–331. https://doi.org/10.1093/alh/ajj019

Navarro, S. (2002). Las voces de esperanza/voices of hope. La Mujer Obrera, transnationalism, and NAFTA displaced women workers in the U.S.-Mexico borderlands. In C. Sadowski-Smith (Ed.), *Globalization on the line: Culture, capital, and citizenship at U.S. borders* (pp. 183–200). Palgrave.

Patton, S. (2017). *Spare the kids: Why whupping children won't save Black America*. Beacon Press.

Perez, E. S. (2020, July 26). Court orders EPA to re-evaluate whether El Paso complies with clean air standards. *The El Paso Herald Post*. https://elpasoheraldpost.com/court-orders-epa-to-re-evaluate-whether-el-paso-complies-with-clean-air-standards/

Pezzullo, P. C. (2007). *Toxic tourism: Rhetorics of pollution, travel, and environmental justice*. University of Alabama Press.

Quintero-Somaini, A., Quirindongo, M., Arévalo, E., Lashof, D., Olson, E., & Solomon, G. (2004). *Hidden danger: Environmental health threats in the Latino community*. Natural Resources Defense Council. https://www.nrdc.org/sites/default/files/latino_en.pdf

Rodriguez, A., Dutta, M. J., & Desnoyers-Colas, E. F. (2019). Introduction to special issue on merit, whiteness, and privilege. *Departures in Critical Qualitative Research*, *8*(4), 3–9. https://doi.org/10.1525/dcqr.2019.8.4.3

Ross, L., & Solinger, R. (2017). *Reproductive justice: An introduction*. University of California Press.

Sadasivam, N. (2018, April 3). Alleging 'environmental racism,' El Paso activists file civil rights complaint against school district. *The Texas Observer*. https://www.texasobserver.org/alleging-environmental-racism-el-paso-activists-file-civil-rights-complaint-against-school-district/

Sadasivam, N. (2019, February. 13). El Paso school consolidation exposes more kids to lead and other hazards, parents say. *The Texas Observer*. https://www.texasobserver.org/el-paso-school-consolidation-exposes-more-kids-to-lead-and-other-hazards-parents-say/

Saldana, J. (2013). *The coding manual for qualitative researchers*. Sage.

Sandler, R., & Pezzullo, P. C. (2007). *Environmental justice and environmentalism: The social justice challenge to the environmental movement*. MIT Press.

Sastry, S., Zoller, H. M., Walker, T., & Sunderland, S. (2017). From patient navigation to cancer justice: Toward a culture-centered, community-owned intervention addressing disparities in cancer prevention. *Frontiers in Communication*, *2*(19), 1–12. https://doi.org/10.3389/fcomm.2017.00019

Sowards, S. K. (2012). Environmental justice in international contexts: Understanding intersections for social justice in the twenty-first century. *Environmental Communication*, *6*(3), 285–289. https://doi.org/10.1080/17524032.2012.700205

Sowards, S. K. (2019). *¡Sí, ella puede!: The rhetorical legacy of Dolores Huerta and the United Farm Workers*. University of Texas Press.

Tarin, C. A. (2019). Fronteras tóxicas: Toward a borderland ecological consciousness. In L. H. Hernandez & R. Gutierrez-Perez (Eds.), *This bridge we call communication: Anzaldúan approaches to theory, method, and praxis* (pp. 31–49). Lexington Books.

Tarin, C. A., De Los Santos Upton, S., & Sowards, S. K. (2020). Borderland ecocultural identities. In T. Milstein & J. Castro-Sotomayor (Eds.), *Routledge handbook of ecocultural identity* (pp. 53–65). Routledge.

Tracy, S. (2013). *Qualitative research methods: Collecting evidence, crafting analysis, communicating impact*. Wiley-Blackwell.

Zoller, H., & Dutta, M. J. (Eds.). (2009). *Emerging perspectives in health communication: Meaning, culture, and power*. Routledge.

Index

Note: **Bold** page numbers refer to tables and page numbers followed by "n" denote endnotes.

For Product Safety Concerns and Information please contact our EU
representative GPSR@taylorandfrancis.com
Taylor & Francis Verlag GmbH, Kaufingerstraße 24, 80331 München, Germany

www.ingramcontent.com/pod-product-compliance
Lightning Source LLC
LaVergne TN
LVHW080653011026
849160LV00014B/1404

* 9 7 8 1 0 3 2 6 6 1 2 6 1 *